Holistic Wellness
in the
NEW AGE

Holistic Wellness
in the
NEW AGE

A comprehensive Guide to NewAge Healing Practices

Editor
Swatika Jain

Compiled By
Sandeep Goswamy

Holistic Health • Wellness • Energy Medicine • Self Help

The LightWorks Publishing
Spirituality . Wellness . Self
TheLightWorksPublishing.com

Published by:
The LightWorks Publishing
G-125 Jeevan Niketan,
New Delhi-110087 INDIA

Copyright © Sandeep Goswamy 2015

All rights reserved. No part of this book may be reproduced or transmitted in any form or by any means without written permission of the author.

First Published: May 2015

Editor's Note

Dear Light Workers!

Yes, you are a light worker!

Wondering how? You picked up this book right now and you reading it, confirms that you are a light worker! A light worker is someone who spreads light through his or her work.

Welcome to the world of holistic wellness!!

In this New Age with its rising challenges and scope for awakening, it is important that we should all be aware of healing modalities because the journey to self realization begins with healing on all levels i.e. body, mind and spirit. Many people learn and work with different modalities and get benefit and yet there are many people who are skeptical and do not fully trust a natural system of healing…for lack of understanding and access millions of people suffer from disease and stress, and this affects us all, it is time we wake up! Now is the time to embrace your inner calling. No healing modality or spiritual path is good or bad. It all depends on what you are most comfortable with and what resonates with your essence. One person may feel Reiki energy to work wonderfully while another person may find Pranic Healing or Angels better suited. You have to find it within you, connect with it and let it flow.

This book is divided into two sections – spiritual-healing modalities and motivational articles. We have strived here to include as many varied and popular healing modalities as possible. Each chapter includes the ESSENCE, the PROCESS and the TECHNIQUE. The technique is something you take back home! The modalities and motivational articles are categorized here under different themes. The themes are: The Wellness Approach, The Belief Approach, The Being Approach and The Body Approach.

We are both blessed and cursed with a tool called MIND. This mind if left unchecked to seek the objects of senses becomes the cause of our ignorance and if we apply this mind to tap the boundless energy and channelize it we can gain lifelong well-being and abundance. This book's purpose is to reveal different ways in which you can attain this goal of healing and realization.

This book can also be your guide in a similar way like the I-Ching. Close your eyes and think of one area of life where you are experiencing a challenge. Once you have a clear picture, keep this book in your hands and keep an intention in mind that this book will give you a message or a way that you need RIGHT NOW. Now open a page. You will surely find the guidance your heart is seeking.

I'll share here an experience that made me realize how the universe talks to us. I was sitting with my nephew Aryan in a beachside cafe, looking at the numbered table Aryan said, "Maasi (Aunt) look! It's 1 and 2". I saw the number which was 12, but for Aryan, who still hasn't learned the number 12, it was two separate digits...the numbers 1 and 2. Both his perception and my perception were different and thus we saw and understood the same thing differently, this insight made me realize how profound the universe's wisdom is that allows a million different ways of understanding and expressing the same truth.

The more awareness we gather, more we understand both the parts and the whole of this picture called cosmic creation. The GESTALT school of psychology says that the whole is greater than the sum of the parts. Mere dots take on a meaning when we can see a circle out of it. Words alone do not make sense until perception creates meaning out of a context. We would never have known the meaning of the world if there weren't an eagle's point of view. I wonder if Einstein and Newton also experienced what we call the "aha" moment, when you realize that what you were looking for was right there all along, all you had to do was change the perspective. And this is what the role of every healer and teacher is i.e. to facilitate a shift of perspective for a patient or a student.

Is it our ultimate goal to find the whole? Isn't that what we're doing all the time, from asking our best friend about relationship advice or seeking knowledge from a guru or seeing our eternity in our children, we are constantly looking for the bigger picture. From where does this seeking for knowledge and love come? And where does it go? The answers as many as there are minds and hearts.

The teacher was once a seeker but in order to teach, he always seeks.

The seeker is both a teacher and a student all through his life. And we are all destined to walk this path sometime or the other. If you have started already, may this book help you in all that you seek and more.

Swatika Jain is a certified clinical hypnotherapist with a Masters Degree in Psychology. Being naturally psychic, she has explored different fields in the domain of spirituality and holistic healing. Through her association with New Age Foundation, she is further exploring her field of knowledge and experience by studying various modalities in depth. Her vision is to complete her journey as a seeker and share her insights for the benefit of all.

Foreword

"The secret of getting things done is to act!" -*Dante Alighieri*

Wellness is the natural state of human beings. Illness is a state where one does not feel well. While quantum physics has opened a new vista in the field of human physiology defined in its wholeness replacing the old definition based on reductionist, mechanistic biochemistry; the world has now come to realize that the conventional definition of health given by the WHO needs change. In this context the IOM, the audit body of US medical establishment, in their February 2010 meeting, had accepted the new definition of Whole Person Healing (WPH) as the future reference for healthcare system.

Wellness (conventionally called health) is now defined as "enthusiasm to work and enthusiasm to be compassionate." Interestingly, this fits in with the time-honored definition of health in Indian Ayurveda, the mother of all medical wisdoms in the world, existing from the time of the Vedas. We have now come one full circle in the so-called scientific medicine with a down to earth holistic definition of health. The man who led the movement for WPH was late Professor Rustum Roy, one of the greatest scientists the world ever had. He was one of the founder members of the IOM.

The marketing and promotion done by conventional medical industry has tricked millions of people into a delusional world of well being where everything has a quick fix, and the harmful effects of these medications are considered for selling another quick fix. And the game keeps on. "Over 40? It is time to fix a date for mammogram and the cost has come down for this holiday season from the 3950 INR to just 1750," reads the prominent headline advertisement in The New Indian Express of the October 9th, 2011 in Chennai. This kind of *disease mongering* efforts, are at the root of all our problems in medical care system. They are based on the wrong science of reductionism. Cancer is not a disease in the true sense. Cancer cells are a bunch of "jobless, directionless, wandering, rogue cells" which remain in the human system for years before they show up as clinical cancer only when their numbers have swollen to millions. Therefore, the so-called early diagnosis of cancer and cancer screening in the apparently healthy populations are only myths, although they make good business sense for the cancer industry.

While I have been writing about this for years, the US government has issued a circular that screening for prostate cancer using PSA test is unscientific and unreliable. Mammogram is not far from that truth. In fact, many places routine mammograms have been given up as mammograms themselves could help generate cancers to grow faster from those wandering cells which otherwise would have died a natural death before they become clinical cancers. Cancer research is an area where the "so called" cancer researchers can tap from a bottom less pocket of the research funds. The research has gone too far from reality into vivisectionist research from reductionism.

This year's Nobel is an example of that last statement. The three people that succeeded in finding out the small receptor on human immune cells have got the Prize. That receptor or its ligand (for making a drug) will not solve any problem. The immune system works as a whole and in association with the other systems of the human being. This has been proven time and again but we do not seem to learn our lessons from our mistakes. Our cloning efforts, our genetic engineering efforts, our stem cell (exogenous) research have all come to naught. In fact, we conveniently forget the efforts of those researchers who have shown us the right path for stem cells research.

Way back in the early 1950s Professor Robert Becker of the New York University Medical School, a great brain in orthopedic surgery, had shown how the body cells, wherever they are, under stress and urgent need, could transform themselves into pluripotent stem cells. This is the body's own effort to produce endogenous stem cells. He demonstrated that the red blood cells at a fracture site under the periosteum of the broken bone could slowly change into nucleated cells and then put out pseudopodia to become real powerful pluripotent endogenous stem cells, which know what to do to heal the bone.

Whereas the stem cells produced by us in the laboratory from any source, when introduced into the human body, need the help of the environment to do what we intend them to do, endogenous stem cells are born with the message to do what is needed. The internal environment for the exogenous stem cells includes not just the body as we see it but the mind. In fact, human body is the human mind seen as a solid body according to quantum physics! The exogenous stem cells could even harm the human system as happened with the first attempts to treat childhood cancers with this method. The original cancer died but a new cancer cropped up! Dolly, the first cloned animal died prematurely as she was as old as her mother (from whom the original cell was used for cloning) and suffered from old age diseases like cancer and joint damage even in infancy! Eric Drexler's efforts to produce self-replicating nanobots, which do not require father and mother, died a premature death before it took off. Drexler made billions from his company shareholders when he claimed that human beings could be made in the laboratory! Venture capitalists poured millions into his kitty without any returns at the end of the day.

AIDS research is another example. While the protean causes of that syndrome are still very vague, researchers make hay when the research funds pour in plenty. They are still going after that poor virus, the HIV, whose original sin was that it was discovered in the bone marrow of that first young homosexual in San Francisco who died of the syndrome in 1981. In retrospect, we now know that any germ could be found in such patients, as their immune guard is very weak. The original paper of this association between HIV and AIDS in the prestigious journal *Science* was only a case history. Based on that case report the author, Luc Montaigner, got his Nobel recently.

Time has come to think afresh in this area of repetitive research in preference to that of holistic refutative research. When we understand wellness and the real definition of health, we would quickly realize that all illness management has to be holistic where the body, mind and environment of the patient are taken into consideration. The era of disease and diagnosis will replace the era of understanding the suffering human being (the patient) in trying to make him whole again. And that is called *healing*. Research must be true "outcomes" research and not research to better surrogate end points as we do now. One example will be in order here. All the studies of cholesterol lowering efforts with reductionist chemicals starting with the original choestyramine to the present statins have only shown the effect of their lowering the blood report of cholesterol levels while they all showed higher death rates in the treated group at the end of the day. Death is the real outcome while lowered blood report is a surrogate end point. The story seems to be similar with our efforts to lower many of the fluctuating biological levels, which we have been labeling as "diseases".

Reductionist chemical molecular therapeutics will have to give place to energy therapeutics as human body is a bundle of jumping leptons and correction of such errors will have to use energy scientifically. Many proven methods of energy treatment have been in vogue for eons in many alternate systems. One more reason why energy methods are better is the speed with which one gets results with energy healing methods. Whereas chemical message transmission happens at a rate of one centimeter per second, energy healing transmission happens at a rate of 1, 86,000 miles per second! Most, if not all, reductionist chemical molecules are alien to the human system and they are rejected by the liver in the first place. (The first pass effect that we teach medical students in pharmacology means that the body is trying to destroy as much of the drug as possible)

The ghost of Adverse Drug Reactions, (ADRs) staring at our face as the biggest cause of death in modern medicine, could be avoided if we follow the holistic management of illnesses to bring man back to his/her state of wellness as defined above. Long live mankind on this planet in good health and happiness. Medical profession is always needed as the doctor is not just a drug vendor but a real friend, philosopher and guide in times of illness. In addition, science has now shown that all the drugs or surgical methods that we use work mainly because of the faith the patient has in the doctor, the so called placebo effect, also called the expectation effect (EE). A good doctor, humane and human, full of empathy, will be God to patients at all times. Basically, a good doctor should be a good human being.

> *"If you want others to be happy, practice compassion.*
> *If you want to be happy, practice compassion." - The Dalai Lama.*

Prof. B.M. Hegde

Preface

Just breathe.

Feel yourself. Our mind, body and soul are all one continuum of energy. For us to fully realize our essence, it is important that these interdependent aspects of our self are in harmony. This harmony when present is reflected in our well being on all levels. When one of these three aspects suffers an imbalance either due to a lack or an excess of elemental energy, it leads to the development of diseases in either mind or body. This is evident from many cases where we can see how a long-term emotional wound leads to a physical disease or when a chronic disease creates mental or emotional unrest.

The right way to achieve holistic wellness is relative to each person's requirements, because we're all unique when it comes to our constitution and our life journey. Each person has specific needs when it comes to healing and each person responds in his own way to a particular treatment. Since none of us is the same, we will each have our own path to achieve all encompassing wellness. But we're not alone in this search for well being; there are experts who can guide us to find out what exactly do we need.

It's been more than 10 years since I started the journey to discover the amazing scope of non-traditional approaches, and working alongside many teachers, healers and other wonderful people, we decided to compile this collection for you. Throughout this book you will learn how to start your own voyage to all-encompassing health through your three gateways.

Which are the three gateways and what do they do, you wonder. To achieve mental, physical and spiritual well being, follow the natural principles, listen to your mind, body and soul and let them guide you to a life that is in perfect harmony with the Universe. Choose any gateway to access and understand the inner workings of your self:

The Mind: this gateway works through the perception of the world around us, as the Law of Attraction dictates: wherever the attention goes, it grows.

To help you change your mindset, following therapies can be beneficial: PSYCH-K®, Hypnotherapy, Past Life Regression and other Emotional Freedom Techniques etc.

The Body: This gateway is an access to our sensory world and it is the store house of our experiences and our responses. Modalities like Massage, Acupuncture, Naturopathy etc. are applied for bringing this gateway in harmony. Our authors have contributed their insights about using different healing practices in this regard.

The Soul: This gateway is our access to our energy and awareness, which is subtle and invisible. Energy Medicine modalities which channelize the universal energy constitute this treatment. Here we utilize techniques like Reiki, Aura Balancing, Chakra Cleansing etc. to harmonize our energy bodies.

You can map your healing requirements by checking out what challenges you have and with expert guidance you can chart out which levels need what kind of intervention. This book will facilitate this process for you where you can learn from the experience and knowledge shared by the wellness experts about different modalities and what best a particular treatment or technique can offer you.

Sandeep Goswamy, founder of NewAge Foundation, is the glue that sticks this book together. He has been promoting alternative and complimentary therapy for the last 10 years. He has also created a network of Holistic Wellness Centres under the banner of "NewAge Wellness World". He is also a publisher encouraging many minds to explore their writing potential.

For details: www.TheNewAgeFoundation.org
www.NewAgeWellnessWorld.com

Acknowledgements

I am extremely grateful to all the wonderful authors who have contributed to this book, especially Dr. B.M Hegde for his encouragement, Dr. Bruce Lipton & Rob Williams for agreeing to be part of this book and blessing it with their contribution. I am grateful to Rita Soman not only for her contribution but for also helping us connect with Dr. Bruce Lipton & Rob Williams. Special thanks to Suresh Padmanabhan for inspiring and encouraging me to work towards fulfilling my dream. Also thanks to Guriya Bhullar, my Reiki teacher, for introducing me to the world of energy healing.

Big thanks to our meticulous editor Swatika Jain for her untiring efforts in editing this book and providing the structure in which this book has manifested to its best.

Sandeep Goswamy

Contents

Editor's Note	*v*
Foreword	*ix*
Preface	*xiii*
Acknowledgements	*xv*

The Wellness Approach

1. Health, Happiness and Harmony in a Time of Love — 3
   Bruce H. Lipton
2. You are Not Stuck! You can Change your Destiny!!! — 9
   Atmyayogi Shri Aasaan Ji
3. It's a YES Universe! — 16
   Lakhwinder Babbu Gill
4. Empower Your Dreams: Practical Steps for Creating Miracles in Your Life — 25
   Suresh Padmanabhan
5. The Willingness Process — 31
   Jane Kirby
6. Ho'oponopono - The Magical Prayer Healing — 48
   Rashminder Kaur
7. The Power of Forgiveness — 58
   Water E. Jacobson
8. Spiritual Healing Through Storytelling — 62
   Dr Amit Nagpal
9. Parenting in the New Age — 68
   Dr. Saloni Singh
10. Holistic Education — 74
    Neha Patel
11. Shifting Paradigm: Healing From Within — 87
    Rucsandra Mitrea

The Belief Approach

12. Origin, history and Introduction of belief — 99
    Naveen Varshneya
13. Journey of PSYCH-K® — 106
    Jurrian Kamp
14. PSYCH-K®-The Missing Piece — 112
    Rita Soman
15. Leading-Edge Neuroscience Reveals Significant Correlations Between Beliefs, the Whole-Brain State, and Psychotherapy — 116
    Jeffrey L. Fannin & Robert M. Williams
16. Reiki and the force called Motivation — 130
    Dr. Paula Horan
17. ThetaHealing® — 139
    Shalin Khurana
18. Aura Healing- The Basis of all Energy Healing — 146
    Nishant
19. Emotional Freedom Technique — 151
    Dr. Rangana Rupavi Choudhuri
20. Serenity Surrender (SS) — 166
    Minal Arora
21. Beyond Self-Sabotage — 186
    Archna Mohan
22. Fitness: The Challenge Within — 200
    Tarini Khetarpal
23. The Four Pillars of Health — 204
    Nandini Gulati
24. Program your mind to a slim body — 211
    Preeti Subberwal
25. Allowing the Magic to unfold: Access Consciousness — 218
    Seema Sharma

The Body Approach

26.	Ozone – Nature's Detox Doctor & Healing Superhero Dr. Paula Horan	229
27.	PEMF – The Fifth Element of Health Bryant Meyers	241
28.	From the Desk of Hermina Hermina Danniel	250
29.	The Art of Acupuncture Dr. Ravi K. Tuli	256
30.	Sujok & Acupressure Amarjit Singh Narula	261
31.	External Counter Pulsation (ECP) - Creating bypass naturally Dr. S.S. Sibia	267
32.	The Magic of Crystal Healing Bindu Maira	273
33.	Breath-Work, The Re-Birthing Process Smita Wankhade	280
34.	Food as Medicine Dr. Ashish Paul	286
35.	Bach Flower Remedies Aryanish Patel	290
36.	Sports and Spirit Theresia Eggers	300
37.	Say Yes to Money Suresh Padmanabhan	303

The Being Approach

38. Healing Through Hypnotherapy *Suzy Singh*	313
39. Integrated Healing Through Hypnotherapy *Anjali Chawla*	332
40. Transformation Through Past-Life Regression *Smita Wankhade*	341
41. Cellular Rhythms in Regression: A new paradigm to healing and integration *Aasha Warriar*	350
42. The Journey™ To Healing *Dr. Rangana Rupavi Choudhuri*	357
43. Working with Angels *Susan Chopra*	367
44. Akashic Records - An Illuminating Healing Journey *Bhavya Gaur*	373
45. Feng Shui *Meenakkshi Jain*	379
46. Colour Therapy *Meenakkshi Jain*	384
47. Astrology - A Tool For Healing Energies *Dipikka Sanghi Gupta*	392
48. Mantra Healing *Ashok Angrish*	398
49. The Wellness Concept *Prof. B.M. Hegde*	404
50. Disinformation in the New Age *Mandy Peterson*	410
51. The Journey of A Seeker with The Power of Gratitude and Birth of A Tarot Reader *Nidhi Chauhan Sharma*	415
52. Spiritual Journey with Animals *Ritambhara Nand*	419
Afterword	*423*

The Wellness Approach

CHAPTER 1

Health, Happiness and Harmony in a Time of Love

Bruce H. Lipton

The Honeymoon Effect: A state of bliss, passion, energy, and health resulting from a huge love. Your life is so beautiful that you can't wait to get up to start a new day and you thank the Universe that you are alive. Think back on the most spectacular love affair of your life—the Big One that toppled you head over heels. For most, it was a time of heartfelt bliss, robust health, and abundant energy—a first-hand experience of Heaven on Earth.

Everyone can remember a time when they were 'head-over-heels in love'. During this dream time of life our perception of the world expands and our eyes twinkle with delight. Our affection isn't limited to our selected partner; rather we are in love with life itself and it shows. We take risks to experiment with our life exploring new foods, activities, clothes and way of being. We listen more, share more and take more time for pleasure. What seems hostile the day before becomes heaven on earth when we're in love. We don't even notice the aggressive drivers that irritated the heck out of us yesterday; today, we're lost in daydreams and love songs.

The "Honeymoon Effect" experience is Nature's premier elixir of life. Through the action of the nervous system, love is translated into physiology, releasing vibrations and chemistry that heal and regenerate the body. The joy and excitement that comes with finally finding the person you believe is the love of your life fundamentally is not the result of chance or coincidence. Insights from frontier science now reveal not only why and how we create the honeymoon experience, more importantly; they also provide a fundamental understanding as to why the honeymoon experience disappears. Knowing how we created the honeymoon effect and the reasons why we lose it, offers an opportunity to create the Heaven on Earth experience every day of life, ensuring an unbelievable happily-ever-after relationship, which even a Hollywood producer would die for.

The honeymoon effect represents the successful fulfillment of a primal *biological imperative*. Biological imperatives are the behaviors of living organisms that assure their personal as well as their species survival. Examples of biological imperatives include the quest to secure water, food, safety, and mates. Imperative behaviors are unconsciously driven by cues provided by the body's physiology. When observed on the conscious level, imperative behaviors are personally experienced as the urges or "desires" that shape our actions.

Our physiology not only initiates imperative-directed behaviors, it also informs the organism as to how well it is satisfying those needs. In assessing an organism's behavior, the nervous system releases certain chemicals that encourage the pursuit of supportive behaviors and releases a different set of chemicals to discourage organisms from engaging in threatening behaviors. Our nervous system translates the body's positive and negative chemical signals into experiential sensations that range from pleasure to pain.

The more an individual's behavior supports their imperatives, the more pleasure and health they experience in their lives. In contrast, based on the severity in failing to meet imperative needs, one's experience can range from simple discomfort to excruciating pain, and even to death. Organisms that succeed in satisfying their basic drives are described as adaptive; those falling short are by definition, maladaptive.

Most of the imperative-directed behaviors we engage in on a daily basis are required for our personal survival. However, to achieve the fundamental imperative of species *reproduction*, it necessitates that we engage with others. For lower organisms, successful reproductive behavior may be nothing more than being in the right place at the right time. Female starfish releases cluster of eggs into the sea, and in response neighboring male starfish reflexively shed their sperm in the vicinity of the eggs. Voilà, reproduction-imperative fulfilled. Primitive organisms, such as starfish, need not attend their fertilized eggs, and each egg will produce an individual that is self-sufficient from the moment it hatches. Simply, there is no need for parental care.

However, as one ascends the evolutionary ladder, the creation of "viable" progeny for higher organisms requires much more reproductive involvement than that necessary to bring sperm and egg together. As species complexity increased, it led to the birthing of individuals that require an extended period of gestation as well as a longer duration of postpartum nurturing before they are able to survive on their own. This is especially true for humans, whose infants necessitate an extended "education" and behavioral skills to enable them to survive and to prepare them to be effective parents for their own offspring.

Nature's design for human successful reproduction is optimally effective if couples maintain a loving relationship for a period lasting about twenty years, and that's if they only have one child. To encourage such long-term relationships, evolution designed the brain to release a cocktail of love potions that reward and encourage honeymoon-bound participants. The experience of falling in love is derived from the secretion of neurotransmitters that provide us with, among others, ecstatic pleasure (dopamine), enhancement of our attraction and attractiveness (vasopressin), exuberant health (growth hormone), and a desire to bond (oxytocin).

To further cement relationship longevity, Nature slips a mickey into the cocktail, by controlling serotonin, the hormone associated with addiction. Once the honeymoon effect is experienced, the brain chemically addicts us to pursue this behavior. This addiction is win-win for both the lovers and for human civilization as well, because of the healthy progeny they leave behind. Of course, the downside of the addiction is the painful depression and withdrawal symptoms experienced when love and the underlying reproductive imperative fail.

Body chemistry in lower organisms is the primary director of what are essentially reflex-driven and unconscious reproductive behaviors. While neurotransmitter chemistry is also an important motivator for engaging human reproductive behavior, evolution endowed humans with a game-changer—consciousness and freewill. Though reproductive behavior is still driven by physiology, what we ultimately experience and what we create with our reproductive imperative is under the control of the mind.

As fully expanded upon in my book, *The Honeymoon Effect: The science of creating Heaven on Earth*, to understand how we create the honeymoon effect and why it disappears requires that we differentiate between the mind's two primary subdivisions, the conscious mind and the subconscious mind. Each mind possesses unique powers, and their interdependent cooperation shapes our life and love experiences.

The conscious mind is the seat of our personal identity, the "home" of our spirit, our uniqueness. The amazing power of the conscious mind is expressed in its creative ability. The conscious mind is the processor that manages our wishes, desires, and aspirations. When contemplating what you want from your life, the answers are derived from the activity of the creative conscious mind. And a fact that becomes profoundly important is that the conscious mind is not time-bound; it can "think" into the future, review the past, or just disconnect from the moment as it processes thoughts in our head.

In contrast, the subconscious mind is a massive super computer, one million times more powerful than the conscious mind that contains downloaded stimulus-response behavioral programs known as habits. Though the subconscious mind possesses a little creativity, it's primarily function is to record and play behavioral programs it acquires from genetics (instincts) and from "learned" life experiences. The subconscious resembles a record–playback device, such as a video camera. Record a behavior and every time the play button is pushed, the nervous system recreates the same behavior, no "thinking" or conscious awareness required.

Operating from the conscious mind, our cognitive activity and behavior are controlled by our personal wishes and desires. However, when the conscious mind is preoccupied with creating the future, reviewing the past or just busy "thinking," it is not being mindful—paying attention to the current moment. At these times, behavioral control is automatically defaulted to the subconscious, loaded with prerecorded programs.

If our minds truly control our life experiences, why are we not manifesting "Heaven on Earth?" Science's answer is profound and empowering, for it explains how we create the honeymoon and why we lose it. Neuroscience reveals that the conscious mind only controls about 5% of our behavior and responses to life. During the remaining 95% of the time the conscious mind is engaged in "thinking," and by default, life is then controlled by the subconscious mind. Simply, the wishes and desires of the conscious mind only control our decisions and behaviors about 5% of the time. The remaining 95% of our lives, essentially all of it, is under the control of prerecorded behaviors in the subconscious mind.

The greatest impediment in creating Heaven on Earth is that the primary behavior-controlling programs in the subconscious mind do not represent *our* wishes, desires and aspirations. Our subconscious behaviors are primarily downloaded by observing *other* people—parents, siblings, extended family and culture. A child can only become a contributing member of a society after it acquires the thousands of rules and behaviors that govern participation. Nature facilitated this need by designing the human nervous system to accommodate a massive download of data between birth and seven years of age. During this period, a child's brain predominately expresses *theta* activity as assessed using electroencephalography (EEG). *Theta* activity, associated with a child's state of imagination, is the operating frequency of a brain in hypnosis.

The child's mind in hypnosis not only records other people's behavior; it also acquires a "self-identity" by down loading other people's opinions as to who they are. Psychologists acknowledge that a majority of the downloaded behaviors and perceptions of "self" are disempowering, limiting and self-sabotaging.

These conclusions are profound—the conscious and subconscious mind, together shape our reality. Consequently, a relationship is based on four minds, two conscious minds and two subconscious minds. The question is which of these minds is running the show? On a daily basis, the subconscious behavioral programs acquired from others control 95% of our lives. It is important to emphasize that because the conscious mind is busy in thought during this time, we rarely observe our own behavior, especially when we are "shooting ourselves in the foot" and sabotaging relationships.

Then how do we create the honeymoon effect? Science has now observed that the conscious mind of people in love does not wander but stay in the present moment, becoming mindful. This means that during the honeymoon period, the participants are controlling their behaviors and actions using the wishes and desires of their conscious minds. Think of it this way, when you are that much in love, why would you let your conscious mind wander when everything you wanted is right in front of your eyes. The result is a honeymoon experience of Heaven on Earth.

The problem that arises for most is that "real" life inevitably intrudes into the honeymoon. The conscious mind drifts off into thoughts about paying the rent, fixing the car, doing the chores. At these times the behaviors expressed and the responses made to partners are not governed by *your* conscious wishes and desires, they are now controlled by the mostly negative behaviors acquired from others. These newly exposed subconscious behaviors were never part of the honeymoon experience, but as they intrude into the relationship, the glow disappears. As more and more, formerly unobserved and negative subconscious behavioral traits are introduced, they continue to compromise the relationship, sometimes to the extent that the end result is a divorce.

With insight and awareness, limiting subconscious programs can be rewritten. What would be the consequence of rewriting negative subconscious behaviors and replacing them with your wishes and desires? A honeymoon effect, that will keep you healthy, joyful and living in harmony the "happily ever after!" way.

Bruce H. Lipton, Ph.D., stem cell biologist and pioneer in the new biology, is an internationally recognized leader in bridging science and spirit. Bruce was on the faculty of the University of Wisconsin's School of Medicine and later performed groundbreaking stem cell research at Stanford University. He is the bestselling author of The Biology of Belief, The Honeymoon Effect, and co-author with Steve Bhaerman of Spontaneous Evolution. Bruce received the 2009 prestigious Goi Peace Award (Japan) in honor of his scientific contribution to world harmony.

www.brucelipton.com

CHAPTER 2

You are Not Stuck!
You can Change your Destiny!!!

Atmyayogi Shri Aasaan Ji

The Ultimate Truth about Human Life is "Your life is not Pre-Determined; you create your Future", only with this simple clarity, you will be able to understand why? With all the unbelievable growth in technology, knowledge, power & money we are still not able to live a life we want or need.

The Divine fact is, your experience with "The External world is nothing but the exact reflection of your Inner World", so the only way to change your world is to change your inner-self. This knowledge will empower you to transform any situation in your life in a way you want because you are no more facing the reality; you are creating the reality of your own choice by changing your inner-self.

A Real Need to Change your Inner-Self

"The Real Change can never happen without changing your Inner-Self"

The Inner self or soul is collections of all your unfulfilled desires & attachment, spiritually known as 'Karma', with scientific perception this can be considered as Psychic Impression & our life is nothing but the expression of psychic impression in the inner-self. The Ultimate purpose of every spiritual practice is to access & alter the psychic impressions & this is possible only by shifting our mind consciousness to higher self "The Divine Frequency "which can be attained by various psychic practice & meditation, at this mental state one can easily remove the unwanted karma/psychic impression & create a psychic impression of their choice. With this explanation one can realize that "Mediation is the only Solution to Redefine your Destiny".

"Life is a Onetime Gift - Gift yourself a Great life!"

As per the Ancient Scriptures & Vedas "Life is not what you have; What you experience with what you have". In human life regardless of your Power, Knowledge, Money & Relationship your experience is determined by Healthy Physical body & a Mind with an Emotional Stability. Meaning there is No point in having a Benz car with a back pain or no point in being a doctor with dementia. So the quality of your experience is directly decided by the quality of your physical & mental health.

Prana-Vritti & Atma-Dhyana thought by Atmayogi Shri Aasaan Ji are meticulously created to experience the Peak of Physical, Mental & Emotional Well-being to enable the practitioner to easily *dissolve the sufferings in the Present & Create a Future free of Suffering & Limitation.* By learning Prana-Vritti & Atma-Dhyana any one can Unlock & Unleash the Ultimate hidden power with in to Manifest a Life Free of Stress & Full of Success, Richness, Wellness & Happiness effortlessly.

"Always remember that YOU are not ALONE- You are ever connected with the divine power which is Everywhere, Every time and in Everyone!!!"

Gift Yourself - A New Life! A New Beginning! - Full of Holistic Health & Happiness

"Prana- Vritti: The Ultimate solution for Total Well-being"

Prana- Vritti is the most powerful method to trigger the Inbuilt Instructions to activate your body's Own Inner Intelligence & Natural Healing power, highly practiced and most recommended by Medical Doctors, Healers & Wellness Therapist for Vibrant Health & Disease Free for a life time.

Prana - Meaning the Life Force or the Vital Energy which is the Reason for the physical consciousness and the existence of life.

Vritti – Meaning an Uninterrupted Circulation and Multifold Manifestation of energy.

The Most Powerful & Effective Self-healing Method & Timeless Energy Technique which are developed after meticulous research by Atmayogi Shri Aasaan Ji which will empower the practitioner to experience the Optimum

Mental and Physical Health throughout the life by increasing the flow of life energy to the total body.

Rediscover Your New-Self

> *"Our Quality of Life is not decided by how long we live, but how healthy we live till the last moment of our breath"*

The state of Total Well-being can be easily achieved by understanding the reality of human body in the first place.

Our Human body is a combination of:

i. **Physical Body** - Meaning *the* Gross Body *or the* Sthula Sariram

ii. **Psycho - Physical Body** - Meaning *the* Subtle Body *or the* Suksma Sariram

iii. **Meta - Physical Body** – Meaning *both* Life-Energy & Light/Divine Body *or the* Prana Sariram & Atma/Teja Sariram

As per the Sarira Dharma in Veda, The Ultimate Secret of Human life which has been revealed by many Sages, Saints & Ancient Philosophers from different parts of the world to experience exceptional health - Is one simple truth,

> *"Till we are in the Human Form, there is no such thing called Nil Effect or Neutral effect"*

"For every food we eat, Action we perform, Thought we think in mind either consciously or unconsciously you will "Experience a good effect or bad effect" in all aspects of your body (Physical, Psycho Physical & Meta Physical Body)"

Prana-Vritti is a Powerful Practice, which will remove all the Ill Effects from the human body & empowers the practitioner to Heal & Prevent from all disease & disorder effortlessly.

POWER OF PRANA - VRITTI
"The Ultimate Power to Regain your Lost Health"

Prana-Vritti increases the Flow of Life Energy throughout the body & promotes the functions of Vital Energies such as Pranan, Apanan, Samanan, Vyanan and Udanan existing in the subtle body which is essential for the Optimum performance of internal organs, Nervous & Endocrine system.

The Real Power & Health of human life is decided by the optimum functioning of the vital energies - Pranan, Apanan, Samanan, Vyanan and Udanan which is essential to purify the 5 Fundamental Elements of the physical body - Earth, Water, Air, Fire & Space which will naturally give the following positive impact & benefits:

i. Increases the Oxygen Supply to every cell

ii. Stimulates the Blood Flow & Purification of the Total Body

iii. Activates the Detoxification process & Elimination of CO^2 effortlessly

Wait "NO MORE" to Change Your Life!

You can make a New Beginning!! It is an ultimate method to Redefine your health & happiness and be Free from Diseases, Disorder & Disability to achieve Success & Peace in all aspects of life.

"Through MEDICINE anyone can increase the life span, but only by DISCIPLINE you can increase your health span"

In reality, almost 87% of human population are not able to achieve their dreams not because of lack of knowledge, lack of money but due to lack of health. By practicing Prana-Vritti you can experience Optimum Physical & Mental health and Unlock the Power within to be diseases free for a life time. It increases the Flow of Life Energy in all Energy centres (Chakra) & Energy Channels (Nadis) which unfailingly improves the functions of corresponding internal organs, Nervous & Endocrine system which is essential for Everlasting Vibrant health. Prana-Vritti is an Ultimate Solution for all Lifestyle Diseases like Blood pressure, Cholesterol, Diabetes, Heart disorder, Psycho-somatic disorders & Chronic ailments.

It is a MUST practice to Experience a Life without Disease, Disorder and Disability

THIS WILL CHANGE YOUR LIFE!!!

ATMAYOGA – The Yoga for Inner-self

Unleash The Power Within You!

AtmaYoga is not a Physical Yoga, it involves no body movement, it's an Attunement of Body, Mind & Atma (Inner self) with the Supreme self to experience the flow of *"Abundant Energy & Divine communion with the universal consciousness"*

ATMA - Meaning the Inner source or the Soul which is the True essence of Peace, Prosperity & the Pure Power within one-self.

YOGA - Meaning Remaining in Union with the Individual self & the Supreme Self.

ATMAYOGA is the Most Powerful Life Transforming Psychic Practice to attain conscious connection with the inner-self and unleash the ultimate power within to create abundance and fulfilment in all aspects of life, which is created by Atmayogi Shri Aasaan Ji.

AtmaYoga is a combination of Unique Deep Meditation (ATMA-DHYANA) & Effective Mind-Tuning Methods where one can activate the 'MahaBuddhi'- The Universal Mind to attain a blissful state & experience total transformation in all aspects of life.

Awakening Your Inner Power

ATMA-DHYANA- Is the Most Powerful Inner-Transformation Technique & Unique Deep Meditation to activate the "MahaBuddhi" the universal Mind, through which you can shift yourlife-consciousness from lower dimension to higher dimension and always be *"Connected to the ultimate source of infinite intelligence and limitless possibilities"*

Atma-Dhyana makes the brain and the body to Vibrate in alignment with Divine Frequency, this will help you gain the power to remove all your negative energy from Past karma & Present life, you will naturally create an inner as well as outer environment with more positive energy which will Effortlessly Accelerate your Consistent Growth & Happiness in all aspects of Life.

By Practicing Atma-Dhyana, You can Unlock & Unleash the Ultimate power within & connect with the supreme energy to experience deep inner peace &

holistic abundance in all forms of life with an unfailing Good Health, Great Wealth, Loving Relationship, Peace & Happiness.

The Real Change can never happen without Changing your Inner-self!!!

If you really want to Change your life & Set yourself free from all the sufferings & limitations, AtmaYoga gives you an exact method & direction to create More Positive energy, Abundance & Fulfilment in all aspects of life right from bedroom to boardroom by removing & protecting you from all the negative vibration that are consciously & unconsciously affecting our peace & growth in life. Irrespective of your present situation one can experience extreme Good Luck & Success to regain your lost Peace, Health, Wealth, Success & Happiness in relationship effortlessly.

Practicing AtmaYoga will make you focus on what you need in life & what is essential to manifest what you really need in life. You will get More Power & Clarity on action you failed to perform in the past being capable and path you must avoid in the future for prosperous living.

In Profound words 'AtmaYoga is an ultimate science to create a Life, Free of Stress & Full of Success, Richness, Wellness & Happiness in every aspects of life'

"Your Present situation is not your final destination"

Prana-Vritti & Atma-Dhyana- created by Atmayogi Shri Aasaan Ji is not aligned to any particular religion or tradition, can be Learnt & practiced by everyone to transform the present life situation in to successful future regardless of their past.

> *One thing that is common in every human is, we all have an Expiry Date; let's take the first step to keep our self Valid & Active till that last moment to Experience Holistic Abundance in all aspects of life.*

> *"If you are reading this - which means, you are having Life in you! I bless you all; in the presence of Divine power to Live your life before it leaves you" with fullest Health & Happiness. - Atmayogi Shri Aasaan Ji, AhamBrahmasmi!!*

Atmayogi Shri Aasaan Ji is a Life Transforming guru who is an Eminent Scientific Philosopher, Inner Science Expert, Master of Holistic Healing & Meditation & a Non-religious Contemporary Spiritual Teacher. He is the creator of Prana - Vritti & AtmaYoga, which has transformed and empowered lives of countless people to regain their lost peace, health, wealth & happiness effortlessly.

www.atmayoga.in

3 CHAPTER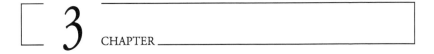

It's a YES Universe!

Lakhwinder Babbu Gill

Life is simple and easy. All That I need to know At any given moment is revealed to me. I trust myself and I trust life. All is well. -Louise L Hay

The Turning Point

The party is in full swing, with music and laughter, some one tells a joke and everyone laughs and someone's laughter is even funnier than the joke!

The pudding is being served, a mango soufflé and a lady beside me declines the pudding saying she is allergic to mangoes. I am surprised and I say to her--- "It's all in the mind." Another lady sitting beside me turns around and asks, "Do you practice mindfulness?" And a little puzzled, I ask, "What's that?" This question brought a momentous change in my life. She mentioned a center nearby at Igatpuri that taught mindfulness and Vipassana meditation and suggested I go and check it out. It was the month of June 1988, and I lived in an Army Cantonment named Devlali, in Maharashtra with my husband and children. Her suggestion came at a time when I was at an all time low in my life. My health was a concern, and my relationships were just not working. I was lonely and sad. I needed a break... I needed to go someplace... And this was the perfect answer. A retreat in silence for 10 days!

Promptly with my husband and my mother in law, we drove off to Igatpuri, to check this center out. The rest is like a dream come true. I fell in love with the sheer beauty and serenity of this place, a haven on earth, the place where I belonged. The management agreed to take me in as a walk in for the 10-day course without prior registration (very unusual). Happily I stayed back; I had gone prepared with my bag and baggage. This was the turning point in my life and ever since that retreat, there has never been any looking back, and life has never been the same.

The Divine Gift

For many years much has been written on the mind, body and spirit connection and of late there is so much information available, I will share my simple yet profound experiences.

> *"Sometimes when things are falling apart,*
> *they may actually be falling into place."*

I can recollect many childhood instances and stories. I have always been intuitive. Before I share these stories, I will preface it all with the fact that I was born to parents who loved me dearly. As I share my experiences at times it may seem that they were unloving but it was completely unintentional. My parents did their best then with the understanding, awareness and knowledge that they had at that time. Children do not come with an operating manual.

As I mentioned earlier, I have always been very intuitive, and somehow whatever I said usually manifested and came true. I was nicknamed- *'Bahen Nanki'* (Guru Nanak Dev Ji's sister). I was blessed to have been born on his birthday. As a little girl, I often spoke with wisdom, beyond my years and whenever I did, my older brother and sister would tease me with *'Nanki...Nanki'*. Soon I grew conscious of every word I said and with time I lost my self-expression. Sadly, a beautiful name became unacceptable for me. Soon I began to paint and make pencil sketches and by the age of 6yrs I was expressing myself through my drawings, making the most beautiful portraits of people around me! I was born a blessed and gifted artist. Thank you Universe.

I remember sitting with beggars and distributing biscuits as a toddler.

Traveling in a car and predicting an accident, and seeing it happen then and there! Predicting my father's promotion all at the age of four and having a near death experience at the age of 13 are some of my memorable experiences that confused and frightened me. My mother was always fearful of what I may see and utter. Amongst the 4 siblings I was my father's favorite but for my mother, I was the unwanted girl child (that's the story and belief I grew up with).

I grew up sensitive to other people's opinions and prejudices and all their negative messages became the truth for me. By the age of 10 years, I was awkward and thin and my French teacher, who also was also our music teacher, never lost an opportunity to remark, "You're too tall and gawky for the school choir." Relatives often compared me with my very fair family, "who does she look like? Her color doesn't match any of you!" I grew up as an angry child with low self esteem who could never rise up to her mother's expectation and I embedded the belief that I am not good enough and am unwanted and an unloved girl child. My life turned into a race always trying to prove my worth! I was sickly and I soon became asthmatic.

I got married at an early age, ready to start a new chapter in my life. I was a successful, creative and gifted artist with a design house and art studio of my own, two adorable sons and a loving and supportive husband. Despite all this, I had this emptiness inside me. This hollow feeling I never understood. A search for something I did not know. I grew up with my share of bruises and challenges.

Realization

How my life's new journey began is very simple, yet powerful. Every challenge that I faced thereafter was an insight with a reminder that "Life is NOW". I got initiated into meditation. On the very first day at the center, rushing up to my room, carrying my heavy bags, I sprained my ankle. My first insight 'Slow down girl, take it easy!' I had to share my room with an elderly lady who snored as loud as a thunder. I complained and requested that my room be changed but I was asked very gently to be tolerant and accepting. Second insight came that of acceptance, giving up judgment and criticism.

On the first day stick in hand and a bandaged ankle, I limped to the meditation hall as fast as I possibly could, the hall was full and as I couldn't walk up to the front easily, I took my cushion and sat at the end of the hall at the back, just next to the entrance at the doorway. I was always a 'first row' person sitting right up in front always. This back end, last seat just didn't work for me at all. I didn't have a choice except to be patient and calm and to surrender to the situation. This seat of mine near the entrance turned out to be a blessing. Each time the teacher and guru ji went past me, they would raise their hand in Aashirwad and bless me with 'Maitri'.

As the course progressed for the next 10 days, there wasn't a moment that wasn't new to me. My Asthma came up during the first session, flashes of childhood experiences flashed through my head. All the suppressed tears, smothered love and pent up emotions arose. The rejection of being an unwanted girl child was painful, the anger and resentment all welled up. The feeling of being unloved wouldn't let me breath until the floodgates broke open and all the buried emotions were released and finally set free. I could see and experience how every thought created a feeling and an emotion and I could experience every sensation at the physical level! Every moment was a moment of arising and passing. Yes, it is here that I experienced and understood the Mind, Body and Spirit connection for the first time in complete awareness.

Life has never been the same ever since that summer in 1988. I released myself of pain and suffocation and have never had another attack of asthma in these years. I saw the need in my consciousness that had kept me stuck all my life, the need to get noticed and to be heard that created this condition.

There was no need NOW in my consciousness for this dis-ease. I took charge of my life. I chose to move from being a victim to a place of power. In my willingness to change and forgive, I set myself free. Never to have another attack of Asthma, ever!

I have been meditating, observing in silence, and expressing my gratitude regularly to the power that created me. I have also been very fortunate to have met SN Goenkaji, my true guru and teacher in a personal meeting and done a few Vipassana courses with him. He is the first person who showed me the true meaning of unattached service, to surrender and just go along with the flow. Be the flow, being present every moment, being mindful of every thought and every sensation arising and passing. I continued this practice at home. I began to see the world with new eyes. Every thing around me was just the same, the people were the same, but I had changed. My relationship with myself had changed. I had altered. I experienced the true meaning of responsibility for everything that occurred around me. I realized the value of moving beyond blaming others. That is the bliss of living in the NOW.

People and resources began to appear on my path that would assist me in healing those wounded parts of myself. I accepted a world of self-discovery, self-love and healing. With this divine surrender, my new journey of self-love and self-acceptance emerged. The connection between the mind and body and the effect of my thoughts on my feelings and sensations intrigued me. As my practice in meditation went deeper, my search for more knowledge and understanding in this field grew as well. I began to read almost everything that spoke about this connection; books, articles, magazines and I began to journal my thoughts. Books became my best companions. I could spend hours in a library or a bookstore!

This is one of my favorite quotes-

> *"I love walking into a bookstore. It's like all my friends are sitting on shelves waving their pages at me."* -Tahereh Mafi

Looking back now, this journey has been not easy. Every challenge that I faced was a life lesson that I needed to learn. My family was happy that I was not 'sick' any more, yet they were a bit confused with what I had become! I had changed, for I was not the Babbu they knew and I am so happy and grateful for this change! My life was truly beginning to feel good. It is during this process that I first saw the little blue book written by Louise L Hay. It had been left at a bookstore in Devlali by a foreign student officer for sale. The slim size, easy to read pages and the name, HEAL YOUR BODY attracted me. This wonderful little book (now my sacred treasure) answered a number of questions that arose in my practice of introspection and meditation.

As Louise L Hay says-

> *"We want to know what is going on inside us, so we can know what to let go. Instead of hiding our pain, we can release it totally".*

When I first read this statement in Heal Your Body, "It's only a thought and a thought can be changed" I never understood it. I never understood that if I was willing to change my thoughts I could change my life! Now I am aware and I know that every thought creates a feeling and emotion. Every thought, determines what I say and what I do. Every thought determines how I feel and that determines my behavior! I now understand that my thoughts create my experiences, my realities. Happy thoughts give happy feelings and unhappy thoughts could create feelings and emotions of sadness, anger, fear, guilt and resentment.

Louise L Hay's philosophy gave language to my silence and introspection.

"Your cells are programmable and instantaneous" -Bruce Lipton. His words kept ringing in my ears after I heard him in a conference in New York. Along this healing journey, I made beautiful friends. Today some of my clients have become my greatest teachers. One among them is my husband and soul mate Iqbal, who has encouraged me from the day we touched each other's life. He has showered me with love, generosity and unconditional support in this journey of self-love and healing.

After individual counseling with clients and conducting workshops and several training programs I have realized that love and forgiveness are the greatest healers. Being a Vipassana Practitioner, and trained in Louise Hay's philosopher, as a teacher and Life Coach, I now have the ability to give language to my experiences and expression to my silence with love and compassion.

There is only one thing that heals every problem, and that is: "Loving Yourself" and the willingness to trust the power that resides within each of us. The point of power is always in the present moment.

"A candle loses nothing by lighting another candle." ~James Keller

Do not allow people's opinions and prejudices to dim your lights. Let YOUR light shine. Our light brings light to others.

It wasn't until I was in my 40s that I learned part of the answer! And it wasn't until my late 50s that I really began to put that learning to use. I learned that other people in our lives are a reflection of how we feel about ourselves. By consciously or unconsciously believing that we deserve to be treated in a certain way, we attract people and situations into our lives that validate our beliefs about ourselves and this belief of undeserved-ness begins when we begin to accept the statements and actions of others as our own truth. Have you noticed how small babies are? They believe they deserve every thing, a toy or to stay up till late? They have not yet accepted someone else's truth about their deserving-ness. Then sometime in school someone told us we weren't good enough; maybe a parent, maybe another classmate, or a teacher and we accepted that truth as our own. We made a choice to accept someone else's truth as our own truth. Once this belief takes hold, it spreads on other area of our lives.

"Average human has approx. 80,000 thoughts / day out of which 98% are negative. Like "I am too old" or "I'll never get ahead" or "I am too fat" etc. Self-criticism will lock us into the patterns we are trying to change.

A belief is only a thought, and a thought can be changed. It would be much better to say "I am always doing the best I can" or "you are really smart at getting things moving". I am encouraging you to initiate a habit of choosing thoughts and ideas that support feeling good and powerful, that elevate you to a higher level of Consciousness."
~ Dr. Wayne Dyer

We have been criticizing ourselves for years, try complimenting yourself, nurturing yourself, LOVING yourself exactly as you are, Right NOW.

Affirm this in the mirror."I love you exactly as you are" Or "I am lovable and worth loving". Keep repeating as often as you can. You may use your phone camera as a mirror. Love others exactly as they are, and they are free to change!

We are selective about the drugs we take, careful, for we know that they could hurt us. Yet are we nearly as careful about the thoughts that we put in our minds?

What is the most powerful medicine we have for healing the thoughts that cause this long list of symptoms? It's called- FORGIVENESS.

Release The Past

Love can heal the world, and forgiveness is the catalyst to make it happen. In addition to loving ourselves it is important to release the past. We cannot change our past, yet we can create our present and our future. If our thoughts create our reality and the way we experience our lives and our physical bodily expression of life then our current experience is the result of the thoughts and beliefs from the last minute the last hour, the last day, the last week, the last year.

When there is distress or imbalance in a relationship, start with forgiveness Just be WILLING to forgive. Remember forgiveness starts as a CHOICE, not as a FEELING. Forgiveness is the greatest gift you can give yourself. Our immune systems become stronger when we forgive. It is the first step to freedom.

Gratitude

Love and forgiveness have seen me through an Ischemic attack, released me of asthma and saved me from a breast surgery. I am grateful!

I am grateful for my breath, that keeps me alive, my parents for being my first guides; my loving sons for the joy I experienced in raising them, my family and friends for always being my support; my teachers and my gurus for making my journey simpler, by showing me the light. Life is simple and I believe that.

Simple secrets for an Inspired Life

Love and Respect yourself, for "what you give out comes back to you."-Louise L Hay

Become aware of the importance of relationships. Relationships are the foundation of life.

Stay Inspired. Use tools like making positive affirmation in the mirror. "Place your orders in the Cosmic Kitchen", as my coach and mentor, Patricia. D. Crane always says -

It is a YES Universe. What you ask, you WILL get. Practice positive affirmations with persistence.

Meditate and listen to your heart and your body. Practice stillness in silence.

Stay inspired. Inspiration is the joyful voice of your intuition fully expressed.

In giving we receive. Service is about giving of self, helping others, being kind and compassionate and making a difference.

Create a daily affirmation, a prayer or pledge, to help you connect with your values and your vision. Post them and paste them, where you can see them to keep your inspiration alive.

Here are some of the physical problems my clients have been able to move beyond by just loving themselves and forgiving themselves and others. Depression, Insomnia, Aches and pains, Stomach aches and ulcer like symptoms Headaches, Back aches, Just to name a few. I myself healed my asthma only through love and forgiveness.

Our immune systems become stronger when we forgive.

"Refuse to allow any thoughts based on your past to define you."-Dr Wayne Dyer

Lakhwinder Babbu Gill is a Vipassana practitioner since 1988. Mindfulness is an integral part of her life. With a perfect blend of the east with the west, she has used Louise. L. Hay's philosophy to give language to the insights she received in the silent practice of meditation. She discovered and experienced the magic of love, the power of forgiveness. She is a certified and licensed "Heal Your Life" Seminar Leader and Life Coach, authorized by Hay House (US) to lead Heal Your Life workshops on Louise. L. Hay's philosophy. As a Metaphysical Counselor, and Self Empowerment Coach, her purpose is to enable people to connect with their inner self, to move beyond their limiting beliefs and thought patterns and be willing to allow the lessons of love and forgiveness to enter.

www.hylindia.com

CHAPTER 4

Empower Your Dreams
Practical Steps for Creating Miracles in Your Life

Suresh Padmanabhan

If you want to find the secrets of the Universe, think in terms of Energy, Frequency and Vibration - Nikola Tesla
(The Greatest Inventor Known To The World)

I started to experiment with the Law of Attraction or Law of Creation or Visualization in my early college days. Thanks to a group of friends who were lovers of the esoteric. We dared to experiment and document our success and failure stories. This was more than a decade before the documentary "The Secret" by Rhonda Byrne made the world aware of "The Law of Attraction". At that time I would not know that many years later I would be taking a workshop "Sankalpa Siddhi- Eastern Law of Attraction".

Logic will take you from A to B, but Imagination will take you everywhere.
-Albert Einstein (The world's greatest scientist)

I believe that the Greatest Human Power is The Power To Create. We all have been doing this unconsciously day in and day out. When I looked at our Sacred Texts, I was stunned by the revelation that the Universe too used this technique billions of years ago. It is said that the Universe was in an Un-manifested state (Shiva State). Maybe it was a rather boring state with Nothing but Pure Consciousness. A thought or a Flash happened; the World got created with a Big Bang. The Un-manifest energy created the manifested visible world (Shakti State). Wow, the whole Universe Just Manifested. So this technique is as old as 13.8 Billion years.

When the human beings evolved, the Universe was benevolent to hand over this same power to us. No other species had access to this Power. From then on we kept on creating. This Great Power has created everything that you see in this World. The huge mountains, the gorgeous waterfalls, gigantic forests, the animals, birds, bees and butterflies all created by The Universe using this Technique. Powerful cars, speed jets and airplanes, fast trains, huge ships, modern technology gadgets were created by the human beings using this power.

Welcome to this Awesome Power waiting to burst out from inside of you.

All of you would want to discover your life purpose, find peace, have great relationships, super careers, be able to afford the best of products, attract money, feel vibrant health, look young, or be spiritually connected. These techniques could help you to have an authentic empowered life.

"Watch your thoughts; they become words. Watch your words; they become actions. Watch your actions; they become habit. Watch your habits; they become character.

Watch your character; it becomes your destiny."

Lao Tzu (world's greatest philosopher 2500 years ago)

Rather than talking about theories let us get into the techniques directly

The Power of Images

Images are the language of the sub-conscious mind. A picture is worth a 1000 words. They are images, pictures, videos, symbols, and anything that is Visual. A very large part of our brain is devoted to processing images. We have been using this since cave times. The world's greatest be it scientist, architects, sculptors or artists were all good in their visualization. They could rapidly see images inside them and simply gave life to them. So if you want to Power your Dreams, you should be good with Imagery. When you close your eyes, the images should feel real. You must have heard that "things are created twice, first in the mind, then in real". Not only you should be able to create images, but you should be able to move them 360 degrees, you should be able to play with images- make them big or small, make them bright or light, make them colorful or black and white etc. This needs years of practice and skill.

So let me share a secret, which will truly help you in doing this. Start with visuals from outside. Imagine you want a car. First be clear about the brand of the car, the color you would love and other details. Take some effort and find a rich image (this is the most important step) maybe from the showroom and hang or paste it in a place where you can see it often.

See it minimum of two times a day, once in the morning because in the morning we are in an altered state of mind, which is the most resourceful state for manifesting. See it once more in the night just before going to sleep. The image goes deeper into your sub-conscious while you are sleeping.

Let us look into images and its practical use for Manifesting

Want to Attract a Life Partner-

- Remove all images, which depict One- Single lady, single bird, single horse etc.

- Substitute it with images, which represent Two -Two lovebirds, a happy couple, Radha Krishna, Rama Sita etc.

- Remove a single bed and substitute by a grand double bed.

- Use the Color "Pink" in some wall of yours, preferable the bedroom, or pink upholstery.

- Get a Rose Quartz, which is a crystal that enhances Love.

- Always keep yourself surrounded by Red Roses

- Listen to Love Songs.

- Each day make an attempt to meet happily married couples. If you can't meet them then see some videos of cheerful couples, happy ending love movies, and listen to talks on relationships that are empowering.

- Attend weddings and appreciate it.

- See Albums of happy couples.

- Buy in advance one attire that you will wear in your wedding.

Want to have your own Cute Baby

- Keep a Photo of a Happy Baby, preferably a big one in your bedroom or where you can see it daily.
- Spend some time with Babies
- Meet your friends who have just given Birth or have children.
- Buy something in advance like clothes for a baby, some rattle or anything associated with Kids. This triggers Faith in Advance that you are welcoming the baby energy into your life.
- Find some temples which are known to have the power to bless couples with child. Tamil Nadu has such Temples.

Want your children to Study Well

- Create a study Room for them with bright pictures of Knowledge.
- Buy them a Study Table and help them to study there only.
- Do not allow them to study in Bedroom, Kitchen or Hall if you have a study room for them.
- If possible let them Study Facing East, next best direction is Facing North
- The Crystal "Amethyst" helps in Studies
- Get them a gadget like the Apple Tablet and load it with apps pertaining to studies
- Get them lot of Books with great pictures. Make their learning Visual.
- Have Bright colors around them
- Ensure they drink lots of water and eat healthy. Almonds (Badam) and Walnuts (Akhrot) helps
- Herbs like "Ashwangandha" and "Spirulina" helps

Want to Attract Money

- Buy a Good Quality Wallet preferably in Red or Green. For guys it could be Brown or Black.

- Keep a Flowing Water Body (waterfall or fountain) in the North East as first choice or in the North.
- Have pictures pertaining to Abundance or Money Flow
- You could keep a crystal of Yellow Citrine and Garnet.
- Be in the circle of people for whom Money Flow is effortless
- Listen to Mantras to Attract Money
- Have a Big Grand Poster of Goddess Mahalakshmi or Lord Balaji
- Attend The Money Workshop

Want to Be Healthy

- Keep photos of healthy people on the wall where you can see daily
- Do not keep medicines unnecessarily in your house unless they are prescribed and you are obliged to take them.
- Keep a Fish Tank, which you should see regularly. This reduces your Stress Levels.
- Learn more about Nutrition, Wellness, and about the mind body connect.
- You could keep a Quartz crystal
- Surround yourself with the color Blue or Green
- Eat Healthy, Avoid Junk
- Focus on Healing and Wellness. Avoid talking about Bad Health or Disease because you attract what you think most.

Want to Buy a Car or a home

- Keep a poster of the car and a resembling home that you Desire
- Take a Test Drive and imagine you are driving your own car.
- Go to the area you desire for a home and visit it regularly if near your vicinity.

- Purchase a Key Chain in Advance. This triggers Faith in Action and soon you will be having your own home or car.

You will Attract Whatever You Give Attention to- it could be positive or negative

Once you understand the principles of Law of Attraction or Manifesting, life becomes Magical. Life becomes Easy. Things are created twice, first in the Mind then in Reality. In this Game you have to win in the Mind before you win in Reality. The whole of the Indian System worked on Mind Mastery- creating powerful states within the mind. It is tough to explain all this in words and needs a personal presence of a master to trigger higher consciousness.

Explore; become interested into this subject because this is the Greatest Power Given to Humans. Why not use it in its full capacity?

Dream Big, Set Goals and Take Actions.

Suresh Padmanabhan is the creator of "Money Workshop", "Sankalpa Siddhi" or the "Eastern Law of Attraction". He is a professional speaker, author, life coach and mentor. He is the author of three books titled "I Love Money", "On Cloud 9" and "Ancient Secrets of Money". His book "I Love Money" ha been translated to 11 languages and is an international bests seller. His talks have been telecast worldwide through Zee Networks; a leading Indian based TV Channel. His aim is to create an impact on millions of people worldwide and raise their level of consciousness in all areas, especially pertaining to Money, Life and Spirituality.

www.themoneyworkshop.com

CHAPTER 5

The Willingness Process

Jane Kirby

"Where there is a will, there is a way."

What an aphorism and The Dalai Lama can teach us…

"Where there is a will, there is a way"…is an aphorism that simply means: Any person, with enough determination, can and will find a way to achieve something!

I would love to share with you a personal story about a meeting I had with the Dalai Lama. It was the second time that I met him, and this time was in 2010. It was a big gathering and there were lots of people, but at the end of the meeting we were permitted to ask questions. There was not much time left, but the assistants said they would choose two or three questions to pass forward.

I had a friend who was visiting me, and he was going through a tough time. He was suffering from intense self-loathing, and I admit I was also a bit worried that he was may be having a real problem with some kind of a substance abuse that he wasn't admitting to.

So my question was: "How does one best help somebody if they are battling with low self-esteem and beating themselves up? What's the best thing that one can do to be of assistance?"

Of course I was asking this question as a friend caring about a friend, and also because being a counselor… this is something that I often have to encounter in my work. But there is a difference between a person coming for professional counseling and someone simply approaching a friend – then one cannot necessarily volunteer assistance, unless the friend is asking for help.

I was lucky enough that my question got passed forward, and the following was The Dalai Lama's reply: **"The first thing that you need to know is that even if Buddha himself came down to assist you with someone. If that person themselves is un-willing to heal, then there is really nothing that can be done to help them."**

I can admit at the time, although his message was clear, I was slightly heart broken. I thought "That doesn't help", but I really got the strength of the message about how *important* it is in any kind of healing, or getting over any kind of fight, whether it's a minor problem or a major illness - that there *is* the reality and essentially it needs our own willingness within that healing process.

The welcomed dichotomy…

It was soon after this meeting I had just begun to facilitate large groups of workshop participants, and this was always in the back of my mind... this willingness.

I began to observe in the workshops, that within the truth of those words of His Holiness that day - was also gifted a beautiful dichotomy, which is that the opposite is also completely true: **When anyone really is willing… then healing can happen, and fights can end, so rapidly that it can almost spin one's head.**

I've seen people come to workshops and shift through and heal stuff that they've been battling with for years and simply get through it within a matter of hours, just in their pure willingness of truly wanting to shift.

Subsequent to this, I started to become genuinely driven by a desire to create a (new) way of conducting workshops. To be able to teach about psychology in a more accessible fun, light way…and so be able to assist people to find their willingness to get past *any* fight or problem.

I was most interested in how to best assist any participant who turns up for a workshop, so that they can tap into their own strength and innate willingness with ease.

Embracing the new...

The result, in 2011, was a new model for teaching, learning and healing called The Willingness Process. It was the fast and effective results, and the poplar response to this model (that involves many interactive exercises and much humor - both essential, I find, for willingness) that led to the kind invitation to contribute to this book. An honor I feel touched by, and reassured by, that this model does have some real merit.

It excites me, as I know in practice that instigating willingness -in anyone of us - *does* have a true effect and huge power.

I am thrilled by the ongoing growth of this model, and of willingness in general in our life time, because I know it really does not matter how much knowledge I may have as a 'therapist' or speaker, (or any of us has as a doctor, teacher, friend or practitioner); it does not matter how much our friends may want to help us. And it does not matter how much we want to help someone in our family. That at the end of the day… it *is* up to each one of us, to tap into what it really takes to *genuinely* shift past our stuff.

Incidentally I am not saying that we *all* cannot be of assistance to other people. We can all be of *great* assistance to all other beings. And particularly of assistance to those of us who may be struggling with being willing to be willing to assist ourselves.

What we can learn from a humorous Dr. of Psychology….

Here, I would love to share with you one of my favorite quotes by one of my teacher's Dr. Chuck Spezzano who often jokes:

"Men have two favorite forms of Personal Growth. The first is _____ (well you can likely imagine what the first is), and the second is when their partner takes the first step forward for them."

How the seemingly impossible is possible…

So often after a workshop, an attending participant will contact me…days or even months later, usually to tell me something that most often reads like this:

"Anyone would have sworn that my partner / my mother / my brother attended the workshop too. I came home and they were somehow different, and the relationship is just so much easier!"

I love hearing these reports as it 100% confirms two things: One which is the *logic* behind why it *is* so worth being personally willing to address an issue or a concern, and the other is a very simple *scientific* reason why this seeming 'miracle' occurs. Being a lover of both logic and science - both reasons and the results enthrall me. I will share these two reasons, in more detail later.

Defining willingness…

At this mid-chapter interim, I would like to share with you a definition of what willingness, in my own words, actually is.

Willingness means: **"To be aware of and acknowledging of the heart - and so of life's effortless ease - and then, actively participating in solutions and resolutions".**

Now that does not sound too horrid or too off-putting does it?

As here is where willingness stands alone as distinguishable from willpower and un-willingness. Exercising willpower and unwillingness usually both require *huge* effort, and usually a lot of strain and restraint. Willingness on the other hand is *much* easier. And likely this is why it suits my (and perhaps your) personal nature. I know it suits me because I am essentially lazy, and anything that requires gigantic effort will always put me off! On the other hand anything that is easy *and* has results - count me in!

The best news here is… All it really takes to shift and speedily work through *any* problem, fight, hurt, or dilemma (no matter how old that 'problem' is) is often just a good dose of self-applied willingness.

Discovering and uncovering your genius…

Willingness I have observed is not only *very* innate within us all, but also inherent in every one of us. In fact, I have not yet met anyone who is *not* a genius and a living master…even *if* they do not *yet* know this about themselves.

Your inherent genius and innate willingness is part of your essential nature. The only question that follows is: **Would you being willing to explore and accept this, as possibly 100% true about you?** It is an important question, as discovering this *is* a truth about you, it can and *will* instantly make your life *so* much easier.

There is one catch though... Exploring and embracing personal willingness *will* make you stop all excuses, any repeating patterns and a plethora of old stories! Can you give that up? **Can you face stopping your own excuses? Of course you can – you're a genius!**

And, of course, you can and may still fall apart at times and fail at times - this is human - and part of accepting what it *is* to be human and not a God!

Here is another question that may assist you in deciding:

Are your 'stories' about what your life is like or was like... killing you, and your happiness, far more than what your life actually is now and could be?"

Whist we consider this, let's talk about *why* when we genuinely embrace willingness and changes within ourselves... *why* others instantly, miraculously, appear to change and become more willing too:

Exploring the logic, the EPR Paradox, and Quantum Entanglement...

The first logical reason why others 'miraculously' seem to change, is because when you / or I change (be it our thoughts, attitudes or reactions) then those around us literally have little to no choice but to change too...as they can no longer relate with whom you were, but now have to relate to who you are!

This is a great and empowering fast 'game changer' - that we all have the innate ability to speed track into place.

When we truly embrace changes within ourselves, then **who we were is just no longer applicable, and soon enough others do realize this...** and their old way of communicating with us either just does not work or - lets be more honest - we have likely become a LOT nicer, clearer and easier to communicate with now.

The scientific reasons why others (particularly those closest to us) do often change, is simply due to the essential nature of all energy and all matter - Energy and matter being one and the same thing really.

This can be best explained by a discovery made by Albert Einstein and two of his colleagues in 1935, called the **Einstein-Podolsky-Rosen (EPR) paradox**... and further expanded upon in 1997 (in a very surprising discovery highly discussed and published at the time) called **Quantum Entanglement.**

I often discuss both of these discoveries in detail in workshops, and for now here is a brief laymen explanation of what these discoveries revealed:

When two energies (in the case of the EPR paradox it was two protons, and in Quantum Entanglement - two particles) **have been in relationship with each other... and are then spilt apart within time and space - they appeared to still be energetically** (and seemingly telepathically) **connected.**

In the subsequently then named 'Quantum Entanglement' discovery, it was noted again that: When the motion or the direction of the spin, of one of the separated particles was altered... then simultaneously the other particle also shifted into *exactly* the same motion and direction. This happened instantaneously... every time they repeated the experiment.

Einstein classically referred to this occurrence as: "Spooky action at a distance"

It is worthy to note here that both science and most people, cannot be fooled i.e. we either change the direction of our thoughts or we do not. If for example, you have not really changed your mind about how you view and perceive a particular matter – do not be surprised if your mother / brother / or seemingly to your 'annoying' neighbor does not appear to change - ever – either!

So why not, rather, take a brave step forward with faith and science (I love when they go hand in hand) and change your spin on life literally... and see what will and *can* amazingly occur. It is worth an experiment of checking it out anyway... even if you do so just to prove Einstein wrong. It won't be the first time he has been challenged!

I encourage you look up these discoveries further. Here is a reliable link: www.en.m.wikipedia.org/wiki/Quantum_entaglement

What learning, unlearning, and everyone can teach us...

The following is what I know to be true - I have observed this within thousands of hours of workshops and hundreds of hours on one-on-one counseling: That healing *any* problem, hurt, situation, story, or illness, is really simply a question of being 100% willing to be willing to do something - *oneself* - about it!

One of my dearest friends – Noma Nontshinga – once said to me, post her single handedly assisting several refugees out of a war torn area into the safety of South Africa; "Well someone had to do something, and my middle name just happens to be 'Someone'."

I am not necessarily suggesting that you too run into war torn areas now, unless you want to. Yes - breathe a sigh of relief. As even just ending the possible war in our own homes is a wise and good place to start, to make a difference.

When we simply choose to become more willingly proactive in our own (and therefore actually everyone's) healing, and not just be reactive to others and to life's ups and downs - which let us be clear, will only keep us all (and life) rocking all over the joint! And it won't be an Elvis jailhouse rock - more like a "Do not pass go, do not collect 200, everyone go to 'heartbreak hotel' jail. Where we all remain stuck - somewhere between a rock and a hard place! *That* does not sound like a fun house party to me!

The first thing to know is - you are the key - and it would be just like you to volunteer would it not? For if you are unwilling to take 100% responsibility and accountability for the state of your own life and your own mind…why should anyone else take care of it?

We are not really here to be each other's mind keepers… we are here to be each other's cheerers, and at the very least what we *can* all do is ensure we come to the table as stable and accountable as we possibly can be!

Secondly: No one is ever past help - not even you, and not even her or even him. The only question is what are you going to do about it?

Looking at life as a smörgäsbord…

There is old wise story about life… that life is rather like a smörgäsbord board, and **we each have our own dish to bring to the table**. We each have our own unique spices, our own ways and our own secret ingredients that make our dish unique and delicious. My dish may not appeal to some people, but yours will. So the most important thing to remember is:

When you don't bring your dish to the table then someone on the other side of the table will go hungry, because they can only eat your dish. Someone else will starve!

So it *is* important that you bring what *you* have to uniquely contribute, as big or as small as that dish may be - if it made love and a big heart that is all that is required! It is in fact what you have come to do – it is one of life's greatest and most fulfilling purposes.

As a facilitator, a lover of change, I find time and again that the more I tap into my *own* willingness…and a willingness *even* to be 100% wrong about how I think or how someone else is, and what any present or past 'fact' appears to be - then others become more willing too!

Embracing a willingness to be wrong…

Herein is an important key to the *huge* transformation that being willing can gift anyone and everyone (including you)… Be 100% willing to be wrong.

It sounds contra intuitive - but it is a gateway to seeing and experiencing new, easier, and faster ways through any upset.

Think of it this way…the need to be right – all the time – is egotistical and rather unlikely! Unless you did write the Encyclopedia Britannica all on your own, and even if you could – shhhhhhh!

Being willing to be a life-long learner will not only enhance your own life – and others lives - it will also make us all not so annoying, more accessible and much more approachable.

Being willing to be wrong, also open us up instantly to a pool of more genius ideas. Many ideas are discovered and uncovered by so many people. I am highly excited by the growing discoveries and even the wild ideas within our time.

As an old but reliable saying goes. "Two heads are better than one", and getting head isn't half bad either! Yes – I just threw that in for the male readers among us.

What our friends and forefathers would say…

And yes they would agree with the above headline.

A friend of mine - Ruth Donald - calls a willingness to be wrong: **Giving up thinking we might be the masters and commanders of the entire universe, and that anyone else is.** And it is what my father would call: Suspending all disbelief. Suspending all disbelief in others and in yourself in particular - will take you far.

There is an old African proverb that I love, that puts this perfectly. It goes like this:

"If you want to go fast go alone, but if you want to go far go with others."

Being from Africa here is some more African wisdom I would love to share with you and it is *very* applicable if you do wish to embrace and access your willingness to transform yourself and the world.

What we can learn from West Africa about willingness....

There is a tribe in West Africa, called **the Dagara**, who **have a very particular way of dealing with conflicts**. Those caught in conflict are called forward to sit, facing one another, in the center of a large outside ash circle.

The entire village community is then gathered to completely surround them. What happens next may not be what you would expect...

First those surrounded are freely allowed to speak about what is going on in the conflict, if they so wish to share... and next (and this is the magic part) **no lengthy discussions follow suite, no blame or judgments are made, no trial to discern the "guilty" and "non guilty"** ... instead the entire tribe simply begins to sing about and directly to those trapped in their conflict.

The songs are specific - and known by heart by every tribe member, of every other tribe member.

The songs on this day are about only those surrounded, and **the lyrics speak only about all that is noble within those individuals:** Of their strengths, their essence and their deepest nature. Of their many noted abilities, and gifts plus the meaning behind their given names... their personal life purpose.

I have been told by a transcriber of the Dagara rituals and tribe, that this particular ritual is 99.9% of the time hugely effective and transformative. I find it very easy to understand why!

In my mind, I envision, an aftermath of two sobbing tribe members in the middle of the circle - touched with humility and care! I've always so loved this ritual of the Dagara Tribe!

In my 18 slow years of studying psychology and my personal experience of facilitating larger groups I have come to notice again and again, that accessing and instigating true willingness is almost exactly like this above Dagara ritual.

Life changing willingness is about remembering who you are, and who everyone is - beyond our fights, beyond our borders, beyond our mistakes that we judge as un-dismissible and unforgivable.

The only 'problem' is when we dismiss ourselves as collectively and individually unforgivable – then we end up missing out on our entire lives… even sometimes taking our own lives and often taking the lives of others. Taking whom you, and he, and she, and we all really came to be – friends and soul mates (not the romantic kind) the real kind… mankind interacting within and being in our full potential.

In the real nature of willingness…as to the Dagara people … **any conflict, be it intra or inter personal is also always viewed as a message to the wider community** and world, that there is also a larger communal conflict in play. And so in reminding the individual of his/her own true nature, in turn each person within the tribe is reminded of his or her true nature and purpose.

Embracing some 'out-lawed' learning…

Malidoma Somë (a Dagara tribesman educated in America) speaks of the time he told his Elders about many of the law practices of The West. They were particularly bewildered and puzzled by the concept of people going to courts and suing each other over a disagreement or a broken agreement. Somë writes that after a short debate amongst the Elders themselves, they had only one question for him:

"How, then - do these people ever learn anything?"

The later catches us more than the former. We can forgive and forget, but **can we truly give up all judgment… and just learn**?

Can we catch that it is, possibly, only our judgments (be it of our selves or of another) that are demanding of us to conceive and perceive that forgiving is necessary and required? Can we realize that to perceive that we must forgive only denotes that we have judged in the first place? I feel the deeper question then becomes, could we rather simply love others and ourselves to let go of our beliefs around the need to judge?

Let us consider for a moment that responding to a mistake or an abhorrent act and being open to seeing beyond it; is not about conceding to the act, but understanding that **responding with an equaled anger or violence -** simply **grows further abhorrence and more mistakes.**

In accepting that the act has occurred, and responding to that in a different way... then assimilates a change, rather than perpetuates perhaps an ongoing problem.

Anyone who has been on the receiving end of TRUE forgiveness - knows this!

And certainly everyone can understand this, even if there is huge resistance to it!

And, yes I know some acts *do* seem so very unforgivable. And I am not condoning those acts at all, I am simple saying when we truly wish to stop such behavior... a different response to those acts is required.

Opening up to the power of non-judgment and defenselessness...

You may find some of the following, challenging to adsorb, and perhaps however just trust me - as someone who has been on the receiving end of what anyone would perceive as an 'abhorrent violation' when I was a very young child (Yes - it was sexual. No it was not a family member), and I do not feel any anger about that... So why, would you?

I know this is a touchy subject for people, which is why I bring it up because it highlights so brightly where we draw our lines. *"No that is the line, do not cross it!"*

Do we stop our own abilities to learn when we meet our lines? Are some of our lines too short?

Why do we have lines?

Do lines not create, and invite predators? Does our defensiveness create our feeling of a need to defend ourselves?

Is defenselessness rather.... the very best defense we could muster, and be brave and wise and willing enough to just develop – fast?

A question is... have I / you / we all matured yet enough to truly see that defensiveness and judgment just simply does not work?

Are you /am I really willing to make a stand for change? Are we really willing to change ourselves or do we just want others to change?

Are you willing to stop fighting in your own home first and foremost? Forget the Middle East for a while, who are we to judge if we're throwing chairs across our own dining tables? Are we willing to stop fighting amongst our own families, our neighborhoods and communities?

Am I truly willing / are you truly willing to also stop seeing another as 'wrong', and stop even perpetually punishing ourselves when we sometimes (quite often - if we are really honest!) get it 'wrong' ourselves?

Does our guilt about when we get it wrong keep us trapped in a projection cycle of fighting and so not seeing and healing our own hurts?

Whilst we consider all this…as yes I realize I have just perhaps jumped way into the deep end of the pool with you... Let's have a joke break. There is always time for a good joke.

OK

A good joke break never goes amiss….

So a builder goes into a bar and hears the most beautiful piano music.

He says to the barman "Wow, where is that music coming from?"

The barman points down to the end of the bar, and there sitting on the bar counter is a miniature man, sitting at a miniature grand piano - playing away.

"He is amazing! Where did you find him?" the builder asks.

The barman points down to the other end of the bar, to a lamp.

"You see that lamp" he says, "It's magic. It will grant anyone who gives it a good rub one wish. I got that piano player!"

"Wow, can I give it a try?" asks the builder.

"Sure, go ahead! But remember you will only get one go!"

Excited the builder rushes outside with the lamp and starts rubbing it frantically. Suddenly millions of ducks start falling down from the sky. The builder runs back into the bar for cover, looking really pissed off.

"Hey this lamp is faulty! I wished for a million bucks, and a millions ducks started falling on top of me?"

The barman looks at him and says, "Hmmmm, yeah I know! Do you really think I asked for a 10 inch Pianist???"

I admit, every time I hear any piano music now, I think of this joke and I smile!

So... back to our conversation about willyness, I mean willingness.

Facing our unwilling and stubborn sides…

If you ever want to witness just how stubborn we *all* really can be… **Just begin to take note of how un-willing you, I, and others can sometimes be at the very suggestion of changing ourselves!**

We are, of course, quite willing to suggest and say, "Oh no, you first, please go ahead. It is after all you who has the problem anyway!"

Even as a facilitator of willingness workshops, I too still sometimes get caught in some of my own unwillingness at times. Yup, sorry not perfect!

And when I do get unwilling… then **beautiful life always gives me a good kick up the backside for forgetting that personal willingness is THE first key!**

A saying by one of my colleagues comes to mind: "A kick up the back side is, at least, always a step forward"

As much as we may kick and scream about how unfair that feels! And oh Yes we can all (definitely including myself) have times may feel so very hard done by, (hold on where's my hard done by hat?) And feel like we have to 'do' *all* the work only, always! (Hold on where's my victim hat?)

Yet, here is the irony…

Don't tell too many people though…Personal willingness IS actually the easy way, and it is so fast… that you will likely kick your own ass the next time forever even thinking another may work faster!

Sure for ALL of us (especially you) it would be so nice if others changed. But for that… are you willing to potentially wait for years /decades to pass perhaps?

If you are anything like me - you are also a bit impatient, so that route will just feel a bit too deathly slow (and in time quite insanely stupid to have even thought up).

Facing the possible inconvenience…

Because here is another inconvenient truth…And sorry to break this one to you, most especially if you are meeting me for the first time via this chapter, or if you know me well (and you may be about to think "hello you're only sharing this with me now?")… Sorry, and the news flash is-

Have you ever, genuinely, considered deeply that it **is quite possible that your spouse / your neighbor / your brother… just may not want to change at all – ever?** More especially not into the way you would prefer!

What if they share with you that they are genuinely quite happy with anyone (including you) thinking they are a 'pain in the ass'? That they do not give an ass about that? It's a free world after all! **Then what??**

Are you then going to get caught up judging them, and in so creating a delay in your own steps forward? Are you, yourself, then going to give up on creating a happier, calmer, and more love-filled life?

Or are you genuinely willing to halt 'wanting others to change', stop complaining about it, and just change yourself?

Don't miss a golden opportunity hidden it that conundrum!

Within all that drama, all that resistance, here is the *fantastic* news (hold on stop the trains) the most superb opportunity about simply being willing to change yourself ...is then, remember 100% of the time, others have to change around you. They have little to no choice, but to! As because you have changed... others can no longer relate to you as to whom you were, but now have to relate to who you are…and who you continue to become.

The bottom line is... **If you want another, or even the world to change** (people love harping on about that one, but I love the huge vision thinking of that!)... Then the very fastest way (avoiding blowing up the planet and starting all over again) always has been, and always will be to change yourself. It's not rocket science really… it's simply being willing to do what it takes to experience real shifts – fast!

In conclusion:

What Mother Nature and you can teach us all…

To conclude to this chapter I would love to offer you one last story – this one is about butterflies, and then I am flying out of here.

When a butterfly is preparing to completely break free of its cocoon… it has already changed from a caterpillar into a butterfly, but it is not quite really yet. No one could do any service to it, in trying to assist it to 'break free' faster than it is doing so on its very own.

In fact, to do so will only injure it, or at least diminish its ability to fly, and in the worst-case scenario: we could even kill it in our hastiness to make it transition at a speed we would prefer to see it change.

Trust is a huge part of life. Trust that most of the time, we need not speed things up. That, in fact, sometimes when we attempt to do so - we can kill what we wanted to nurture!

The struggle for a butterfly to break free is exactly what prepares and empowers that butterfly to one day fly with elegance, beauty, and great strength. Likewise… **when living with yourself and with others - do not force anything faster than you or they can appear to move.**

Trust your life. Trust others. Believe in yourself. Believe in others! And then *trust* again – that **everything that has happened so far,** for you and to anyone else - **has happened, or is happening, at exactly the correct pace** for you, and them, to know how to truly fly one day.

The even better news is... when we are on the cusp of change, breaking free of all our old constraints (both mental and practical) - change can, will and does occur very fast!

There always comes a time in every butterfly's life and in every human life - when left unforced that the end of all struggle becomes both inevitable and evitable.

So don't give up hope, and don't force. Just allow and remember that everyone you see is a master, we just don't all know that yet!

The crystal key to all healing is very simply not to judge - not yourself – or anyone else! For we can either judge or we can help, but we can never to both at the same time.

Self-forgiveness ironically ends up being far more difficult than ever forgiving anyone else. Life asks of us to extend compassion to everyone – including ourselves!

Truly feeling and extending compassion with, for, and to everyone is the heart form of deep willingness. Your heart and your willingness will always give back to you, and others, far more than it ever asks of you.

Without extending compassion all the time to everyone (again including to yourself) - No matter what 'story' or 'proof' wants to tell us otherwise - why we could and should not be compassionate.

And then we get stuck in thinking that some should suffer or deserve to struggle, and some of us don't. And we miss the very point of life - why we are really here... to remember we are already whole, and that we all come from one source. Even if we may disagree on what that one source is - it remains unaltered that we all started at the same point at the beginning of all time.

It is only when we forget this, and choose to judge each other (and ourselves) instead, we also miss out on the great mastery present and offered to us *all*, in any struggle.

Dissolve all barriers of 'right' and 'wrong', 'us' and 'them'… and you will release yourself from all war (and the acronym for war, if you did not know this already, is: We Are Right)

The butterfly does not fight to be right… it struggles only to break free of all its constraints. Just as we do as humans. Judge not the fight…simply watch and learn.

People often do *huge* service for us in showing us in which direction we do not want to go. It may be hard to watch, but it is still a service for all to observe, and all to learn from!

Be patient with everyone. *Everyone* you ever meet is already a master, is already a son, or daughter or living being of one original source.

We cannot ever really get it 'wrong', we can only sometimes be quite slow in coming to remember this! And time is irrelevant. Time as science has shown us, and mystics speak of, does not really exist.

So breathe… Learn, allow, and let yourself fly…and in doing so you may be surprised how many around you also begin to experience flight.

In conclusion, remembering only this… at heart, you are already perfectly whole and innocent – as is everyone – and if you are willing to remember this, you are actually already flying.

I wish you huge personal willingness, gigantic happiness, and nothing less!

Jane Kirby is a qualified therapist, international trauma counselor, and the creator of The Willingness Process modality. She works full-time as a counselor, public speaker, master workshop facilitator, author, and master trainer at the NewAge Foundation India and International. When Jane is not traveling conducting live seminars, she lives in Zambia with her husband Chad.

www.janekirby.info

CHAPTER 6

Ho'oponopono - The Magical Prayer Healing

Rashminder Kaur

The Essence

If there is something that transcends all boundaries of culture and creed and unites humanity, it is the practice of prayer. Prayer is much more than a religious ritual and its essence when understood becomes the very purpose of life itself. As Rumi says, *"After all, the purpose of The Prayer is not to stand and bow all Day long. The purpose is to possess continuously that fragrant state which appears to you in prayer."*

We all pray and we all know how prayer brings solace, faith, courage and strength to persevere in our aspirations and the challenges. Prayer when done with consciousness can enlighten our life path and turn our mundane existence into a beautiful melody. Prayer is the most personal experience that we have; it is an inner journey and yet due to cultural conditioning, prayer is often reduced to perfunctory chanting or ritualistic worship.

Prayer sets the stage for genuine healing. And when we truly learn how to pray, we never fall apart in life. Wisdom and love emerge and help take us on the journey to full awakening. Prayer is an essential element of man's divine aspiration to know the meaning of life and his own self. And prayer becomes a seeker's first and last resort on this journey.

As a child I used to do our religious prayers everyday and I did it quite religiously for years, I asked for protection from nightmares, I asked for a good life, I asked for relief from my sufferings and the list went on. However, at some point, I realized that I never truly understood what genuine prayer means and what the real focus of prayer should be. But with time I learned some precious lessons about praying. It was through Sufi poetry and the works of poets like Khalil Gibran and Rabindranath Tagore that I began to get a real clue.

Though I have been praying every day, I never considered that prayer could act as a healing method until I came across Ho'oponopono. This practice and its essence have changed my perception of prayer and today I use this practice whenever I face any challenge. Not just that, I do Ho'oponopono even when I am completely fine as I find that it is the simplest way to return to your true self. Ho'oponopono is a manifestation of the highest aspect of love and freedom that we are, and its essence is infinitely inspiring.

I am glad to share my perception of this wonderful prayer healing. In my last six years of experience as a holistic healer, I have worked with many people who come to me with their problems including physical ailments, emotional traumas, painful life experiences or spiritual chaos. For many years I have used Reiki, EFT and sometimes other remedies like diet, music, color therapy etc. to help them, besides offering them counseling to shift their perspective.

Having seen varied shades of human suffering both in my own self and through others I had a quest to understand and eliminate this suffering that ultimately led me to explore Non-Dual Awareness. However, it was as a part of this quest that I came to know this wonderful healing practice called Ho'oponopono to which I was first introduced in one of the workshops led by my teacher Dr. Paula Horan four years ago.

I was amazed by the simplicity of this practice and its innate wisdom of oneness; however I did not practice it much in the beginning. But when lost in a desert, you look for an oasis! And so it was that a year ago, I encountered a particularly challenging life situation and I realized that I only had prayers to my aid. We normally take refuge in prayer when no physical action is possible or effective in a situation. However with Ho'oponopono I realized that prayer should be the primary course of action as the insight revealed through it can lead us to take the right action, thus saving us from being erroneous in our effort to resolve a problem.

Ever since my own experience with this form of prayer healing, I am using it with every patient and every time its benefit is verified sometimes through miraculous results and sometimes through revelation of much needed insight into a problem. Whatever be the case, I feel Ho'oponopono is the dark horse of healing. A practice that looks too simple to be truly effective, but when done with persistence and real presence, can open doors to true wisdom and love.

I am sharing here a brief insight into Ho'oponopono and its various aspects. As much of the general information is available through many resources, my focus here is to offer my perspective on this practice and how it can be applied and understood for the best result. Though my journey with Ho'oponopono has not been a long one, time never defines the expanse of an experience and so I feel that despite my not so old encounter with Ho'oponopono I can share some amazing insights and healing experiences I received through this practice.

The Process

What is Ho'oponopono?

Ho'oponopono is a prayer healing which has been practiced by the ethnic people of Hawaii. There are many different forms of this prayer healing which are practiced across many Polynesian islands as well. We have seen how ethnic communities rely on either natural elements or divine forces for healing and reconciliation and how shamans and priests play a great role in such communities offering counsel and acting as a medium between the man and nature.

Ho'oponopono has also been practiced in a similar way where a priest or elder of the family would offer prayer along with the members of the family for a conflict resolution or healing of physical illness. In traditional practice the healing or resolution is also celebrated with a ceremonial feast. When studied closely we understand how wise and holistic the people of these ethnic civilizations are, as they truly understand the cause of suffering and work on it in a way that eliminates ego and isolation and brings our awareness closer to oneness. It is this very essence of Ho'oponopono which I admire and I often take refuge in this prayer healing whenever I face a crisis and my awareness is under the smog of suffering.

The meaning of Ho'oponopono in Hawaiian is 'mental cleansing'. Ho'o is similar to 'To' as it appears before a noun in English. And 'pono' is defined as goodness, correct, well being, welfare, true condition or nature, righteous, just, beneficial, successful, in perfect order, accurate, relieved, necessary, eased, fair, virtuous etc.

Ponopono is defined as "to put right; to put in order or shape, correct, revise, adjust, amend, regulate, arrange, rectify, tidy up, make orderly or neat". And this is what any healing is focused at.

The prayer comprises of four phrases: Please forgive me, I am Sorry, I love you, I thank you. Ho'oponopono is done by repeating these four phrases continuously, keeping the person or problem in mind. And this practice is done repeatedly for days or weeks until the healing or resolution takes place.

What looks like a simple chanting of some phrases has a profound effect when done from a heartfelt space. And that is why it is important to understand the correct perspective you need to have while doing this practice, without which it will only remain a superficial chant and one would not receive its benefit.

Thus the right perspective is the core of this practice, because the prayer in itself is simple and can be learned and memorized in less than a minute. However, what it takes a healer to work with Ho'oponopono, is the awareness from which you send the prayers.

History of Modern Ho'oponopono:

Ho'oponopono in its traditional form was primarily used for reconciliation among families by the natives of Hawaii, by offering forgiveness, acceptance and gratitude in the form of prayers done under the guidance of a priest or a family elder.

Ho'oponopono as we have learned and practiced it today has come from Morrnah Simeona who is regarded as a healing priest or kahuna lapaau. Simeona adapted the traditional Ho'oponopono and applied it as both a general problem solving process and for psycho-spiritual self-help. In accordance with the Hawaiian tradition she emphasized prayer, confession, repentance and mutual restitution and forgiveness. However her application of the practice is also said to be influenced by her Christian education as well as her study of Eastern philosophers and Buddhist influence which comes from the Chinese and Japanese immigrants to Hawaii which has also permeated Hawaiian culture.

The first modern teaching of Ho'oponopono started with Pacifica Seminars founded by Morrnah Simeona in Germany. After Simeona passed in 1992, her former student and administrator Ihaleakala Hew Len, co-authored a book with Joe Vitale called 'Zero Limits'. The success of this book marked the entry of Ho'oponopono into the western world. And since then this healing practice is spreading across the world as millions of people experience its graceful impact.

Dr. Hew Len has a very inspiring story of how he healed the inmates of a mental asylum just by using Ho'oponopono perseveringly for 4 years. The result of his magnanimous effort has been one of the most astonishing stories of alternative healing. It was precisely this story that stirred my heart and propelled me to learn more about it. I have found that just doing Ho'oponopono in difficult times brings my composure back within minutes.

I recommend people read about Dr. Hew Len's work to receive more insight into the history and practice of Ho'oponopono.

The Technique

With any practice, if you understand the essence, you never go wrong in your application. And it is the same with Ho'oponopono. The application is only an extension of the essence and thus in my own work I focus on delivering the essence of a practice in its entirety. In the same way, if you learn the basics of car driving, you can drive any car with ease, if you learn the basics of healing you can utilize any healing practice to its utmost efficiency. And Ho'oponopono reflects the essence of healing in its simplest and most subtle form.

The essence of Ho'oponopono is the manifestation of three key aspects of universal love. These are –

- Acceptance
- Forgiveness
- Gratitude

Universal love, which forms the very fabric of creation, from which all matter and spirit evolve, is embodied by these attributes of Acceptance, Forgiveness and Gratitude. When we focus on these attributes and integrate them with our full acceptance of responsibility for whatever problem is occurring, we easily manifest the universal love, which cleanses faulty patterns from our consciousness and fills us with awareness.

Thus Ho'oponopono is not energy based, but consciousness based practice and that is why it is devoid of any visual or energetic experience but it brings healing through awareness.

Another key aspect of Ho'oponopono is that it helps us to cultivate responsible Love. In his experience with the inmates of the mental asylum, Dr. Hew Len has shared how it was not the inmates whom he healed; rather it was a part of his own consciousness that had created the reality of the inmates, which he healed. This is very profound, because in truth, whatever we see in our environment is a projection of our own inner imprint. And thus it is not the patient alone but the healer as well, that needs the healing.

While doing Ho'oponopono, the healer or the person doing it, needs to cultivate a loving acceptance and a sense of responsibility for the whole condition of the situation. And then seek forgiveness from the imprints that cause it and offer gratitude for the lesson and the final release.

Thus, Ho'oponopono works at the very root cause of any suffering or disease, which is a false pattern or wrong imprint caused by our negative belief. To rectify this error in consciousness one has to first accept it, take responsibility to correct it, seek forgiveness for the error and be grateful for its release. This approach is what needs to be embedded in any healing practice, and that is why knowing and practicing Ho'oponopono elevates the understanding and perspective of a healer to a great degree.

During my experience in the Core Empowerment retreat with Dr. Paula Horan, I realized the significance of responsibility in healing and spiritual evolution. Without taking full responsibility for ourselves and all of our actions, for our life and for everything that we see, hear and face, we cannot attain freedom. Escape is not the way to nirvana, owning up is.

Ho'oponopono propels us to take responsibility not just for ourselves but also for others, as they are part of our own reality and thus not separate from us. This also points to the realization that Non-Dual awareness gives us; that we are the creators of our own reality and only by taking responsibility, can we change reality for the benefit of all.

Ho'oponopono like Reiki connects us to the source, which is not any force or entity outside of ourselves, but to our own awareness. The prayers are offered to this source with request to correct what is not in place, to discharge the memories that create bondage and suffering.

With this approach, Ho'oponopono also eliminates the feeling of 'doership' in a healer. It frees the healer from attracting any ego identification and thus the practice creates a more holistic awakening into greater awareness.

Ho'oponopono also allows us to see the oneness in everything, and that is evident as we intend the healing toward the problem, encompassing it as our own erroneous projection. When we integrate the love, forgiveness and gratitude in us toward the problem, we heal our internal projection of the problem and thus it changes the outer reality. It is beautiful to see how this practice dissolves the boundaries of inner and outer reality, of our self and others around us and gives us a glimpse of oneness.

It is true that we all take refuge in prayer and it offers an anchor to our faith and gives strength. However many times the prayers in our daily routine are a form of pleading for desire fulfillment and the true perspective of prayer is not reflected in it. But Ho'oponopono immediately turns our attention toward awareness, toward universal love and a sense of oneness with all that is. Our ego identification then dissolves as we immerse ourselves in the prayer state.

Some interesting experiences

My first miraculous experience with Ho'oponopono happened after I parted ways with a friend and was very upset, because we had not talked for more than a week's time. One evening after I finished my work, I was relaxing in my room and I thought about how I was contributing to the separation and not taking the needed step to bridge the gap. Immediately I sat down and started praying. I poured my heart into that healing and surrendered to the emotions that came up. After sometime I felt light and I stopped. I resumed my work without wondering what will happen. But within 5 minutes I received a message from my friend. We broke our silence and the bitterness from the argument was erased. Slowly we resumed our friendship and the hurt feelings were repaired.

Another incident happened when I was doing a Ho'oponopono session on a train journey. I prayed for various aspects of a problem to be healed, I prayed and prayed for two hours at a stretch and then relaxed. Suddenly I realized that my ego had tricked me. While doing the treatment, I had looked down upon other people involved and had a superior feeling and was directing the healing to happen as I wanted it to be.

A dark cloud of guilt loomed over my head and I was deeply disturbed. Two hours of prayers were wasted and I wondered how much wrong I might have done instead of creating harmony in the situation. I asked for forgiveness and prayed again and cleared my ego's projection in the situation. I was relieved that I received the insight to see this and rectify it. Ever since this incident, I am always more attentive to the thoughts and emotions that emerge during the practice.

The fact is, we have little control over our thoughts and emotions and they come in accordance to our resistance to, or incompleteness of an experience. We then try to fill the gap with our desired projections, however, this creates an egoistic barrier and the awareness of oneness and feeling of universal love goes missing. It is important that we keep our identification in check and do not fall into this trap.

A dear friend of mine, who had been going through a difficult phase in her marriage, also had some amazing results with Ho'oponopono. She did the prayers for her husband when he was in a very depressed state and she saw how he always felt better after the prayers and their fights ended in peace.

Another experience I often have with Ho'oponopono is that as I begin, I slowly feel the pain and agony of the person or situation. As if I become that person and situation and I can see it from all aspects. This enables me to find out where prejudices are coming from and what is missing in the picture that is creating the suffering in the first place. Sometimes it is difficult to do treatments with such intense emotional immersion, however one always feels light at the end and the calmness that comes is very healing in itself, as you feel a deep sense of resolution with the issue.

I truly feel that by doing Ho'oponopono, although it looks very simple, it has a very profound effect on our awareness, if we do it consciously. Because it is a prayer with four simple phrases, it can easily turn into a mechanical, automatic action if you don't allow yourself to be present and become unconscious.

The book 'Zero Limits' by Joe Vitale and Dr. Hew Len illustrates how by doing Ho'oponopono, we go into a zero state with no identity, no memories and thus no limits, a state in which we have infinite potential to manifest. This can be experienced by practitioners as they refine their practice day by day.

Ho'oponopono can be a great tool for healing however we should not expect miraculous results in every session. Life has its own design and a treatment session done now, can show its effect in a future event. In cases where many aspects are involved, it is suggested that the practice be continued for a longer period of time without seeking any immediate benefit. This is especially for people who are facing severe life challenges and going through a very complicated crisis.

In my view, Ho'oponopono complements the teachings of Non-Dual awareness and when integrated it can give even greater benefit and better understanding of the subject matter as well. If done in unison, practices of Non Dual awareness and Ho'oponopono can help us clear our Karma as well. As being aware allows us to disengage from ego identification and Ho'oponopono can help us complete our unfinished karma by offering love, forgiveness and gratitude.

I have always been in search of the most simple tools and teachings, as I believe that simple is divine. Nature accomplishes most complicated tasks with the simplicity of its design. Ho'oponopono, just like non-dual awareness is simple and grounded in the eternal principles of creation.

Necessity in today's time

Ho'oponopono is indeed a necessity of our time as we are all facing a major transition as many of our own shadows are being exposed to the light of awareness, through the individual and larger chaos that we are all enduring. It can offer peace, composure and awareness to overcome each of the challenges that arise. And because as a wise man once stated, "We are creating 97% negative karma in every moment (even people with the best of intentions), it behooves us to constantly be clearing our karma every day."

Also as violence, natural calamities and other social and economic upheavals are rising; people can practice Ho'oponopono to bring peace to the environment. It is said that the family that prays together stays together, and Ho'oponopono is the most altruistic prayer to offer in service to that, which is divine in all of us. It is not essential that we do Ho'oponopono only when there is a problem. We can do it for peace and harmony to prevail on earth.

Ho'oponopono reminds us of the eternal light of oneness. Its practice prepares us for our evolution where our existence reverberates with the energy of love, gratitude and forgiveness in every moment. It gives us the soil to sow the seeds of harmony and reap a life of grace and beauty.

It is my wish that the essence of Ho'oponopono and its practice reaches all sentient beings and the source of endless love opens for all.

Rashminder Kaur is a Reiki & EFT teacher and a student of Non Dual Awareness. Living in Ahmedabad, India, she offers healing and counseling services, and leads workshops to raise awareness in both social and spiritual domain. She is also working for a fitness center chain in Gujarat, offering creative consultation. In her spare time she offers volunteer service for nonprofit organizations that are working for the cause of organic and sustainable living.

rashmi_mimi@yahoo.com

CHAPTER 7

The Power of Forgiveness

Water E. Jacobson

Forgiving others is an act of compassion. We know this. Nonetheless, oftentimes we don't do it. We want those who hurt us to suffer for what they did. By withholding forgiveness we think we are punishing them. We think we are keeping them stuck in a prison of guilt and shame. But the fact is we're just punishing ourselves.

We're prolonging our own suffering. We're withholding from ourselves our own peace of mind. We're, essentially keeping ourselves locked in an emotional prison cell that is of our own making. We victimize ourselves long after having been victimized by our offenders.

Anger Hurts, Forgiveness Heals

Although anger has value as a signal device for survival, to alert us to danger so we can respond appropriately, most of us hang onto our anger long after it has served its purpose, using it to assault and manipulate those who have hurt us. Unfortunately, when we do this, we are hurting ourselves more than anyone else in the process.

Anger deprives us of inner peace and joy. Anger diminishes our capacity to give and receive love. Anger is hazardous to our health. Anger stimulates the release of stress chemicals that wear down our bodies. Anger raises blood pressure and increases our risk of heart attacks and strokes. Anger depresses our immune system, makes us more vulnerable to diseases and cancer, and makes it more difficult for us to recover from illnesses and injuries.

Anger causes us to be emotionally imbalanced, sometimes to the point of making very impulsive, irrational, reckless decisions that have dire physical consequences for ourselves and others.

Forgiveness decreases our anger, healing us emotionally and physically, it's a no-brainer that the smart money is on forgiveness and that to hang onto anger is the real sucker play.

There is absolutely no advantage to staying angry. We can take care of ourselves and protect ourselves and our interests just as well, if not better, when we are calm and non-reactive.

If we understand the danger our anger alerted us to, we'll know what to watch out for in the future for our safety and security, and we won't need to continue attacking ourselves by hanging onto our anger. And so it behooves us to consistently remind ourselves that anger hurts us and forgiveness heals us!

When We Forgive Others We Free Ourselves

Forgiveness decreases our anger, our depression, our stress and our anxiety as well. We sleep better. We have more energy. We're more at peace with ourselves. Our general attitude is more positive, optimistic, hopeful and joyful.

All of this maximizes our potential to attract people, places and circumstances into our lives, which will support us, synergize with our goals and propel us towards the fulfillment of our dreams.

Consequently, it is always in our own best interests to forgive everyone. Unconditionally. Without exceptions. Regardless of how they're behaving or what they have done to us.

What To Do When We Resist Forgiving Others

When we are having difficulty forgiving others, we focus on our blessings and on being grateful for what we have in our lives despite what has been done to us. This can take the sting out of any offense and make it easier for us to let go of our resentments in order to forgive.

When we are having difficulty forgiving others, we remind ourselves that "but for the grace of God go I," that under other, less fortunate circumstances we might have found ourselves in desperate situations doing unworthy and unloving things to others, out of fear and a belief that they were necessary for our survival.

With humility, we remind ourselves that stressful circumstances can make fools and devils of us all, such that good people do bad things, and, therefore, that it's best to put our harsh judge's robe in the closet and don a cloak of graciousness, compassion and mercy instead.

When we try to walk in another man's shoes, to get a sense of the difficulties he's endured, how he's been damaged in his life, and how he's been programmed from childhood experiences to take and not give, to attack and not love, and to withhold and not share, it provides us with the opportunity to see the offender in a more compassionate light, which then enables us to turn down the intensity of our anger over what has been done to us, and allows us to be more empathetic, and practice forgiveness.

For example, if we know someone was abused as a child that can make it easier for us to understand his or her bad behavior and forgive it. Along the same lines, if we're aware of the current circumstances in the offender's life, such as being unemployed, having no savings, about to be evicted, with a wife and two children to care for, that can make it easier for us to understand why they behaved badly, and to forgive them.

It doesn't mean we're condoning or excusing their behavior, or suggesting they not take responsibility for their bad actions. It just means that we're choosing to see them from a more sympathetic viewpoint, and to let go of our critical judgments.

Humanize Rather Than Demonize Others

It can help us to forgive others if we perceive offenders as part of God, despite their ungodly behaviors. Martin Luther King, Jr., once said, "We love men not because we like them or because their ways appeal to us or even because they possess some type of divine spark; we love every man because God loves him."

If we don't believe in God, we use other labels and tools to see the humanity in people despite the errors of their ways.

It's easier to forgive others if we can find some meaning, some wisdom, some benefit born of the assault and the suffering we experienced. If we can do this, if we can find a way to learn and grow from what has happened to us, if we can discover a blessing in disguise, our perspective changes, we feel less angry, less victimized and damaged, and it gives us permission, so to speak, to not resist extending our compassion and forgiveness.

Ultimately, when we have difficulty forgiving others it is best that we repeatedly remind ourselves: "I forgive others for my own peace of mind."

When we are having difficulty forgiving others, we focus on our blessings and on being grateful for what we have in our lives despite what has been done to us. This can take the sting out of any offense and make it easier for us to let go of our resentments in order to forgive.

Walter E. Jacobson MD, Psychiatrist, therapist, spiritual advisor, mastery of life mentor, author and speaker, motivates audiences to break free from self-limiting concepts and negative behaviors getting in the way of their happiness and success. He inspires commitment and change, increases self-esteem and self-confidence, and improves efficiency and productivity. He emphasizes on the power of spiritual techniques and cognitive tools to generate happiness, well-being and material success. He is the author of Best-Selling Book "Forgive to Win".

www.walterjacobsonmd.com

CHAPTER 8

Spiritual Healing Through Storytelling

Dr Amit Nagpal

A participant in a workshop asked me recently, "Is storytelling a luxury, a comfort or a necessity?" I had to reflect for a moment and I replied, "Sometimes storytelling is a soulful luxury, sometimes it comforts your mind by bringing out your perspective and sometimes life leaves you with no option but to tell that 'straight from the heart' story."

So the question arises, how can we use storytelling to heal ourselves of the past and unburden our soul? In my opinion, the process requires the following five steps: -

- Get Conscious of your story-The Consciousness
- Deciding to what extent would you share-The Content
- Turning wounds into gifts-The Cure
- Look at tragedy as if it were comedy-The Comedy
- Become a witness to your story-The Context

I have developed the above '5C framework' to simplify the process and represent it in a memorable and simple way. In the first step, we develop the consciousness of our story and understand & trust that there is a gift behind all the pain and suffering in our life story. Once you get conscious about your story then only you can leverage its power in your life's work (purpose or deep passion).

In the second stage, we take a well thought and conscious decision of how much of the story to share and with whom (which depends upon our evolution, courage and social culture). We may share part of our story with the world, more of our story with a coach/counselor and keep a part with us, which makes us feel too vulnerable. This part can be shared too at the right time and can be healed by writing or expressing in private (in a personal diary for example) till then.

In the third stage we look deeper into our story to find the cure to our wounds by realizing that true gifts emerge from our wounds only. In the fourth stage, we shift our perspective and look at life as a drama and even tragedy as comedy. This shift of perspective further helps us in healing and unburdening our soul.

In the fifth and final step, we understand that we are not our mind and body, but we are the awareness (or soul), which is watching the drama. This helps us in detaching ourselves from our life story and becoming witness or audience to the drama of life and mind.

Let us look at each step in detail now.

The Process

Get Conscious of your story

Start your journey with a reflection on, *"What is the life riddle you are trying to solve and how does this riddle relate to your own pain, suffering, and confusion about the world?"*

Silence and contemplative practice are useful to connect with our deeper selves and become aware and conscious of our story. Once I had posted on Facebook, "Passion is easy to discover but deepest passion requires deepest connection with self." Silence is the best way to connect with our inner selves. It may take time and effort but it is worth it because we come to know our deepest desires, our life purpose and what do we truly want out of life. A cluttered mind or a pressured mind just running the rat race will never even find out what its true desires were.

Once your consciousness level goes up with regular contemplative practice, you have more inclination for personal growth too. You will start looking within for things gone wrong. You will realize that the locus of control is inside you and not outside you. Spirituality says we write our own destiny with our thoughts and actions. Once you start believing this, you will make an attempt to control negative thoughts and avoid negative actions. Since the blame game is over, you will start a new game, where you are the captain, the skipper, the person in charge. And you are ready to take charge of your life and your story.

It's only when you get fully aware or conscious about your story that you can leverage its power in your life's work.

To what extent should you share?

I had posted once on social media, "Some stories are shared with the world, some only with close friends and family and some stories are best shared with your own soul." No one knows your circumstances and no one can decide how much of story you need to share. It is best to ask your own inner voice.

I personally believe in the sharing of story in installments. Share the portion of the story, you feel comfortable sharing. Many factors can influence your decision of how much to share such as culture, age, community and so on. For example, a young person is more likely to be laughed at by sharing vulnerabilities while a middle-aged person has lesser probability.

From healing point of view here are few options and suggestions:

- If you feel very vulnerable in sharing a family trauma (incest for example), I would suggest that you write your complete story and tear it later. It will still help in releasing the pent up emotions and trauma.

- Share your story with coaches/counselors. The probability of a story leaking is less as the coach has professional commitments, as you become a client. It is better to share as much as possible. The more you share, the better counseling you will be able to get.

- Share your stories publicly when you have healed yourself of a certain issue and your struggle has become a victory. This will inspire others and since you have healed the past, you need not bother too much now.

- Michael Margolis, Founder & CEO, Get Storied says, "It's out of our wounds—the stories we are most afraid to tell—that the true gift emerges." There is a popular saying in USA these days, "Vulnerability is the new black." Or in other words, it is beneficial to be vulnerable, yet I have my doubts about the practical side of such openness in eastern cultures (as the family and community loyalty often gets precedence over the individual).

Turning wounds into gifts

Irrespective of how much of story, we want to share at what point of time, it is good to introspect about our wounds, our suffering and emotional baggage. The genius has often emerged out of a difficult pain or struggle. The more an arrow is pulled back, the longer distance it travels after all.

Michael puts it aptly, "Your greatest source of untapped power is the place in your story that needs to be reconciled." It becomes important to reconcile yourself to the deepest suffering in your story and tap its power for personal and professional growth. At the same time, it is important to remember to take charge of your story, as we need to move on from the stories we are born into, to the stories we choose to live. Don't we?

Look at tragedy as if it were comedy

In this stage, we shift our perspective. There is a famous saying, "The troubles of today become the jokes of tomorrow." And if you reflect, you would find most of the time it is true. In fact, Michael points out, "Is your life a comedy or a tragedy? Just depends on how you write the story." If our wounds hold the true gift, then the wound is a gift too. In fact contemplation and spiritual practice can help in this change of perspective.

Isn't life just a make-believe story? In a way we all live in our own make-believe worlds because our beliefs make and break our worlds. So our story twists, based on what we are able to make our mind believe. Scott McPherson points out in his poem beautifully,

> *"You use words to ask where can I find the end of suffering*
> *And I say there is no end of suffering*
> *But there is gratitude-*
> *For even the suffering,*
> *For without it,*
> *You could not find your way to peace."*

I have personally evolved from brutally honest to kindly honest. Here is an interesting anecdote, I wrote based on my life experience: -

I am 22 and my life Catch 22

The disciple, "Guruji, I have always suffered personally and professionally because of my habit of telling the truth. I may have been brutally honest and ruthlessly frank at times. People are not ready to listen to the bitter truth and I don't want to tell lies. I am 22, my life Catch 22"

The Guru, "Tell true stories to give hints and mask the characters, if required. A signal is sufficient for wise (and the fool will not understand, even if you beat the drums). Bare truth is like an ugly skeleton sometimes, so dress it up as a story."

He added further, "Most of the people have not evolved enough to listen to the truth. We are insecure, frail, weak and vulnerable beings. It is more important to be kind than true under such circumstances. Yet, professionally, learn to be, "Kindly honest, politely frank."

Become a witness to your story

The final step in human evolution is to completely detach ourselves from our life story. As the famous quote of Pierre Teilhard de Chardin goes, "We are not human beings having a spiritual experience; we are spiritual beings having a human experience." If we are spiritual beings and we identify our life as a temporary experience, the perspective automatically shifts. In a Skype chat, Michael put it beautifully, "Transformation requires a witness; which is why we have to tell our story."

We become a witness when we reflect, and there's a different story altogether, when one sits in the emptiness.

The Tip

The Universe designed us for storytelling and story listening. Our hearts connect to stories, our brains are wired for stories and our ears want to listen to stories. We want our stories to be heard because our experiences are stories, our complaints are stories and sometimes the biggest burden on our soul, are our untold stories. Great legends leave behind legendary stories; great souls write inspiring stories and great angels in our life keep to themselves our embarrassing stories.

Beliefs are the stories tattooed on our mind, thoughts are the stories we tell ourselves, words are the stories we tell others and actions are silent yet the most powerful stories in our lives. And as Gooch's paradox goes, "Not only, things have to be seen to be believed, but also things have to be believed to be seen". No wonder 'Miraculous stories' happen in lives of those who believe in miracles.

Richard Stone points out in his book, "The Healing Art of Storytelling- A sacred journey of personal discovery" that by restoring our lives we can access tools for building self-esteem, learning from mistakes, affirming personal values, and celebrating the miracles of everyday life. I strongly feel we can. Do you?

Dr Amit Nagpal is Chief Inspirational Storyteller at AL Services. He is a Social Media Influencer, Author, Speaker/Trainer and Coach. His special interest and expertise lies in inspirational storytelling, anecdotes and visual storytelling. AL Services offers content development/story writing, consulting, training and other services in the area of brand storytelling.

www.dramitnagpal.com

CHAPTER 9

Parenting in the New Age

Dr. Saloni Singh

The Essence

"Your children are not your children.

They are sons and daughters of Life's longing for itself.

They come through you but not from you.

And though they are with you yet they belong not to you.

You may give them your love but not your thoughts,
For they have their own thoughts.

You may house their bodies but not their souls,
For, their souls dwell in the house of tomorrow which you cannot visit,
not even in your dreams.

You may strive to be like them, but seek not to make them like you.

For life goes not backward nor tarries with yesterday.

You are the bows from which your children as living arrows are sent forth.

The archer sees the make upon the path of the infinite, and He bends you with His might that His arrows may go swift and far.

Let your bending in the archer's hand be for gladness.

For, even as He loves the arrow that flies, so He also loves the bow that is stable."
- Kahlil Gibran

"What a journey parenting is, one of the hardest one you shall ever do but also one of the most rewarding one, the one that teaches you the meaning of love, of life itself."

Parenting is considered as one of the most challenging work of our life. Though some of us might feel parenting is just a part of life, children grow naturally, what is the big deal. Though very few parents realize the impact parents make on their child's entire life and are fortunate enough to receive the quality guidance required to raise a child. Due to that, invariably enough we end up passing our subconscious deficiencies and incapabilities onto our children, inspite of the fact that we love our children the most and always try to do our best as a parent.

So how we can break the chains of old patterns, drop expectations and let love and care come through us rather than projecting our parent self from a fixed mindset of raising an 'improved second version of our own selves'.

To raise a child is to raise oneself!

Most of the time, as parents we are not even aware of all the damaging effects our lack of self-control and patience, our impulsiveness and indiscipline have on our children, also all the positive influence our attitude and actions could have on them.

Whatever it is we wish to see in our child; whether it is respect for self and others, self-control, self-confidence, good listening and understanding; we need to imbibe that first. Remember that there are no guarantees in this path, but the chances are you shall make a positive long lasting impact.

So in reality, to earn our children's respect and trust we have to be worthy of that respect and trust in every moment and that will require a good deal of self-inquiry and introspection. A good question to ask ourselves is - do I earn trust or fear, respect or resentment by being authoritative and demanding from my children.

As parents most of the times, we believe because we are elder in age than our children, we know better. Hence we should tell them what to do; which is the basic flaw with parenting. While the true foundation of parenting or any kind of guidance, is the fact that the child is innately wise and want to learn naturally. The more we trust this fact, the more we can be true guide and light to our own children, rather than imposing our knowledge on them. As a parent our job is to pass information we have and that too, in a way that is understandable.

The Process

In my work as a parenting coach, parents bring lots of questions to coaching sessions and group workshops.

Let's look at some of them and explore some answers –

How to inspire children to have a balance of freedom, discipline and responsibility?

When we loosen our perception of how the child should be, we provide the child with a sense of freedom, which cannot be explained.

We live in a modern information age where young children can get any information they want and can be more knowledgeable (in terms of information) than their parents. Whether we like it or not, in modern age parents cannot expect unquestioned obedience and respect from their children as they might have given to their parents as a child and if tried, it usually ignites short-term compliance followed by rebellious blasts later on and can also lead to lack of self-esteem and decision making in the child.

Let's start with some reflection; what happens when we try to teach responsibility and discipline to a child by telling, lecturing, scolding or hitting, we are just doing it from a place of personal reaction to their mistakes or our own beliefs of how they should or should not behave. And the child sees our weakness, our lack of self-control and discipline, she/he is hurt and fearful but not inspired to improve on the mistake. They might change because of that fear but the change is usually superficial and temporary.

It's not only our children who grow, parents do too. As much we watch what our children do with their lives; they watch us what we do with ours. We can't tell our children to reach for the stars or moon; all we can do is reach for them, ourselves. When we remember those eyes are watching us every moment, we can strive to be the more of who we are, more loving, more respectful and more compassionate.

Holistic Wellness in the New Age

So how do we bring the balance in our children in this fast, modern age – the fact is there are no set rules. Every moment one must endeavor to stay, be and act from a place of one's higher self. We all are in that place some times when we can calmly listen, understand our child and also help them to understand. The more we practice, the more we can operate from that place.

To inspire your children, start with a belief that your child innately is balanced and it's our focus on certain things and outer world conditioning that makes us and them see and behave otherwise. Then train your mind to accept them without any judgments, look what positive behavior they are already exhibiting and start acknowledging that. The more you trust and acknowledge their wisdom, the more they will do too and regain the balance they are born with.

"Our kids require us most of all to love and accept them for who they are, not to spend our whole time trying to make them into who we think they should be. Also they need our love the most when we feel they deserve it the least"

How to help children improve at any thing?

Have you got any clue where did human ever get this crazy idea, that in order to make children or anyone do better, first we have to make them feel worse? Think of the last time you felt humiliated or treated unfairly. Did you feel like improving, cooperating or learning to do better?"

When someone recognize your little self as big self, celebrate your tiny triumphs, of even trying to do better, empathize and be there with you when you couldn't do better, accept you just the way you are; that's when you really feel like improving and working harder to achieve more.

Human brain is inclined to get attracted towards negative; the things which are not completed, jobs not being done, the place being messy and so on… It is time for parents to retrain their brain to find the positives about their children; the treasure already hidden there. The more they find it, the more it grows everyday.

"When parents take the time to actually listen, with humility, to what children have to say and share, it is amazing what they can learn and provide a valuable gift to their children.

"You cannot keep on doing the same things over and over again and expect a different result; so now is the time to change your approach."

How to help children prioritize, learn self-control and set limits?

To teach anything to your children, first you need to earn their unshakeable trust and faith in everything you do and say. Let your children feel and learn from your attitude that they are so important to you, more significant than anything else. Let them know your trust in them is unshakeable. And if you think they already know, you are mistaken dear friend.

Many surveys show that children feel unloved or loved conditionally, untrusted and insignificant in the modern age because they feel work, money, status, society, even laptop and phone calls and other things are more important to their parents than them.

What is the reason they should listen, set limits as parents want and learn self-control if their own parents cannot. Parents cannot teach their child what they have not learnt themselves.

Model good prioritizing habits; can you avoid the phone calls in family time or when talking to your child if it is not an emergency call. Can you control the urge to check your emails or social media status more than necessary and set limits around things you would like to achieve, like exercising or healthy eating?

"The Best and the only way to help your child learn anything is to model that yourself. Children are natural mimics; they learn and do what they see around them."

How to help a child realize his/her true potential?

PLAY. For a child, life is a playground and that's how they learn most of the things. If we cannot understand the world from a child's eye, how is it even possible for a child to understand what we try to teach them?

Be a playful parent; play with your child as often as you can. Stretch yourself beyond your comfort zone; play things your child likes, even if you might have never played before. Show courage, show confidence and bring the child within you alive. Your child will deeply connect with you and in turn with himself.

Accept him/her; encourage him/her for who he or she is. Be kind; don't try to convert them into some ideal. It can be a rough world, and your child, like everyone else, is fighting to survive. Be a happy parent who is balanced and strive for excellence, without being overly attached to the material achievements. And you shall see your children being grounded with strong roots and fly with wind underneath their wings.

"My mother and father gave me the greatest gift anyone could ever give to another person, they believed in me and I soared."

What is the best way to inspire the children towards their purpose, their own deeper calling in life rather than influencing them to live the parents' dream or tread the beaten path?

Inspire means 'in spirit'; go soul to soul versus role to role. Start reflecting on your ability to see your own divinity, your true purpose, your spiritual existence and you will start communicating at soul level. You will experience your interactions will be naturally more joyful, nurturing, inspiring and truly loving.

Experience deeply that the essence of who you really are, is most beautiful, creative, loving, eternal, unlimited formless spirit made of divine essence. As you truly observe other human beings (especially children), you will be able to experience that. Create a family where normal interaction is soul to soul and not role to role; where you can see the beautiful divinity of others and they can then see it for themselves too.

The Tip

"Be a person in whom they can have full faith beyond any doubt. When you are old, nothing else you have done will have mattered as much."

So now if you want a parenting mantra, it would be as simple (or may be not so simple) –

"Bring the qualities in yourself that you want to see in your child – Be the person you want your child to be and feel the magic."

Dr. Saloni Singh, a medical doctor turned qualified Life and Parenting coach is working with parents and couples to enhance their relationship with each other and their children and bring joy and harmony in the families. www.salonisingh.com

CHAPTER 10

Holistic Education

Neha Patel

The Essence

Children are pure, innocent beings who come into this world with a clean slate and the ability to live in the 'now'. They absorb all that they observe and experience. Somewhere along, due to the ways of the contemporary world, they start losing their natural inborn balance and tend to get entangled with behavioral patterns, which are based on manipulation, fear and guilt. They get conditioned to think negatively and perceive the world to be unfriendly, competitive and stressful. The education today focuses on academic excellence and does not give enough importance to the emotional and spiritual growth of the individual.

Our vision is to give children the platform to recognize and enhance their own unique abilities; use their inner intelligence effectively and live with compassion for others and respect for nature. We endeavor to be a widespread global movement, by reaching out to children, parents, teachers and communities; through workshops, summer camps, after school programs, teacher training programs, online learning, parenting support and eventually full-fledged schools.

Experiential academic learning, enhancing the emotional and spiritual quotient of the child, applying the multiple intelligence paradigms and helping the child excel in that in which his strength lies; are some of the highlights of these programs. For these children, education will be inspiring, creative and supportive. Some of the vehicles to achieve these objectives are innovative use of art forms, ancient teachings and wisdom along with contemporary methods and techniques, which will empower children to be psychologically, socially, spiritually and academically well balanced individuals at the forefront of human evolution.

We have already sown the seeds of our Holistic Education Model in the form of the 'Little Buddha' program and the non-profit organization called Reform Education For A New World (RENEW)

The Process

Why Holistic Education?

Children come into the world with innocence, some genetic information and an inner innate intelligence. They have hope; they are ready to go with the flow. These children grow up to become the future of the present world. But their future depends a whole lot on what they are exposed to as they grow up. The variety of information that they get from their parents, family, society, school, culture and their country, all have an impact on them.

So what are we exposing the innocent unassuming child to? Well, we are all aware of the state of the world as it is today. There is immense depletion of human values, respect and basic integrity. There are rapes, violations, killings, scams and so many other atrocities that are carried out.

They have gotten woven into the fabric of the society creating greed, hatred, indifference, power play, manipulation, guilt, fear and apathy. There is a huge loss of freedom. Materialism is emphasized. Insecurity and suspiciousness are at large. There is loss of trust and peace of mind. The point is that are the children of today and citizens of tomorrow aware of how to deal with all of this? Are they aware that they have a choice and that they can choose to create a different life and reality for themselves?

In most cases the children are trained to buy into this disruptive state of the world. They come to believe that it a dangerous tough place to live in where you have to fight to survive. Their natural instincts are curbed and their inner knowing is not allowed to surface. Their inherent knowledge takes a backseat and most children end up getting on to the factory belt of conventional education and conditioning, being packaged for the material world ahead of them.

We are living in a world where at the macro level we face rapid depletion of natural resources with no alternatives and yet we continue being wasteful, creating a world of scarcity. Environmental issues such as global warming, harmful effects of pollution, radiation, weapons of mass destructions, poverty, terrorism, etc. continue to haunt us.

At the micro level, we live in a society where a "more is better" mindset prevails, leaving people dissatisfied with what they have. Today's highly structured environment leaves many individuals lacking the very skills needed to live with ease and joy such as creativity, adaptability, communication and resilience. The way of living, places emphasis on high level of competitiveness, which is cut throat at times, the pressure to perform is so great that many collapse under it, leading to depression, anxiety and physical ailments.

Such exposure has negative effects on the child's mind wherein they implicitly learn to trust only a few, learn that the world is a bad and dangerous place. What we don't realize is that these implied thoughts, beliefs and feelings create an imbalance in a perfectly balanced child, by triggering their sympathetic nervous system and thus they are constantly on a high alert and behave selfishly to "preserve" themselves. This behavior rather than being helpful in emergencies has become the child's first nature in today's times. Thus, the person is always on the fight-or-flight mode.

In my practice whenever a child is brought to me for therapy by the parents, more often than not, the child turns out to be the most functional in the dysfunctional family he or she belongs to. The child's behavior, which is seen as an emotional disturbance or as disruptive by the parents, is actually a reaction to the dysfunction in the family. When this is brought to the notice of the parents they often tell me that we cannot change so you get the child to change. They don't even recognize or admit how their behavior and patterns are leading to the difficulties the child is facing. But how will the child adjust and change his reaction when day in and day out he is exposed to the same dysfunctional behavior in his home? Then he has the choice of joining in and becoming like them or becoming indifferent or rebelling or caving in under the pressure. The child ends up living in a vicious circle, the parents are disillusioned by the world and its systems so they believe in fighting to live, this is passed on to the child and the child indulges in the same behavior as he does not know any better and the cycle continues.

Holistic Wellness in the New Age

In this fast paced world where on one end technology has increased comfort it has also decreased the frustration tolerance. The individual's environment is changing rapidly occupying most of his attention and leaving no time for introspection. This has created progress externally but regression internally.

We often don't understand our feelings. For example, when we're feeling sad, we say we're just bored. When we're angry we say we're just tired. We have lost access to our feelings and neither do we want to accept them, if they arise. We seem to have found a way to advance at lightening speed yet at the same time have dropped to new levels of low.

These loop holes are not unknown to society nor are they ignored, but whenever an individual or organization has tried to bridge the gap, it hasn't been as successful as they would have liked to be. This is due to our own resistances. The society is not ready to move out of their comfort zone and face the unknown. The bandwagon effect is so deeply entrenched in the masses, hampering to bring about the change.

It is therefore time to question: What would it take for us to make sure we create a conducive and free environment wherein the children are allowed to blossom?

What would it take for us to work towards a better future for our children?

How can we together work towards this?

What can we do and change now? What will be the effect of this change 5, 10, 15, 50 years from now?

The Vision

The first 8-10 years of the child's life are the most influential ones. It is at this time that they develop their perception of the world and their surroundings. Every aspect about living and the way of being gets fitted into their psyche. The core beliefs that they acquire during this period play a significant role in the choices that they make during the course of their life, which in turn shapes their future.

What if we could present to the child universal wisdom and the techniques to imbibe it just like we present to them and make them aware of history, geography, chemistry, physics and biology?

There is a movement around the world where people are waking up to the present situation and shifting towards a holistic way of living, working and being. They are awakening to the necessity of getting in touch with their own core being and living life with authenticity. The need of the hour is for an extensive movement to create a wide shift in the present situation.

Our vision is to have a holistic system of education, which includes the emotional, spiritual, psychological and intuitive aspects of the child along with the academic information that is made available for the child. A system in which the child learns from within; has intrinsic motivation; where the emotional health of the child is given as much if not more importance than the academic performance. A system where students are not just learning to get the grades or marks, but learning to understand and apply; they have the freedom to express themselves; they are able to relate to nature and are able to use their creativity at every point.

The idea is to educate the children using multiple models, techniques, applications drawn from the world wisdom and weaving them into the academic and non-academic training that the child receives so that education is inspiring, creative and supportive.

Some of the significant aspects of Holistic Education are:

Experiential Learning: The children are given opportunities to acquire and apply knowledge, skills and feelings in an immediate and relevant setting. It is a direct experience of whatever is being studied.

We need to let the children live with the question, let them explore and find the answers. In this way various faculties and abilities are put into use and the connections between different topics becomes apparent to them.

Every topic that is covered in the curriculum is converted into the project format and clubbed together with various techniques that interests students and help them ingrain the subject matter.

Being in Balance: extremes of any sort create an imbalance in the functioning of an individual or society. The holistic education model believes in allowing the children to enjoy all aspects of life but with awareness, balance and their values in place. In the process they will learn to make choices that work towards their own highest benefit as well as that of those around them.

Some of the areas where extremes are experienced are competition and praise.

Healthy competition is known to be conducive for the growth of a child and helps them to reach higher levels of their potential. Unfortunately the present systems undermine the positive learning climate in schools leading to unhealthy and extreme competition. Creating a balance enables a child to get an opportunity and allow his/her uniqueness to flourish. Holistic education encourages children to improve themselves rather than improving themselves compared to others.

Praise on the other hand if given in extreme, leads to the child having to live up to the expectations of others at all times. This leads to undue stress, pressure and feelings of inadequacy. Too little praise tends to be de-motivating for a child. So parents and teachers too need to learn to keep a balance.

Acknowledging Individual Uniqueness:

Children come with their own distinctive abilities and intelligence. Moving away from the general practice of fitting the children into pre-cast dyes of how they should be learning. The Holistic Education Model encourages and provides children with the means and opportunities to explore their own uniqueness, to learn, and to develop in the way that suits them the best. We apply the Multiple Intelligence Paradigm by Howard Gardner, which acknowledges the fact that humans have varied intelligences and they function using a combination of them.

For example, If a child has been indentified as being high on musical intelligence, he is given specialized training to develop it further. Not only that, this ability of his is used as a modality to help him learn other topics too.

Mindfulness Training: This is one of the most important aspects of Holistic Education. Mindfulness is defined as "the awareness that emerges through paying attention on purpose, in the present moment, and non-judgmentally to the unfolding of experiences moment by moment" (Kabat-Zinn, 2003, p. 145).

The children would be trained in being mindful and incorporating this training in every aspect of their lives.

Research suggests that training in mindfulness has the potential to enhance children's attention and focus, and improve memory, self-acceptance, self-management skills, and self-understanding. (Hooker.K.,Fodor.I)

Expressive Arts: Another very important aspect of the Holistic Education Model is Expressive Arts. Children experience art from the beginning of their life. . Art is a powerful resource that is built within each individual.

The rhythmic beating of the heart, the rocking movement that the child experiences comfort from, the different facial expressions they see, are all forms of art. Art forms are not only taught as formal dance, drawing or music training. Going beyond that, art forms are included in every aspect of the program to express, experience and put forth their creative abilities in all areas of their lives. For e.g. a poem in English would be sung to music and dramatized. That way the child doesn't simply learn it 'by heart' but understands the true essence of the poem.

The different art forms included in the model are dance and movement, drama, music, visual arts and crafts, storytelling, play, pottery etc. There is immense amount of research done and information available on the usefulness of art forms for the overall development of a child at all levels-psychological, spiritual, physical, emotional and academic.

Spiritual Intelligence:

Holistic Education focuses on tapping into and developing the Spiritual Intelligence of the child. It aims at bringing up and enhancing the abilities of the child to be compassionate, self-aware, non judgmental and loving. Living with integrity, honesty and equanimity, connecting with the deeper intelligence within, respecting self, others, nature and humanity are encouraged. Conscious living is taught where caring for nature and its resources is emphasized. Their intuitive abilities are sharpened.

Unique Assessment System

The Holistic Education Model has a flexible assessment system and yet is in line with mainstream education. We believe children should have equal opportunities to excel in whatever they are learning irrespective of the style of delivering it. Evaluations are done not to pass or fail a child but to make sure that the child has understood a concept. Instead of tests, project and research formats are utilized and the children are assessed on the basis of that project such as the language aspect, the aspect of science, research the methods used, their understanding of the outcomes. We believe in individual abilities of each child and one child may excel in a particular ability while the second in another. Instead of pitting students against one another, the child gets a qualitative feedback for their performance on a project, task or activity and is given the guidance on improving in it if required.

Enhancing Emotional Intelligence:

Emotional intelligence refers to an ability to recognize the meanings of emotions and their relationship and to reason and resolve the problems based on this understanding. Emotional intelligence is involved in the capacity to perceive emotions, assimilate emotion-related feelings, understand the information of those emotions, and manage them (Mayer, J.D., Caruso, D., & Salovey, P., 1999).

We believe that the emotional well being of an individual is very important and can take them far ahead in life. The Little Buddha Program, which is a major component of The Holistic Education Model, works towards helping the child enhance his/her emotional intelligence.

The Little Buddha Program and Workshops

The program helps children in understanding emotions, and expressing them constructively, creating a balance in their thoughts and actions. It works towards enhancing the already built-in intuitive capacities of the child. It teaches children to keep the highest good of self and others around them in perspective while taking any action. It teaches them to recognize others as well as their own uniqueness, appreciate it and set comfortable and achievable targets to better themselves. It builds the frustration tolerance of the children and helps them become resilient. It embeds gratitude, trust, humility, compassion, honesty and respect into their way of being. It teaches them to be self-reliant, responsible and taking initiative for self-growth.

The Little Buddha program is a *non-religious* program, which works towards the psychological, emotional and spiritual growth and wellbeing of a child. Through different activities and sessions coupled with their inner understanding and intelligence the children incorporate everything they experience in the program into their way of being.

The word Buddha comes from the Sanskrit word 'Buddh' which means being awakened and enlightened. Our vision is to help the children become aware beings who live their life to the fullest with balance and integrity. This program aims at bringing out a 'Little Buddha' in every child.

The program is designed for children between the ages of 3-16 years. It is divided in to 3 groups of ages, 4 to 6, 7 to 11 and 12 to 16. It makes use of Art Based Therapy techniques, meditation, role-play, visual imagery, Emotional Freedom Techniques, Access Consciousness and many other modalities. Through different activities and sessions coupled with their inner understanding and intelligence the child incorporates all they experience in the program into their way of being.

The Little Buddha Program, Some Highlights:

- Works towards enhancing the already built-in intuitive capacities of the child and helping the child to use them effectively

- Teaches the children to keep the highest good of self and others around them in perspective while taking any action.

- Teaches children not to compete with others, instead recognize their own uniqueness, appreciate it and set comfortable and achievable targets to better themselves. Teaches them to be non-judgmental of others. It helps them see others perspectives and points of view, thus accepting self and others for their own uniqueness, helps children understand emotions, and express themselves constructively creating a balance in their thoughts and actions.

- Builds the frustration tolerance of the child and helps them become resilient.
- Helps the children break out of self-imposed limitations and let go of limiting ideas, beliefs, thoughts and feelings.
- Weaves gratitude, trust, humility, compassion, honesty and respect into the fabric of their life.
- Teaches children to value and appreciate all that they have and be conscious
- Teaches them to make conscious choices, enhance their self-confidence and self-worth.
- Encourages assertiveness, team-work, understanding boundaries, empathizing with others, prioritizing effectively, dealing with bullies and peer pressure, respecting gender differences, and forgiving self and others.
- Teaches them to be self-reliant, responsible and taking initiative for self-growth.
- Aims to improve their concentration and focusing skills.
- The children are allowed to be themselves, without any judgment. They are allowed to express themselves and they feel totally accepted just the way they are.

The environment influences the child and evidently plays a big part in his/her perception of everything within and without. Parents play a very significant role in their life. Therefore, it is important that these significant people also enroll into the Little Buddha concept for the child to benefit completely from it. To achieve this there are group sessions and individual sessions conducted with parents of each child. These sessions intend to promote unrestrictive parenting which benefits the child by improving parent child relationship. The parents would be able to see their child in a different light and understand his/her uniqueness and needs. This will further help the child carry forward whatever they learn in the program and also imbibe it into their own lives.

Some of the techniques and modalities we use while conducting the Little Buddha Program are:

- Arts based therapy techniques such as drama, singing, dance and movement, visual arts, music, story telling and free play.
- Guided Imagery
- Visual Meditations
- Role play
- Emotional Freedom Technique
- Mindfulness Training
- Metaphors
- Affirmations
- Access Consciousness fundamentals
- And many more

So I ask all the conscious beings reading this;

What would it take for us to believe that a change is possible?

What energy, space and consciousness can we be to co-create a different reality for the children and for us?

How does it get any better than this? What else is possible?

Lets all contribute to make this world a better place, for you, for the entire human race.

The Tip:

- Children are to be appreciated for who they be and not only for what they achieve academically.
- Keep the Balance in your life and it will be reflected in your child's life. Balance in every aspect is important.
- Be smart about praising your child. Too much praise leads to the child having to live up to your and others' expectations at all times. This leads to

Holistic Wellness in the New Age

undue stress, pressure and feelings of inadequacy. Too little praise tends to be de-motivating for a child.

- Encourage your children to work towards improving themselves rather than trying to get better than the other.
- Include a practice of meditation daily for yourself and your children to tune into their own awareness and intuitive abilities and their true potential.
- Inculcate being mindful and aware as a way of life for your family.
- Refrain from projecting your own limitations, conclusions, judgments, issues, expectations on to your child. Remember that the child has come into this world through you but to live his/her own life.
- Be the change yourself, and the rest will follow, if it's for their highest good.
- Give your child a chance to make choices.
- Encourage and help the child develop his/her own uniqueness.
- Your child will definitely teach you a few lessons, so be ready to learn.
- Trust in abundance.
- In every situation, say to yourself "How Does It Get Any Better Than This? And the universe will follow up on that.
- Listen to your child. Truly Listen.
- Include art forms into your life. Just for the fun of expressing yourself.

Neha Patel comes with 19 years of experience working with children and adults as a trainer, counselor and psychologist. She is the Founder of Sharnam Therapy and Healing, a centre for psychological, emotional, spiritual and occupational wellness. She is also a trained Arts Based Therapy (ABT) Practitioner. She is a certified Clinical Hypnotherapist, and has trained in Emotional Freedom Technique (EFT), Play Therapy, Transactional Analysis (TA), Rational Emotive Behavior Therapy (REBT), Skills for Adolescents (SFA) and many other techniques and modalities.

She believes that to sow the seeds of positive emotional health in childhood is to reap a harvest of healthy well-balanced adults. With this vision in mind, she created the

Little Buddha program for children, which focuses on the psychological, spiritual and emotional enhancement of the child. At a global level she has co-founded the Reform Education for a New World (RENEW) program in order to provide a complete and holistic education system for the children. She shares her learning and experiences through articles and quotes in English and Gujarati publications, and appearing on television as a guest speaker for several shows.

nehapsychologist@gmail.com

CHAPTER 11

Shifting Paradigm: Healing From Within

Rucsandra Mitrea

Healing starts within and in the present moment. It does not happen in the past or in the future and it does not occur through acquiring recipes for health and healing. In order to access the innate capacity for healing that we have been endowed with, we must be able to look inside ourselves and be present with what we see and feel. There is however one formidable force that will prevent us from connecting to that inner essence that holds our inherent healing power: FEAR.

Healing cannot occur in the presence of fear and any healing process requires the full release of fear, with its many layers and deeply seated authority. Fear is the energy that impedes and stops true healing. Most people are afraid to look within, at the magnificent and sacred place inside themselves that holds the key to health, abundance, joy and love. They are afraid because fear is the only field that they have been trained in, sequentially and consistently every single day throughout their lives.

Fear is an intrinsic part of our lives and can be categorized as follows:

1. Sociological fear
   - Societal fear
   - Familial fear
   - Individual fear
2. Perceptual fear
   - Factual fear

- Imaginary fear
3. Universal fear
    - Abandonment and Separation
    - Low Self-worth
    - Lack of Trust

Understanding that fear defines our limitations will give us the tools to unleash the force of inner healing.

I will explain these categories, one by one.

1. **Sociological fear**
    - **Societal or Collective Fear**

        We are the children of our society and we have been forged and conditioned, taught and chiseled by our forefathers' beliefs, rules, accomplishments and fears. This would be all good news if our society were based on love, compassion, understanding and respect. Unfortunately it is not. With maybe a few isolated and small cultures around the globe, otherwise we live in a world shaped and defined by fear.

        Society has been very effective in teaching us to live in fear: fear of war, of cancer, of financial crisis and depression, fear of God, of heart disease, of terrorism, fear of going to hell, of not having the right job, fear of other people, of other nations and other customs, fear of being too fat to be considered beautiful or too weak to become successful, of illnesses and viruses and epidemics.

        We live our lives in various gradients of fear without even being aware of it. We are imbued with fear in all its colors, flavors and intensities.

        Fear is everywhere. People take their first dose of daily fear with their morning coffee, while watching the news, reading the newspaper or listening to the car radio on their way to work. They start to feel the fists of fear in their guts right after brushing their teeth in the morning.

The truth is that fear sells. It is also true that for every sad and disconcerting thing that we hear about in the news, there is a beautiful, uplifting and empowering thing that is happening somewhere in the world. Unfortunately, that would not sell, so the accent is put on what sells: tragedy, pain, and fear. A continuous stream of fear-creating news is bombarding us all day long.

Scientists study the effects of fear on individuals and society. Dr. Deepak Chopra and Jim Clifton in their article entitled "The Fear Factor: How Scared Are People?" say:

"Over the past decade the word "fear" has become all too familiar. After 9/11, critics of the war on terror called it fear mongering. After the financial crash of 2008, living in a climate of fear became the lot of millions of people who lost their jobs, retirement accounts, and homes. In the face of such violence, the prevalence of fear can have a profound effect on the health, well-being, and economic development: if a society is in a constant state of fear, it won't produce anything good."

Fear is a phenomenon with a strong grasp on our society.

- **Familial Fear**

Familial fear is what we are exposed to on a smaller scale, in our very own families.

For example, if a mother is afraid of germs and getting sick chances are that her children are afraid of the very same things. If they were brought up into her way of thinking, they too will believe that germs are scary and that it is extremely easy to get sick.

If parents or primary caretakers were afraid of other people, afraid of life in general, their children learn a specific behavior that they believe will keep them safe. Fear, distrust and living their lives in small doses created an inherited behavior with deep repercussions for their quality of life.

These are familial fears; they are familiar, so most people do not even question them. Until they are released, life will be shaped by them.

- **Individual Fear**

    Individual fears are based on a person's own past experiences. If something did not turn quite the way it was expected and that caused suffering, we are now afraid of doing it again.

    For example, falling in love only to end up being rejected and hurt might create the fear of meeting new prospective partners. Going along with the dream to start a business and doing everything to make it happen, only to fail, might lead to the decision of playing it safe by not following the call of inner desires ever again.

    These are individual fears. The first layers are embedded in our cells even before we were born. When we were formed as new life potential in our mother's womb, our continuously growing number of cells was nestled at the core of the mother's body, surrounded by her cells. What this means is that our cells were already experiencing the emotions and feelings of joy or despair, fear or love that the mother felt.

    To sum it all up, from a sociological point of view, we are drenched in fear. We are first soaked in family fear, even preconditioned before birth; societal fears are attaching weights to our ankles and fogging our minds on a daily basis; and then our personally created individual fears stop us from living.

2. **Perceptual fear**
    - **Factual Fear**

        Factual fear is based in real life and is related to things that are indeed dangerous, without dispute; like being on the path of a developing tornado, or close to a raging forest fire, or going for a walk bare foot in a snowstorm. This is the healthy energy of fear that allows us to remain safe and it is embedded in our DNA.

    - **Imaginary Fear**

        The very opposite of the factual fears, the imaginary fears are not based in reality. They are fabricated, knitted, colored, inflated, expanded, manufactured, embellished soap bubbles created with our thoughts. Questions such as "What if I fail?", "What if this goes wrong?" or

"What if I will be alone for the rest of my life?" create an imagined fear, because they are not anchored in reality. We do not know with certainty that we will fail, that our plans will not succeed or that we will not find a partner to share our lives with. Imaginary fear stems from thoughts directed towards a future that we couldn't predict. The negative "What if?" questions have the power to paralyze us and stop us before we even start.

The third category of fears has been identified by the great visionary Gregg Braden. He says that these three Universal fears are at the base of all the fears and behaviors that are present in ourselves and others.

3. **Universal Fears**

These three basic underlying fears are the root of the sociological and perceptual fears. With few exceptions, our experiences of pain, suffering, illness, disease, and emotional trauma have their roots in these core universal fears.

In his book "The Divine Matrix", Gregg Braden wrote: *"The root of our 'negative' experiences may be reduced to one of three universal fears (or a combination of them): abandonment, low self-worth, or lack of trust."*

- **Abandonment and Separation**

    The fear of abandonment and separation stems from the ancient fear that we were abandoned by our creator without explanation or reason. As a result of this perceived separation we feel alone in the world and in the Universe. This fear is manifested in our lives through the relationships we create with other people. We are devastated when they fail or we leave them in order to avoid getting hurt. The truth is that relationships do not fail; they cannot fail. They are taking their course as energy streams between people; they are the creations of people's beliefs, fears and expectations.

- **Low Self-worth**

    The second Universal fear is the fear that we are not "good enough". Almost every person in our world has experienced low self-esteem.

The professional, friendship or romantic relationships in our lives will match our expectations and our beliefs of not being good enough. When we don't feel worthy of our most cherished dreams, we create our relationships and experiences from the standpoint of low self-esteem.

- **Lack of Trust**

  The third universal fear is the lack of trust in life. Most people believe that this world is not safe for us to live in, and the processes of life are unsafe, scary and threatening. This fear is expressed as the inability to surrender to our experiences and relationships. These relationships mirror our projections of this world being unsafe and unworthy of our trust.

Louise Hay says:

"Fear is a lack of trust in ourselves, and because of this, we don't trust Life. We don't trust that we're being taken care of on a higher level, so we feel we must control everything from the physical level. Obviously, we're going to feel fear because we can't control everything in our lives."

The universal fears are deeply embedded in the collective and individual consciousness and create the core of our fear-based life. It is no mystery that we are afraid and that fear is a well-accepted state in our society, in our families, amongst our friends and inside ourselves. Our inherent capacity for healing is deeply buried beneath all these layers of fear; therefore in order to access it we must release them all.

Underneath all the fear there lays our very essence: powerful, magnificent and whole.

How do we release fear so that we can heal our bodies and our lives? How do we let go of the fear so that we can connect with who we truly are? How do we deal with fear?

Dr. Wayne Dyer says:

"The only way to deal with a fear is to face it directly. In the book A Course in Miracles, it says there are only two emotions: love and fear. When you're in fear, you have left love behind; meaning, you have left your belief that there is a divine source

that will guide you through all aspects of your life. Reconnect to your source, know that you're not alone, or, as the Course says, "If you knew who walked beside you, at all times, on this path that you have chosen, you could never experience fear again." Trust in yourself, and you're trusting in the very wisdom that created you."

The only way to deal with fear is to face it openly, to remain still in its presence, to breathe and allow it to wash over us and be present while feeling it; by doing so we stop resisting it. By releasing our resistance, fear releases its grip. There are no corners to cut and there is no running in circles: the only way to deal with fear is to face it fully, without resistance; feeling the layers of fear snapping at our heels and instead of running away from them, choosing to turn around and face them straight in the face.

A Practical Guide for Releasing Fear

After reading this article so far and finding about all the different categories of fear and feeling it more acutely in your body, you might be asking now: how about me and my fears in this very moment?

Here's a fragment of my "Sacred Oak Tree Meditation" that will teach you how to release any emotion or fear that troubles you. The **Oak Tree Visualization** is a powerful emotional cleansing technique to use when you are afraid, emotionally overwhelmed, stressed out, unclear or drained.

Here it is:

Imagine an old, beautiful and majestic oak tree. See yourself becoming this imposing and strong oak. Feel its strength in your body and feel the deep connection you have with it. **You ARE this tree.**

Your strong and powerful roots go deep into the Earth. As you become more aware of them they grow deeper and deeper. **The deeper they go, the stronger and calmer you feel.**

Now allow your fears to come up one by one, bring them to the surface and feel them fully. Do not dwell on them and the reasons why you feel you might be right to be afraid. Just let them come to your awareness and look at them, feel them as they come; all of them. Don't hold back. Be ruthlessly honest and courageous.

Breathe calmly. Now, from this place of strength, allow yourself to let go of all that is not serving you and that is not in your best interest: old fears and feelings, new fears and emotions. **You do not need to name them one by one, just intend them to release from your system right here and now.**

Allow all the things and situations you are afraid of to come to your awareness. Choose one of them and sit with it. Allow it to become as big, as strong, as fearful as it is in your awareness. Sit there. Feel it. Look at it. Allow it. Breathe. Do not move. Breathe deeply and sit in that fear. You are strong, calm and nothing can make you move.

The calmer you remain, the weaker the grip your fear will have on you. And after a while, it will dissolve. Once the fear is gone, only YOU, capital letters YOU will remain.

Streams of old and stuck energy are leaving your body through your deep and powerful roots. Let it all go: named and unnamed fears, old or new, small or large. They are being released through your roots deep into the Earth. The Earth will clear and transform them into neutral, uncharged energy.

You can finally let them all go. It is a light and easy process. **All your fears are being drained from your body and from your energetic field with ease, with no resistance.**

You can feel the cleansing taking place as the last streams are leaving your system. **There was great strength hidden behind all that you let go of. Your strength and clarity return and you feel powerful and peaceful.**

Breathe. Thank your roots for helping you through this process. Return your awareness to here and now.

Feels great, doesn't it?

The more you practice this visualization exercise, the faster you will feel a great sense of relief and re-balancing taking place. This great tool can be used every day and in every situation, in order to release fear and restore your authentic self.

Practice it as often as you can. It gets more powerful every time.

The Oak Tree Visualization is one technique that you will use every day:

- You are ready to go to a meeting and you're not sure about what to say, what others will say, or you might be afraid and a little apprehensive. Clear yourself with the Oak Tree technique first and then go into the meeting.

- You are going to spend time with family and you are starting to worry, judge or be afraid of what might go wrong. Become an Oak Tree first, release everything that troubles you and then go meet your family with a clean slate.

- You are concerned about your finances or your job. When you feel the first sign or concern or fear, use the Oak Tree Visualization to release it all. Over and over and over. The less afraid you feel, the more you can see opportunities and invite the right people in your life.

These are only a few of the instances in which this technique will clear your energy and will help you release fear right then and there. You will feel better immediately, and if you feel better you are more authentic.

How will you know what the effects of using this technique really are?

You will feel them. You will start to deal with everything from a powerful stance of authenticity and will not be guided by fear, but rather by your essence. In turn, every situation will resolve with more ease. You will find that people will come to you with solutions and responses and your relationships will improve.

You are as strong as your Inner Sacred Oak Tree and fear cannot lead your thoughts and actions anymore!

In his novel "Dune", Frank Herbert offered us the magnificent and formidable "Litany against Fear":

"I must not fear.
Fear is the mind-killer.
Fear is the little death that brings total obliteration.
I will face my fear.
I will permit it to pass over me and through me.
And when it has gone past I will turn the inner eye to see its path.

*Where the fear has gone there will be nothing.
Only I will remain."*

In the absence of fear, only we will remain.

We will turn around and look deep inside ourselves and see our own magnificence. In the absence of fear the answers to our questions will arise from deep within our divine essence and healing will take place. In the absence of fear we will access the strength and the power to heal ourselves, our families, our communities and our world.

Rucsandra Mitrea is a healer; her work with countless clients over the years has earned her the title "The Body Whisperer". Her mission is to teach her clients that their capacity for healing resides not in other people or in the outside world, but within themselves. She teaches them that physical healing becomes possible when they accept the emotional, mental, energetic and spiritual aspects of who they are. Rucsandra is the founder of leading edge Mitrea Wellness Centre located in Toronto, Canada. The Centre's emphasis is on complete and lasting transformation of body and mind.

www.mitreawellness.com

The Belief Approach

CHAPTER 12

Origin, history and Introduction of belief

Naveen Varshneya

In the beginning, there were two types of human being. One who accepted existence of self and went on to survive by discovering food. He is called 'Survivor'. The other one questioned his existence and went deeper in the forest to discover the meaning and the purpose but more than that attempted to know what is life and who am I? He is called 'Mystic'.

Origin of 'belief' lies in the journey from 'I Survive' to "I Exist'. Else, there was no reason for man to care for his own existence and try to survive by discovering food and protecting himself against dangers of the nature, unless he was driven by need to survive. Hence Belief is originated from the realization of "Need" i.e. "Need to survive". This 'need to survive' became the origin of belief, which in turn became mother of all belief for humanity to evolve. Need to survive is indifferent towards existence of higher self, cosmic power or God as Survivor had no clue about it. There was no way, need to survive and evolution would have happened, had humanity known existence of God because with that, would have come the paradigm of being "taken care of" or "being provided for".

The biggest hurdle for survivor was uncertainty posed by death, dangers of nature, search for food etc. And to reduce uncertainty, he created institutions which were rulebook be it marriage, monogamy, family or social. It was to ensure higher degree of certainty. However desire to chase certainty did not happen without the birth of emotions which gave optimism and hope for tomorrow and man wanted to look forward to it. If not for emotions, man would have lived his life in each moment after discovering food and sex and knowledge of death which he has no control on.

3 meals a day was not created as a need of the body but to ensure certainty for food. Like wise, humanity had to cultivate monogamy to ensure survival. It was also built to ensure food is available. Monogamy was essentially the first contract ever signed between a man and a woman to ensure that if woman stayed back and did not search for food, food was to be provided by man in return of sex. After the birth of child, it got further imposed more strictly as man wanted to take limited responsibility of being a provider of food, which by now included his own self, his woman and children. Clearly, he did not want to hunt for food for months to come back and discover that he has to provide for one more child which is not his own. Hence sex and food were interwoven and traded. Monogamy or loyalty were natural outcome of this trade contract but were never the reason for men and women to agree to monogamy in that pre contractive era. Same were the reason for woman to ensure that her man remains loyal to her and continue to provide food and certainty and shall not build another home. If not for food and non-availability of contraceptives, humanity would not have agreed for something as un-natural as monogamy. This is what west today is experimenting where food, safety and sex is available, hence people are breaking formal family and social institution.

Hence loyalty, commitment, security were invented through marriage and that is how interdependency was cultivated which gradually was scaled to build a connected community. Survival through food was not a challenge for men and women as they both were capable of finding food for themselves. If not for sex, birth of child and emotions, interdependency would have not have developed.

Life was still quite mechanical till this point and wheel of time and space was just beginning to move for him, through hunger, sex and uncertainty, they had some sense of emotions but survivor did not know how to react to it till procreation happened which gave birth to emotions. Birth of a child gave birth to 2 distinct emotions. Curiosity and Wonderment. This was the beginning of birth of mystic in a survivor.

In wonderment, he discovered himself merging in the flow. He turned more an explorer and danced to the tune of nature and began to recognize sunrise, sunset as much as laughter or cry of a baby. It triggered hope, optimism and desire to experience life. But this was still not enough for him to dig deeper into life as

Holistic Wellness in the New Age

it generated no such need to know higher self. Hope and desire thus created through wonderment further pushed him to reduce degree of uncertainty and mind was developed to work to ensure that food and sex are taken care of to ensure rhythm of wonderment to be continuous.

It is through unknown nature of death, fear of survival for himself and family, disruption in his joy and wonderment gave birth to pain and forced him to become curious about life. Thus through the development of mind, as he applied curiosity to discover deeper layers of emotions, he had the desire to discover the same question asked by Mystic. In essence, His questions about life kept growing to understand the human spirit and evolution on the planet so that he can better prepare for tomorrow and be certain. However hard he resembled his quest by now with that of a mystic, there was one clear difference in mystic and survival. Survivor wanted to know answers of deeper questions to be more certain and survive, while mystic had no such assumption in his quest. Hence, his quest for deeper secrets was to gain more certainty.

With these questions, survivor then happens to interact with Mystic who had very little knowledge about the needs of physical body, responsibilities, needs, commitments, loyalty, and belief. It had no idea of human emotions from survivor's perspective and only knew about the spirit of humanity through revelation and self-actualization in meditation. It knew bliss and knew there is something deeper about human life then just actualized by the survivor. Mystic knew no suffering, pain or certainty or death as they saw life as continuous rhythm beyond the presence of physical body and for them everything was an experience.

Mystic faced one big challenge in showing that light to the Survivor to alleviate their sufferings and make them understand higher meaning in life. Mystic failed in explaining, hence focused on helping Survivor experience the mysticism through which they will discover the cause and cure for their suffering. Initiation into connecting with the inner self to implore required that survivor believes that some infinite invisible force but has design of the life and has power to help us alleviate from our suffering. Hence invention of rituals, techniques and process to help humanity acknowledge existence of higher self took place, which gave birth to faith and all these rules were put together to keep faith intact, which later on became religion. Intent of the religion was never to turn a survivor into mystic but to make him better at surviving. It was only meant to a) develop faith in life so that curiosity rests and give peace by parking his quest and hoping that someone out there will help and b) become gateway to connect with mysticism and begin to have same revelation as mystic had to experience truth.

This brought paradigm shift in evolution. Birth of faith which gave hope, raised vibratory level of the survivor to look beyond his own selfish survival needs and leave heritage on the planet in hoping of getting to see god after death if not in the life time. Objective of meeting god was to experience life beyond sufferings and explore possibilities of the choices, heaven and hell along with god was created by mystic to further give a form to their faith. Possibilities of choice that were rather limited for the survivor now through revelations became possible and Survivor began to evolve their belief about what is possible for human being to achieve more degree of certainty. Clearly they had to create punishments for people who break these rules and breaking the rules meant threat to survival of society and to family and then to individuals. This is how morality was born to safeguard survival.

That is how faith became the driver of human belief system. Choices showed that more is possible and that got mind thinking of exploring more. Through mythological stories, Heroism was created with the intent to expand horizons of human mind to break his limitation and create hope that more choices can be exercised to feel empowered.

Like the first contract between man and woman to have loyalty and commitment, He created rules at each level. Marriage had one such rulebook and then they expanded it to create rulebook to build a society to live together. These rules were consciously developed for mutual survival and were passed on to the next generation. Over the centuries, no one questioned them, but they were passed on as way of life. They became belief and got coded in the subconscious of coming generation which gradually became human intelligence over a long period of time before getting passed on in the DNA. So, an experience when classified as essential for survival becomes belief, it gets stored in consciousness and over a period of time, gets pushed into sub consciousness and then finally becomes part of the DNA and gets passed on in genes.

Every moment is an experience and if we have a choice to live that moment in wonderment of nature but we also have a choice to call it good or bad. If we label it, we create a belief. So, if you look at a flower from the window of your car on the roadside, you can wonder how nature has created so many colors and smells, turn curious to experience all such colors or think how dirty that flower is and how much you love roses. If you choose to live in wonderment and develop curiosity, your energies will automatically begin to observe all such wonders of the nature thus making you live a life in bliss. But when an experience is not lived with degree of wonderment, thus curiosity, it generates an emotion and a thought which is what a belief is. By developing mind to like or dislike an experience, we are tuning ourselves towards certainty. We just did not like color and smell of a new flower and we wanted certainty of our emotions when we see a flower and that is fixed in our mind as to what comes from Rose. Hence mind was cultivated to ensure certainty and direct our energies towards the experience, which we have known. This is how belief works by creating patterns, which ensures certainty of the experience.

A belief has 2 components to it and that is emotion (Yin) and a thought (Yang), which is generated, based on an experience. Together they become electromagnetic field as per quantum physics, which says everything is vibrating and nothing is fixed in the universe. So, when we form a belief, we begin to limit range of frequencies in which known experiences which validate our belief become prominent rather than expanding our frequencies range in case of living in wonderment which opens us up for new experiences.

Parents pass on to us all the belief, which ensure that we are safe and can survive. Hence parenting is done not in a manner where child is allowed to explore life and its own path but to ensure that child survives based on best of the knowledge available to parents. So, if you are an engineer, safest bet for you is to see that your son is also an engineer and that way, you have fulfilled your responsibility towards your child. However it has to be very loudly realized that such type of parenting operate at bare minimum fulfillment of the responsibility and has being obsessed with self than realizing the true, infinite potential of the child.

Belief is for human life what operating system is for computers and cell phones. It is an environment which support certain type of human experiences and thus creates a domain within which journey of human life operates. So, how can an application meant for Windows environment work on other OS? If your operating system says, all men are stronger than us and that life is a compromise, how could you experience anything other than this belief, which is your own personal truth, either acquired or developed? So, if you went through abuse in the hand of men in your childhood and formed a belief that men abuse, you will either always work towards protecting yourself thus turning aloof in your growing years or always finding a situation which witnesses that belief as often as you seek validation of your truth.

And this is the irony. We human beings have this constant need to experience our existence (in absence of a mystic component in us). It is our need to prove that we are surviving. Our survival is dependent upon how we see life, which is nothing but belief. Hence we would always have those experiences, which validate our belief. So, when a partner cheated me, it confirmed to my belief that partnership shall not be done. I had gone outside my belief to enter in partnership and that is why it fell flat to bring me back to my stable point of belief.

Hence, though, we could go out of our belief but that creates so much of uncertainty that we get unstable and instability shakes the basic belief of "Need to Survive" and system automatically works towards creating events in which we feel safe and surviving.

If we wish to break limiting belief given to us since thousands of years which are stored in our subconscious, we have no other option but to integrate a mystic in us to open up to infinite possibilities and through that we will be able to attune ourselves to the CODE written in our subconscious for the purpose of our this life time. This means, begin a shift from "Survivor" to "I Exist" and this means really defining your minimum needs for existence. So, here is how you can do it:

Make 3 circles: innermost circle carries need for breathing, food, shelter and health: When I did it, I found that I can exist with bare minimum money and move to a village. This took away all the compulsion to live in large city, facilities etc. It just vanished when I found that I could exist through my life.

Second circle: choose the intimate environment, which will support your existence: In my case, it was my family, nature and free harmonious expression.

Third circle: This is the circle in which you have all the compulsions which in absence of connectivity to inner self, create an illusion that it is real and put you in constant chase:

After making a list of desires and ambitions, I turned inwards to innermost circle and remained there and purpose of my life unfolded on its own through series of mystical experiences including clairaudience. Once found it, automatically I saw changes happening in this circle of people, relationship, surroundings and work. This process will trigger deep-rooted emotions, belief and you shall begin to ask why, do I need to experience all this. This is the beginning of integrating Mystic in Survivor giving you joy of life fulfilling purpose of life.

Though it is a detailed process and often may require guidance of a coach, but then there is always an Eklavya in us, if we believe in it.

Naveen Varshneya is a Founder, Life Coach & Healer- NV Life Treatment Centre- Treatment based on quantum physics and techniques are taught to heal self in 'Science of Life' Workshop program.

About NV Life: In year 2010, New Delhi, through a series of coincidences and divine intervention, first patient of Schizophrenia stopped hallucinating using simple principle of balancing electromagnetic field. Through word of mouth, as patients suffering with various disorders began to get relief, they established science of illness and cure, which found its base in Quantum Physics. These principles were then applied on various issues from chronic diseases to boardroom problems and found validation of the principles. Objective was to establish a science, which can be passed on to people to help them cure themselves. This led them to come out with a program called "A course in Science of Life", which is now taught as treatment in their clinical practice and taught as self help and wellness program in workshops so that people can begin to reverse their disorders and sufferings. They presently operate from Bangalore and focusing on teaching the science of treatment as self help program.

www.nvlife.in

CHAPTER 13

Journey of PSYCH-K®

Jurrian Kamp

This article was published in the international magazine The Intelligent Optimist, a magazine that focuses on the people, passion and possibilities changing our world for the better. Find out more on theoptimist.com

EVER SINCE HE SAW DISNEY'S animated classic *Fantasia* as a young boy, Rob Williams had dreamt of being a magician. Now, a half-century later, he has become one. Williams doesn't use magic to clean the kitchen, like Mickey Mouse does in *Fantasia*. He cleans something far more important: the subconscious, which drives most of our behavior and experience. There is no shortage of personal growth gurus today. Yet many of the techniques they offer fail when conscious commitments fail to overwrite self-limiting subconscious beliefs. Changing the subconscious is precisely the focus of Williams' PSYCH-K® method, which he developed almost 25 years ago. PSYCH-K® offers a simple, direct process to overcome self-sabotage.

Rob Williams didn't set out to become a psychotherapist. After studying philosophy in college, he took a job in the backpacking industry, inspired by a powerful experience in nature he had as a teenager. He later moved on to executive positions in the energy management and telecommunications industries, until one day he realized that his work was not fulfilling. So he got a master's degree in counseling and began a career as a therapist. He quickly discovered that the worlds of business and counseling were far apart. In business, he had always learned "to get results, no matter what"; in therapy, he discovered that it was all about the process. "The process is the end itself," he says. "You just *need* therapy." That dichotomy felt unsatisfying, so Williams took courses—in neurolinguistic programming, hypnosis and touch for health, educational kinesiology and reiki—in search of more effective treatments to help clients make positive changes in their lives. "I was also frustrated by the limitations of the old counseling formula of 'insight + willpower = change,' Williams says. "Many of my clients, up to their eyeballs in insights about how and why they had become the way they were, were still not experiencing the satisfying lives they sought." Then one very frustrating December day brought Williams the answer. He had spent the day putting together a mailing to promote his counseling services and encountered all the maddeningly familiar printer and photocopier challenges. When he finally gave up, he fled to his garden and sat on a half-frozen lawn chair. Still fuming, he said out loud, "Okay God, if you don't want me to do what I'm doing, what *do you* want me to do?"

Not considering himself susceptible to spiritual experiences, Williams didn't expect an answer. But to his astonishment, he recalls, "Within minutes, the details of a pattern for changing subconscious beliefs showed up in my head, like on a teleprompter." He ran to his computer and typed what he had seen, most of which was new to him. That was the beginning of PSYCH-K®. We meet in a San Francisco hotel that looks out over the bay. In the distance is Alcatraz, once the site of a notorious prison. Today, the spooky empty buildings are a popular tourist destination. Staring in the direction of Alcatraz, Williams says: "Many people are prisoners of their own beliefs. PSYCH-K® is all about breaking out of these prisons." He is an articulate and rapid-fire speaker, still more the can-do executive than the counselor comfortable with long pauses. But there is also warmth and passion in his eyes and voice. After almost 25 years, Williams is proud to have trained about 40 PSYCH-K® facilitators around the world. There is no aggressive PSYCH-K® marketing machine, no desperate attempts to get publicity. The therapy and training are available for those who find them and are ready for them. Authenticity and sincerity are hallmarks of Williams' approach. PSYCH-K® works with sets of paired statements, such as "The universe is a friendly place" and "The universe is an unfriendly place" or "I love myself" and "I hate myself." Research has shown that the subconscious directs the body's motor functions and controls muscle movements, so PSYCH-K® uses the musculature to communicate with the subconscious. It's the same idea as behind lie detectors, which measure skin conductivity. When someone is lying, they become tense, which raises their blood pressure, then makes them sweat, and thus increases skin conductivity. Measuring differences in muscle tension can lead to similar results, such as whether someone really agrees with self-reverential statements like "I respect myself" or "I do my best, and my best is good enough." The goal: to discover which self-limiting beliefs individuals might subconsciously be holding. "You can repeat affirmations until you are blue in the face," Williams says. "It seldom makes any difference. Most of the time, it's not about positive thinking. It's not about, 'Oh, cancel. I don't want that thought.' You already had the thought. So until you change the basic software of the subconscious, your hard drive, your life won't change." The problem is that our subconscious 'records' experiences from our earliest moments onwards. "We are brought into this world into various cultures that have a whole bunch of mindsets already in place for us" Williams explains. "We start internalizing those even before we are out of the womb. Your parents start to treat you in a way that fits the society's norms and their own beliefs. By the time you're 12 years old, generally speaking, you are quite asleep at the wheel of your own life because you are 'inculturated' by whatever your culture and your parents say is true and right. That's not all bad. But you want to change the beliefs that are not serving you, that are limiting you in some way."

When muscle tension reveals a disagreement between your conscious desires and your subconscious beliefs, the process of reprogramming can begin. For this, it is critical to "speak the language of the subconscious," Williams says. The subconscious mind thinks literally, he argues, so the simple thought, "I want to be happy" is too vague. You have to specify the details of your goal, and you have to do so in sensory-based language. What will you see in your life when you have accomplished your goal? What will you *hear* other people saying about you? How will you feel when you have succeeded, and where in your body will you feel that? PSYCH-K® also uses what Williams calls "belief points" on the body. These acupuncture points from Chinese medicine relate to specific organs associated with certain emotions: the heart for love, the lungs for self-esteem. Addressing these points helps release the physical blockages associated with self-limiting beliefs. Still, there is something magical about the experience, Williams says: "Magic is possible in the world, but you don't do it until you are wise enough to use it properly."

Williams first tested his new approach on himself and a few close friends. "I felt physical changes in my body," he recalls. "I was astounded, because I'm not that sensitive. I don't feel things in my body, but I did then." He vividly remembers his first major case with a client, a woman addicted to smoking and drinking who came to him from a rehab center. She also had Crohn's disease. After about 45 minutes into her first PSYCH-K® session, on a massage table in Williams' office, she said: "I don't know what, but something just happened." "I said, 'That's great, I don't know either,'" Williams recalls. "A few months later, I heard from the woman that the doctors who had diagnosed her Crohn's disease couldn't find it anymore. New tests and X-rays didn't show anything. The doctors said that they must have misdiagnosed because Crohn's is an incurable disease. This was my first major indicator that I was onto something." Williams explains how he believes the healing works: "All these supposedly 'incurable' diseases aren't so incurable after all. That 'incurable' really means incurable from the outside. If you want to interrupt a physical process called disease, you need to leverage belief systems that will activate biological responses that will trigger a self-healing response.

PSYCH-K® does not heal anything. It is a catalyst for the body to heal itself. The mind is the doctor. The pharmacy is in your head. With the right instruction by the mind, our bodies produce all kinds of things that are similar to the drugs that are made by the pharmaceutical industry. "It is very simple: If you have a disease, and all of a sudden you have an altered subconscious belief that your body is in perfect health, a dynamic tension arises. That tension has to be resolved in favor of the consciousness because that comes from a higher energy dimension. And consciousness will use all the magnificent resources of the mind-body system to make that new reality come true." IN ABOUT 80 PERCENT OF CASES, THE changes are long lasting, according to Williams. He compares the process with a word-processing program on your computer: "You change a document and you press the save command. That's the version that remains. You don't open the document the next day to find that is has changed to an earlier version. It's the same thing with PSYCH-K®. There is literally an edit and a save command in the process. You can take that same thing that you have done and overanalyzed for years and you write some new 'software', and then that becomes what you boot up with in the morning." Where PSYCH-K® fails is mostly in terms of what Williams calls "secondary gains." "Somebody may say: 'I want to get well and get back to work,'" he says. "And then, when they do, they find that they are missing something. They were getting attention, for instance, when they were sick. A disability was also ability for them to get something else. In such cases, people may fall back to old behavior."

Listening to Williams I realize that while we are listening to dysfunctional political debates in most Western capitals and read about the damage done by big business to society, we are also on a high-speed track toward a healthier and wiser world. Just think about it: If more people embrace opportunities for personal transformation offered by programs like PSYCH-K®, more people will become happier and more aligned with their own life's mission. Many of us are changing and because of that the societies around us are bound to change too. Williams also focuses on the business community. "Most of the business people making decisions that are trashing the planet don't want to do that," he says. "They just do not know any other way. In order for them to get out of these destructive patterns, they have to be able to change their subconscious beliefs." He pauses, and then adds, "In today's society, money management is the most important skill. That's wrong. Mind management is the most critical skill. If you manage your mind, you will always be in a good state." There are big books that describe the different psychological disorders. I think there is really only one disorder: I call it 'the illusion of separation'. If you believe you are separate from the source of all that is and separate from each other, you will have all kinds of problems in your life. The illusion of separation gives us the idea that we can harm somebody else and not harm ourselves at the same time. You can't bomb another country if you realize that these kids are our kids. You cannot make a decision in New York City or São Paulo to destroy a rainforest if you know that forest is part of the eco-system that your life depends on.

Ultimately Williams sees PSYCH-K® as an instrument for spiritual growth: "I think we all have one purpose and that's to manifest our full divinity while we are incarnated in physical bodies." At the same time, he observes that few people pursue this highest of goals: "I think the biggest misuse of PSYCH-K® is that people settle for too little. All they want is money or health or the right partner, all those things that people think they want. But if they get them, they find they are hopelessly inadequate to get what they really need. These things don't produce the stuff that really counts—love, joy, purpose, satisfaction and peace. In fact, they are often distractions to that." Someone may say, 'I want $10 million.' But if you delve deeper you will eventually come down to an emotion, an intangible. That person wants to be happy. People think they need tangibles to get to the intangibles. They think they know what they want; seldom do they know what they need.

Laughter and music rise from the street beneath the window of the hotel. San Francisco is enjoying summer. My thoughts go back to the wizard in *Fantasia* as Williams concludes: "Deciding what's worth wanting is a lot harder then getting what you want. I can teach you how to get what you want. If you believe you are separate from the source of all that is and separate from each other, you will have all kinds of problems in your life"

Jurriaan Kamp added a missing piece to his subconscious and watched **Fantasia** *for the first time while writing this article.*

The Intelligent Optimist (formerly Ode) is an independent international media platform focused on solutions, possibility and inspiration. We present optimism as the most effective, efficient and by scientific research confirmed strategy to drive the innovation and creativity that are necessary to solve the problems and meet the challenges that people and society face.

The Intelligent Optimist was founded as Ode in 1995 in The Netherlands by Hélène de Puy and Jurriaan Kamp who left the world of mainstream journalism because of its never ending focus on whatever goes wrong. Since 2004 the platform is led from twin headquarters in Rotterdam, The Netherlands and San Francisco in the US.

The Intelligent Optimist publishes a daily selection of solutions-news online, webinars to support the optimism lifestyle and an award-winning quarterly print magazine in which we point to groundbreaking innovation and the people leading the way. We also offer our readers the chance to connect with these pioneers of possibility and deepen their learning and understanding in interactive online events and courses.

www.psych-k.com

CHAPTER 14

PSYCH-K®-The Missing Piece

Rita Soman

Neuroscience reveals that we run our lives with our creative, conscious mind about 5 percent of the time. Ninety-five percent of the time, our life is controlled by the beliefs programmed in the subconscious mind. You may hold some positive thoughts but that has very little influence on your life because of the limited amount of time you actually run with your conscious mind. We are not locked in to fate, because we have the freedom to change the way we respond to the world. We are the masters of our genetics rather than the victim of our hereditary traits. Our fate is really based on how we see the world or on how we have been programmed to experience it. So whatever we programmed into our minds, those beliefs will shape not just our genetics but our behavior to conform to those beliefs as well. If we have positive beliefs built in our minds, then our behavior and our genes will lead us to health and happiness, says Dr. Bruce Lipton, author of book, The Biology of Belief.

"The 'secret to life' is BELIEF. Rather than genes, it is our beliefs that control our lives." --Bruce Lipton, Ph.D Cellular Biologist, author of Biology of Belief

The good news is that we can reprogram our subconscious mind with positive beliefs. Using PSYCH-K® process that was established in 1988, by Robert Williams, you can easily rewrite beliefs that have been affecting you your whole life in a matter of just minutes. Psychoanalysis and psychotherapy may have brought a better understanding to why we behave as we do, but rarely succeed in fundamentally, changing our lives through these methods. Another reason why psychotherapy does not work is because it addresses only 40-bit processor (i.e. the conscious mind). While the enormous power of the 40 million bits processor, (i.e. the subconscious mind) is largely un-utilized. Helping clients

Holistic Wellness in the New Age

change self-limiting beliefs into self- empowering beliefs would greatly benefit them.

Research has shown that the subconscious directs the body's motor functions and controls muscle movements, so PSYCH-K® uses the musculature (kinesiology) to communicate with the subconscious. PSYCH-K® process has been successfully used for over 23 years by psychiatrists, psychologists, social workers, hypnotherapists, counselors, energy healers, professional performance coaches and general population. It is a whole-brain integration process, which increases the communication between both brain hemispheres that supports the subconscious mind in the change process. This whole brain therapy gets to the root of embedded problems, limiting beliefs. Since the challenges we experience in our lives are really a result of an embedded problem with self-esteem or shame or guilt or grief or holding resentments, when you use this process you get to the source and heal that. The problem is solved for good and people are able to live freely and happily. It's very quick.

"Whole-Brain State is a significant contributor to human evolution. From a neuroscience perspective, it allows greater efficiency in the brain and enhances both conscious and subconscious processes. From a quantum perspective, it is the gateway to higher consciousness." says Dr. Jeffrey Fannin, Director for Cognitive Enhancement.

PSYCH-K® is a profound and energizing experience. With this process people are able to tap into their core self-definitions. We do that with a series of new suggestions, new definitions. It's almost like post hypnotic suggestions where these new definitions replace the old ones. With this process we get to the embedded anxiety, that place of fear where they have a conflict on some unconscious level that's triggering the anxiety to continue with their self-sabotaging behaviors. We get to that. We heal that. Now, their conscious mind which wants to succeed, be happy, have healthy relationships, be prosperous and self-confident, is linked up with their subconscious mind which no longer sabotages them and is totally in alignment with the plan to achieve their goals. It is a way to once and for all get you to the root of the problem, and not replace one symptom with another which can happen in traditional therapy. With this process we resolve the core of the problem so people are not doing symptom substitution. They actually heal themselves.

I am truly grateful to PSYCH-K® process. It has helped me to break-free from past limitations. Utilizing it as the foundation of my practice, allows the synergistic blend of many modalities including traditional psychotherapy to benefit my clients' transition from a belief of being powerless to being empowered. This process makes sense, makes scientific sense. If you do not treat the underlying cause of problems you cannot expect positive, long-term results.

The power of the mind, the power of our beliefs is the platform to 'curing' diseases. Self-defeating beliefs and behaviors are like being imprisoned behind iron bars with the door left ajar – all we need to do is walk through the door but our mind thinks it is impossible to 'escape.' Our clients have sought us out to change how life occurs for them. They rely upon us for the answers to release them from their life sentence. There is an epidemic of addictions and physical and mental health related issues and it will continue to ramp up if we do not intervene with methods that can bring them positive and long-term results.

This is what I would tell my peers. If you have a technique which actually heals people where they've internalized really healthy, spiritual and cognitive and therapeutic messages, it is great. If you can really heal people and send them on their way and then they lead fulfilling lives, excellent. But if there are limitations to what you can do, if your clients aren't able to go out from therapy and be independent, then maybe you should look into PSYCH-K®.

Ignorance can kill us or, at the very least, kill our spirit. It is incumbent upon us, as professionals/healers to educate ourselves with the latest technologies, methods and processes to help those who come to us with great hope.

"Heal thyself" is not just an adage. I am living proof of the long-term and positive results PSYCH K® creates. Every day is a gift and I am grateful for the wonderful life I have created with my husband. It is my honor to share this highly effective process with those who are ready for a 'real breakthrough' in life or want to help their clients/patients more effectively. This message brings hope and excitement to those individuals who have been feeling powerless and living in fear.

"I am a perpetual student…. I'm always open to acquire knowledge and learn new tools to help me on my life's journey. I found PSYCH-K® to be of tremendous benefit for me not only personally but also in my business. What I especially appreciate about PSYCH-K® is its simplicity. The techniques although simple are extremely effective. I

was very surprised at how quickly (5-10 minutes) and easily my limiting subconscious beliefs could be shifted to support my goals rather that work against them. PSYCH-K® works!" – Susie Park (Actress)

Rita Soman, MA, CADC III, is an Addiction Treatment Specialist for 26 years and Internationally Certified PSYCH-K® Instructor. She has recently co- authored two books, The Thought That Changed My Life Forever and Thank God I Am An Empowered Woman. Rita is from Delhi, India. She has been residing in Portland, Oregon, since 1987. She works with local people from her office in Portland and others living at a distant by phone and Skype. She will be in India in December for six weeks, to teach Basic PSYCH-K® workshops. She will be available to do private sessions during her visit. Dr. Bruce Lipton has endorsed Rita for her commitment to help the powerless become empowered!

www.ritasoman.com

15 CHAPTER

Leading-Edge Neuroscience Reveals Significant Correlations Between Beliefs, the Whole-Brain State, and Psychotherapy

Jeffrey L. Fannin, Ph.D.
Robert M. Williams, M.A.

The latest understandings in neuroscience are revealing important information for psychotherapists. This article is designed to inform you about some of the key elements of those new understandings, including the importance of subconscious beliefs, the Whole-Brain State, and the basic mechanisms of the mind/brain interface. All of which can assist you in being more effective with your clients.

Let's begin by defining two key terms in this article. The first is *belief*. The dictionary defines belief as, *something one accepts as true or real; a firmly held opinion or conviction.* From our perspective, the origin of beliefs can be traced back to conclusions drawn from past experience, i.e. fire can hurt me because I have had an experience with fire that demonstrated that truth! Beliefs can be both conscious and/or subconscious. The second term is, *Whole-Brain State.* This is a state of coherency in the brain, marked by a bilateral, symmetrical brain wave pattern, allowing for maximum communication/data flow between the left and right hemispheres of the brain. So, what do these terms have to do with psychotherapy? The surprising answer is…*everything*! If we accept that the overall goal of psychotherapy is to produce fully functional human beings, then being able to optimize belief systems and brain function is a major factor in accomplishing that goal. Consider the role of beliefs in our lives. Beliefs are like filters on a camera. What the camera "sees" is a function of the filters through which it is viewing its subject. In other words, how we "see" the world is a function of our beliefs, and profoundly influences our personality. As a result of our beliefs, we define ourselves as worthy or worthless, powerful or powerless, competent or incompetent, trusting or suspicious, belonging or outcast, self-reliant or dependent, flexible or judgmental, fairly treated or victimized, loved or hated. Your beliefs have far-reaching consequences, both positive and negative, in your life. Beliefs affect your moods, relationships, job performance, self-esteem, physical health, even your religious or spiritual outlook. Most psychotherapists deal with one or more of these issues on a regular basis with their clients. Clients are often plagued by beliefs that are self-limiting. Consequently, the ability to help individuals change self-limiting beliefs into self-empowering beliefs is of great value in a psychotherapeutic environment.

Beliefs can be conscious and/or subconscious. We are using the word *conscious* in its ordinary sense, as awareness of the environment. We are using the word *subconscious,* as awareness *below* the conscious level. Like a hard drive in a computer, this is where most of the belief-system "software" is stored. And, like a computer memory, the data are stored, not *in the central processing chip* itself, but rather *in the energy field* that surrounds and interpenetrates the chip. There is an analogous relationship with the brain and mind, respectively. This "software" is largely responsible for our habitual thoughts and behaviors. Advances in neuroscience have provided important information about the subconscious mind. For example, in a study cited in Harvard Professor Emeritus Gerald Zaltman's book, *How Customers Think*, neuroscience reveals that at least 95% of our thoughts and decisions originate at the subconscious level of the mind. That leaves a very small percentage of our decision-making capacity for the conscious mind to exercise. These subconscious beliefs create the perceptual filters through which we respond to life's challenges. So, while we may be mostly unaware of their influence on us, our subconscious beliefs largely 'direct' our observable actions and behaviors. They form the basis for our actions and reactions to each new situation in our lives.

Another important quality of the subconscious mind is its processing capacity. In his book, *The User Illusion, Cutting Consciousness Down To Size,* author Tor Norretranders, provides important information about the processing capacity of the conscious and subconscious minds.

As remarkable as it may seem, the conscious mind processes information at an approximate rate of 40 bits of information per second. While the subconscious mind processes approximately 40 million bits of information per second. Ironically, most standard approaches to psychotherapy address only the 40-bit processor (i.e. the conscious mind). While the enormous power of the 40 million-bit processor, (i.e. the subconscious mind), is largely un-utilized.

What about the Whole-Brain State?

A great deal of research has been conducted for decades on what has come to be called "brain dominance" theory (also known as split-brain research). The findings of this research indicate that in general, each hemisphere of the cerebral cortex tends to specialize in, and preside over, different functions, process different kinds of information, and deals with different kinds of problems.

The LEFT Hemisphere	The RIGHT Hemisphere
Uses logic/reason	use emotions/intuition
Thinks in words	thinks in pictures
Deals in parts/specifics	deals in wholes/relationship
Will analyze/break apart	will synthesize/put together
Thinks sequentially	think simultaneously
Identifies with the individual	identifies with the group
Is ordered/controlled	is spontaneous/free

It should be obvious from the qualities and characteristics described above, that ideal brain functioning would be the ability to simultaneously utilize both sides of the cerebral cortex. However, life experiences often trigger a dominance of one side over the other when responding to specific situations. The more emotionally charged the experience (usually traumatic), the more likely it will be stored for future reference, and the more likely we will automatically over-identify with only one hemisphere when faced with similar life experiences in the future. As a psychotherapist, the ability to help clients achieve a balanced identification with *both* hemispheres of the brain, (i.e. the Whole-Brain State) with respect to past traumatic experiences, is paramount in helping them to achieve a new perspective of their past. This new perspective can free them from the habitual perspective, held in the subconscious, which can make a *past* trauma into a *current* nightmare. By re-perceiving a past traumatic experience with new Whole-Brain "filters," clients can be freed from the automaticity of past perceptions, which limit their happiness and wellbeing.

In addition to its usefulness as a tool for dealing more effectively with life's challenges, past, present, and future, the Whole-Brain State has another major benefit. It can be used as a foundation for quickly and effectively changing self-limiting subconscious beliefs. The research that follows, utilized PSYCH-K®, a popular system for subconscious change. This system has been used by psychiatrists, psychologists, social workers, professional performance coaches, and others, for over 23 years. This is a testament to its versatility. In the hands of a professionally trained psychotherapist, it is an effective therapeutic tool. In the hands of a sports performance coach, it is as a way to dramatically enhance sporting ability. Used as a tool by educators and parents, it can significantly help students achieve academic success.

Healer Heal Thyself…and Your Clients too!

The powerful influence of the Whole-Brain State was demonstrated in a study reported in 1988 in the *International Journal of Neuroscience*, by researchers at the Universidad Nacional Autonoma de Mexico. It suggests that synchronized brain states significantly influence nonverbal communication. The study was done with thirteen paired subjects. The subjects were tested in a darkened and soundproof Faraday cage (a lead-lined, screened chamber, that filters out all outside electromagnetic activity). Each pair of subjects was instructed to close their eyes and try to "communicate" by becoming aware of the other's presence and to signal the experimenter when they felt it had occurred. The brainwave states of the subjects were monitored during this process.

Experimenters reported that during the sessions an increase in similarity of EEG (electroencephalogram) patterns between the pairs of communicators developed. Furthermore, the experimenters noticed, *"The subject with the highest concordance [hemispheric integration] was the one who most influenced the session."* In other words, when you are in a Whole-Brain State, your brain wave pattern can automatically affect your client in a very positive way, even before you communicate verbally!

These conclusions support the allegation that our thoughts, even nonverbally expressed, can influence others. In fact, the more whole-brained *we* become, the more we influence *others* toward that state of being as well. The therapeutic benefit of this kind of influence on therapists, as well as their clients is self-evident.

QEEG and the Whole-Brain State

Our research gathering documented one hundred twenty-five (125) cases, with data gathered over 12 months in three different locations, utilizing different EEG technicians, using two different types of EEG equipment; the result of this investigation produced a pvalue of <=0.010.

A baseline of EEG (electroencephalogram) data was established for each case. Three baseline readings of five minutes each was recorded; five minutes eyes open, five minutes eyes closed and five minutes with the brain on task (silently reading a magazine). A Certified PSYCH-K® Facilitator, used standard PSYCH-K® (corporate version is identified as PER- K®) practices. This is a *process for subconscious belief change* to achieve the *whole-brain state*. Following the intervention of the PSYCH-K® change process (aka a *balance),* a post-intervention EEG was recorded in the same manner as the EEG baseline stated above. The *balance* took approximately 10 minutes to complete.

Raw EEG data was artifacted to eliminate eye movement, tongue movement, swallowing, or other unwanted disturbances in the EEG. NeuroStat, a function of the NeuroGuide program from Applied Neuroscience, performed statistical analysis. NeuroStat allows for individual independent t-tests to be performed. The following is an example from the base of 125 cases examined for the whole-brain state. The independent t-test compares condition A to condition B and shows if there are differences in the dominant brain function, when we consider Shannon's method of statistical analysis [4], we understand that when we measure two groups, A and B, (such as pre-balance and post-balance) each of them having a well defined probability distribution, respectively, as well as a joint probability distribution, then the mutual information between A and B is defined. The concept of mutual information can easily be extended to quantum systems of entanglement. This leads us to understand that having quantum mutual information, which, for a general state of either A and/or B is now defined and provides the basis by which the relationship can be understood, a sample depiction of the whole-brain state seen in below:

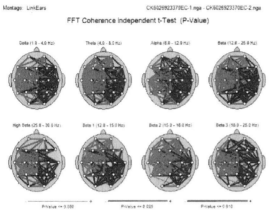

Figure 1:
Following a PSYCH-K® balance, this person demonstrated a statistically significant shift in hemispheric coherence patterns, which were reflected behaviorally in increased access to emotional resources and integrated, "whole-brain" behaviors and relationships.

To better understand the scientific significance of this report, understanding the significance of pvalue will help to put this research into perspective. In statistical significance testing, the p-value is the probability of obtaining a test statistic at least as extreme as the one that was actually observed. When the result falls at 0.05 or 0.01 is said to be statistically significant. In the case of the Fannin-Williams research a very high degree of statistical significance occurred, <=0.010. This indicates that the relationship between the two phenomena is highly significant and not a function of chance. The colors on the independent t-test show phenomena A (dominant brainwave pattern)

BEFORE the PSYCH-K® *balance* is depicted in RED, left side and phenomena B (dominant brainwave pattern) AFTER the PSYCH-K® balance was facilitated is depicted in BLUE, right side. The *whole-brain state* is considered to be the combination of RED, left side; condition A, dominance prior to the *balance* process, and condition B, right side, dominance after the *balance* process was facilitated.

Due to the space restriction of this article, it is not possible to provide a comprehensive treatment of this subject, or the numerous changes that a majority of subjects in this research experienced. However, the volume of data collected, and the unique properties it represents, afford us the opportunity to evaluate and continue to understand what the data means, as well as providing intriguing hints as to the nature of its potential. Singularly, the most significant information to come from this research, in 98% of the cases measured, presented very high statistically significant correlations, demonstrating the difference between baseline measures and the presence of the *whole-brain state* after the intervention occurred. As mentioned above, just because the whole-brain state is present does not mean that it is being continually activated, so the person can take full advantage of it in a given situation. Sometimes secondary gain issues come into play, or other subconscious belief patterns that may need to be addressed in order to effectively activate and/or allow the person to fully use the whole-brain state.

The whole-brain state is better understood with some education regarding a few of its more unfamiliar components. Figure 1 uses the term *coherence*. This is an energy signature. In physics, *coherence* is a property of waves that enables stationary a temporally and spatially constant to brainwave function. More generally, coherence describes all properties of the correlation between physical quantities of a wave. This is important in order to understand the physics of resonating wave patterns in the brain, its connection to the whole-brain state, and how it impacts our behavior.

An additional component to the whole-brain state is identified as *constructive* and *destructive* interference patterns. If two waves are interacting with one another in such a way that they combine to create a wave of greater amplitude than either one by itself, the result is called *constructive interference*. Constructive interference is said to occur when waves are in-phase with one another. However, if the waves interfere with each other in such a way as to diminish the amplitude of the other, a *destructive interference* pattern is created. In this case, the waves are said to be out-of-phase with each other. Phase is important in brainwave patterns, just as it is in other principles of physics. That is to say, two waves are said to be coherent if they have a constant relative phase. The degree of coherence is measured by the interference visibility, a measure of how perfectly the waves can cancel due to destructive interference. Cancellation is virtual or local since a wave cannot have negative energy.

Holistic Wellness in the New Age

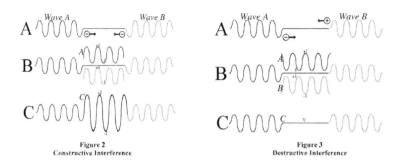

Figure 2
Constructive Interference

Figure 3
Destructive Interference

Constructive Interference as seen in Figure 2, for example, would be like two sets of ripples moving across the surface of water toward each other, as seen in depiction A. Both wave A and B are moving toward each other with their ripples in-phase, in this case both waves are leading with their negative amplitude. Their cycle patterns are aligned. The waves merge together at the interface where two ripples meet. The consequences of this merger, the waves are drawn with one above the other as seen in middle depiction B. The common expression of, *being in rapport, or in sync, or on the same wavelength* with someone, is an example of how this concept is relevant to therapist/ client relationships.

Destructive Interference, as seen in Figure 3, for example, the ripples might be best understood when thought of as waves created when a pebble is dropped into water. Wave A in depiction B, are moving from left to right. Wave B in depiction B, moving right to left, wave B represents the ripples from a second pebble dropped shortly after the first. Since the pebbles did not enter the water at the same time, the waves will not be aligned when they merge they will be "out of phase." The physics of a destructive interference pattern has wave A is leading with negative amplitude and wave B is leading with positive amplitude. Where they meet the waves are a mirror image of each other. As shown in depiction C, the amplitude values of each wave cancel each other out[5].

The significance of this principle of physics is fundamental to the coherence of the whole-brain state. Allowing brainwave energy to be more focused and effective at resolving problems and accessing information with ability to not only resonate properly to influence brain function, but also interact with subconscious beliefs.

Emotional Engagement and Subconscious Beliefs

From a neuroscience perspective, the basis for understanding why we experience particular emotions is centered in the relationship between the *anterior cingulate cortex* (ACC) and the *amygdala*. The amygdala, usually thought of as the fear detector, also detects all other emotions. It responds to fear because it processes emotions in order of their significance. So, when fear is the most significant emotion in the brain, the amygdala will respond [6]. When fear is the most dominant emotion in your thinking, it taxes the subconscious mind, which does most of the fast processing of information.

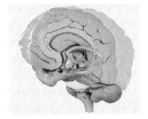
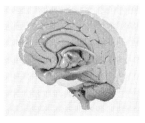

Figure 4:
Anterior Cingulate Cortex (ACC)
Front part of the Cingulate Gyrus

Figure 5:
Amygdala – Thought of as the fear detector

For example, if a person who left a secure job to pursue her dreams, started to read statistics about how unlikely it was to be a successful entrepreneur, the amygdala would likely have been stimulated, making her more anxious. As a result, her *subconscious fears* would be active even when she was thinking about other things. Scientific experiments found that when fearful facial expressions were shown so that people did not know they had seen them, the amygdala was still activated.

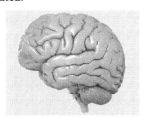
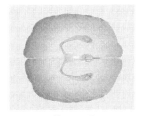

Figure 6:
Prefrontal Cortex (PFC)

Figure 7:
Amygdala

The amygdala is connected to multiple brain regions. One of those regions is the frontal lobe, where many important decisions are processed. If the amygdala is activated, the activation affects various regions in the frontal lobe, particularly the *prefrontal cortex* (PFC), and thereafter affects decision-making, as well as emotional centers. We can recognize that we are vulnerable to fear and anxiety in such a way that it compromises our own abilities to attend to relevant content. The impact of this is that it consumes our *thinking resources*. We should also understand that the amygdala is the *emotional relevance detector* rather than just a fear detector. The amygdala-PFC connection is important because a part of it acts as short-term memory and another part as the "accountant" in the brain calculating risks and benefits of our thinking. Subconscious threats over-activate the amygdala and lead to a decline in thinking and productivity when we focus on negative statements such as:

- "How am I ever going to keep up with everything? What if I fail?"
- "What if I can't afford food, gas, healthcare on what I make?"
- "The government is not doing much to help me or my family, so the odds for success are stacked against me.
- "What if I get laid off?"
- "I'm not smart enough to be successful."

These kinds of negative thought patterns can create what could be identified as an *amygdala hijacking*. The amygdala kicks into action in preparation for "fight or flight," creating unacceptable levels of anxiety and fear at a subconscious level that negatively impact our behavior and productivity. This subconscious patterning becomes part of the default network and will keep us focused on looking out for danger. The authors of this paper contend that entering into what we call the *whole-brain state* will move the brain out of the negative default mode and allow access to more resourceful thinking processes.

High-speed mindset change taught in PSYCH-K® and/or PER-K® is an effective method for identifying and changing the conflict between the conscious and subconscious beliefs.

Worry is another component related to normal brain function. It is the brain's response to fear, it is thought of as a response of the brain to block out negative emotions that reside in the subconscious. Some neuroscientists have suggested that worry is a strategy of cognitive avoidance in which internal verbalization acts to suppress threatening emotional imagery. It is believed that worry leads to missing important negative information such as risk that may be relevant to making optimal decisions. This information is mostly subconscious. Worry disrupts the "brain-bridge" (corpus callosum) and slows the transfer time across from the left to the right hemisphere.

Taking additional time for processing without creating a solution to the problem. People who are constantly worried, often see this worry as an attempt to find a solution, but may in fact be stuck in worry. That usually keeps productivity to a minimum. The whole-brain state increases communication between the left and right hemispheres of the brain, and speeds up the transfer of information across the corpus callosum, thereby diminishing the capacity to worry without excluding or ignoring important information leading to a productive behavior.

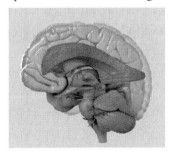

Figure 8: Corpus Callosum, "the brain-bridge.

The authors of this paper point to the research herein, which suggests that, the Whole-Brain state allows access to the inter-hemispheric activity connecting to more efficient brain function. Further, we would have you understand that from the research presented here we identify the *whole-brain state* as a bi-lateral, symmetrical brain wave pattern allowing access to positive mood and cognitive openness.

In conclusion, we suggest that this research demonstrates a significant connection between beliefs, (especially at the subconscious level of the mind), the Whole-

Brain State, and high-speed mindset change, as well as their relevant utility to psychotherapists.

The data presented here strongly suggests a correlation between the state of mind of the psychotherapist and the state of the mind of the patient/client. Hence, the relevancy of doing psychotherapy from a Whole-Brain State, with the appropriate subconscious belief systems, in order to be optimally effective as a catalyst for change.

References

1) Zaltman G. (2003). How Customers Think: Essential Insights into the Mind of the Market. *Harvard Business School Publishing.* Boston, MA 02163.

2) Nørentrander, Tor. (1991). *The User Illusion – Cutting Consciousness Down to Size.* Penguin Books.

3) Ferguson, M. (1988*). The Brain Revolution and Brain.* Universidad **NacionalAutonoma de Mexcio.** *International Journal of Neuroscience,* **vol 13, 10a, 148.**

4) Claude Elwood Shannon (1916-2001) was an American mathematician, electronic engineer, and cryptographer known as the "father of information theory." Shannon is famous for having founded information theory in 1937, when as a 21-year-old master's student at MIT, he wrote a thesis demonstrating that electrical application of Boolian algebra could construct and resolve and logical, numerical relationship.

5) Lipton, B. H. (2005). *The Biology of Belief.* Santa Rosa, CA: Mountain of Love/Elite Books. p. 116.

6) Whalen, P. J., et al., (2001). A functional MRI study of human amygdala responses to **facial expressions of fear versus anger.** *Emotion***, 1 (1): p. 70-83.**

7) Morris, J. S., Ohman, A. and Dolan, R. J. (1999). A subcortical pathway to the right amygdala mediating 'unseen' fear. *Proc Natl Acad Sci.* 96 (4) p. 1680-5.

8) Williams, M. A. and Mattingley, J. B. (2004). Unconscious perception of nonthreatening **facial emotions in parietal extinction.** *Exp Brain Res* **154 (4), p. 403-6.**

9) Whalen, P. J. et al., (1998). Masked presentations of emotional facial expressions **modulate amygdala activity without explicit knowledge.** *J Neurosci* **18 (1), p.411-8.**

10) Rhudy, J. L. and Meagher, M. W. (2000). Fear and anxiety: divergent effects on **human pain thresholds.** *Pain.* **84(1): p. 65-75.**

11) Mohlman, J., et al., (2009). The relation of worry to prefrontal cortex volume in **older adults without generalized anxiety disorder.** *Psychiatry Res* **173(2): p. 121-7.**

Jeffrey L. Fannin holds a Ph.D. in Psychology, an MBA and a Bachelor of Science degree in Mass Communications. He is the founder and Executive Director for the Center for Cognitive Enhancement and Thought Genius, LLC. He has worked in the neuroscience field, mapping and analyzing the brain for over 15 years. Dr. Fannin has extensive experience training the brain for optimal brain performance working with Attention Deficit Disorder (ADD/ADHD), anxiety disorders, depression, and trauma recovery.He has appeared on Quantum World TV, recently as presenter at the World Congress for Quantum Medicine; also on Gaiam TV, You Are Not Your Brain. His work has been featured in local media, international media such as the Wall Street Journal, Fox News, Business Week, London Financial Times, in Singapore's Weekend Edition, BBC radio, and many more.

Rob has a Bachelor of Arts Degree in Philosophy from the University of California, at Los Angeles, and a Masters Degree in Counseling and Personnel Services from the University of Colorado. He is President of The Myrddin Corporation, and Director of the PSYCH-K Centre International.

For the first 14 years of his career, Rob was a direct participant in the U.S. corporate world, holding management positions in the backpacking, energy management, and telecommunications industries. Experiencing a spiritual awakening during this time, he moved out of the business environment into a life of service as a profesional psychotherapist. Finding the accepted counseling philosophy of the day lacking in spiritual essence and overall effectiveness, he studied many non-standard modalities for change, both ancient and contemporary. Out of his studies came a series of intuitive insights that became the body of work called PSYCH-K.

Originated in 1988, PSYCH-K is a simple and direct way to change self-limiting beliefs at the subconscious level of the mind, where nearly all human behavior originates, both constructive and destructive. Its overall goal is to accelerate individual and global spiritual evolution by aligning subconscious beliefs with conscious wisdom from the world's great spiritual and intellectual traditions. The practical application of this wisdom in our personal and professional lives brings a greater sense of purpose and satisfaction, mentally, emotionally, physically, and spiritually. PSYCH-K is taught world-wide by Certified PSYCH-K Instructors.

www.psych-k.com

Chapter 16

Reiki and the force called Motivation

Dr. Paula Horan

May all beings have bliss and the cause of bliss
May all beings be freed from suffering and the cause of suffering
May all beings never be without the supreme bliss which is free of all suffering
May all beings reach the limitless equanimity, which is free of near and far,
Attachment and Aversion. -The Four Immeasurables

The Essence

Reiki, the hands on energy healing practice has been a vital part of my work in the last 25 years. When I embarked upon this journey of healing and self-exploration, I did not know that I would reach this far in my understanding, had it not been for Reiki and its touch of gentle awareness, I would not have found the insights that led me to accomplish my work as a student and teacher of Non Dual Awareness.

Reiki is simple yet mysterious like the creation itself. And it is a blessing that this energy is available to us today to guide our way through the chaos of the planetary transition. I have shared my extensive experience and understanding of Reiki in my books, but here I will share something, which is not just limited to Reiki practice, rather it applies for any spiritual or creative pursuit that you might be having.

For any effort to sustain and bear fruit, for any practice to become a way of life, for any essence to become fully manifested one needs to learn the art of self-motivation. Hundreds of seminars, books and other educational content are created on this subject and yet we all know how difficult it is for our mind to become attuned and focused with a practice, bringing consistency and intensity in the effort.

Motivation cannot be fostered without cultivating the right perspective about the practice and our role as the practitioner. To know the strengths and weaknesses of our mind, to know the pitfalls in the realm of thoughts and emotions, to realize the amount of effort needed to cultivate discipline, for all this we need to understand the highest aspect of Motivation. If we try to control or tame our mind, try to enforce discipline it does not work in the long term, only by natural spontaneous motivation driven by a higher purpose that itself is evolutionary and makes our awareness expand, only such a motivation can sustain itself and help our practice to become immaculate.

Motivation is a force for all our endeavors; however this force also needs a subtle force to work on it, which is the realization of the purpose. Reiki or Universal Life Force Energy when practiced with right perception and clarity brings this much-needed realization and thus the spark of highest motivation is ignited.

When this motivation is present inside us, it propels us to practice everything that is in accordance with our evolution. It helps us attain a holistic view of life and an awareness of our potential to manifest our fullness of being.

Had it not been for Reiki, I also would not have had the motivation to do the work that I have done. Reiki's presence and influence in my life is the cause for successful journey that I had as a teacher and guide. So, I am sharing here an excerpt from my book 'The Ultimate Reiki Touch' which elucidates the mutual relationship between the practice of Reiki and the force of motivation. Each fosters the other and takes us forward into a fulfilling life.

Motivation is a very important aspect to understand and work on if we are serious about anything in life, because everything in our life is decided by the level and quality of our motivation. A life without motivation is stagnant and sick. So it is important that we learn about this essential element of every practice and what better way than to study it in the context of Reiki practice, as Reiki fosters motivation. I wish that this excerpt completely conveys the significance and true understanding of motivation and its role in any practice, so that the readers may be inspired to cultivate this perspective and make progress on their path.

"The most desirable motivation in life is to be helpful and responsible. It is also the most fitting motivation for Reiki. When we approach Universal Life Force Energy with the intention of helping ourselves and others, this altruistic impulse supports us in remaining open and receptive. When we are open and receptive, we do not tend to narrow the potential of the energy by trying to make it fit our perceptions and short sighted imagined needs, even treating ourselves with such openness is altruistic, because it deflates the selfish control of the mind by exposing it to the vastly beneficial presence of Universal Life Force Energy.

Reiki blossoms and flourishes at its best when we take responsibility for our own well being. In fact, through the practice of Reiki, we express our firm conviction that, as vessels of Universal Life Force Energy, we ourselves are the creator and therefore responsible for our own health, happiness and welfare. Step by step, the more we venture into the healing powers of Reiki, we also cease being the victim of circumstances. Instead, we continue to grow into taking full responsibility, first for our physical health and emotional balance. Later we also learn to take responsibility for our entire life and all the circumstances we attract, never again blaming any outside force for whatever may occur.

This responsibility has nothing to do with an ego-inflated sense of false grandeur. Rather it amounts to a gentle surrender to the greater power that we truly are. It all begins with the simple wish to be helpful and responsible in our everyday lives. Over time, Reiki then naturally, influences us to wish for ourselves and all sentient beings, bliss and the cause of bliss, and to be freed of all suffering. Simultaneously it influences us to efficiently apply ourselves to the manifestation of that same intention.

The Process

Healing Begins at Home

If we are drawn to Reiki or are considering learning and practicing the Usui Method of Natural Healing, by the very power of this wish, we kindle the spark of the supreme motivation in us to heal and be healed. If we act on this intuition, it follows easily that we will then be moved to cultivate the universal human qualities of love, compassion, joy and equanimity. At first, this motivation may seem to last for only a split second, to come and go like a flash of lightning in the darkness. However brief it may appear to be, if we fan this spark, it will not only plant but also strengthen the seed for a desire to liberate both ourselves and others from physical illness, mental stress and emotional conflict and turmoil.

Holistic Wellness in the New Age

To fulfill the purpose of healing, we don't have to be immaculately selfless, either. Selfless motivation does not require that we think only of others. It simply requires that we focus on whatever is wholesome. If we wish for healing, for love, compassion, joy and equanimity for all sentient beings, this wish has to begin at home, with us. In fact, if we truly wish to heal anyone, we first have to heal ourselves.

At the highest order of understanding, healing is not an issue, because from this perspective there was (and never will be) anything wrong or out of order to begin with. However it takes time and skillful observation to fully appreciate the true silence and completeness of all beings, including ourselves before it can be expressed as wholeness and healing in the human body. Only after we have had glimpses of such wholeness in our human body can we inspire similar experience with others. That is why it is so important to experience this ever-present wholeness in us first.

To heal our families and us is part of Reiki tradition. Mrs. Takata was quite adamant about the correct order of things, when she stated something to the effect: First, heal yourself, then heal your family, only after that go out and do healing sessions outside of your immediate circle of family and friends. Of course, we can follow all three approaches simultaneously. We can practice self-treatment, treat members of our family and share additional treatments with others (If we indeed want to be of consistent help to ourselves and to others). It is important, however to take into account our own resources and not spread ourselves too thin. Notwithstanding all of the above, during the initial first twenty-one days of Reiki practice; it is essential to treat as many different people as possible in order to gain confidence in our own ability to convey Reiki.

Liberation from Hypnosis by Beliefs

Although the day-to-day world is not the real world, but a dream or fiction projected by the mind, we still have to take into consideration the effect of this dream's hypnotic power over us. From the fact that everyone is by group consensus hypnotized into believing in this world of restriction, we have to conclude, that for the hypnotized, restriction is very much a reality. Limitation and restriction are therefore the codes we are led to live by, as long as we are subject to the hypnotic influence of the body/mind's acceptance of the collective unconscious so-called reality.

To give an example: As everyone unquestioningly subscribes to the arbitrary and even downright destructive and exploitative rules of today's so called 'economic realities', we cannot empty our bank accounts to give away every last penny to the needy. If we did what the Native Americans sometimes did, by giving away all their material possessions in a ceremony they called the 'great give away', we would very soon be stripped of any means to help either ourselves or others. We would bankrupt ourselves in the process. This is because humans over many centuries have been mass hypnotized into the belief that 'having' is better than 'giving': that lack is more real than abundance.

If we lived in a society that valued a woman or a man for what they gave away rather than for what they kept in excess, we could give much more freely. Energies between humans would be exchanged in a much more natural flow than they are now. Everyone would then not be conditioned to grab as much as they can and hang onto it for as long as conceivably possible – that is until death do us part.

As long as we remain identified with our human body, we inevitably become a part of the mass hypnosis of our particular culture. We are compelled to operate within the beliefs of that same culture, however silly or ridiculous they may be. After all, we can only give what we perceive ourselves to have.

Through the practice of Reiki, over time, more and more limitations fall away. We are then able to give more, for we begin to recognize in truth the vast abundance already available to us. The motivation to fend only for oneself, transforms to encompass the omnipresent 'beingness' that we and all others ARE- and the imagined little 'self' falls away.

Reiki is not an Ego Based Pursuit

The belief in human limitation, lack and loneliness begins to dissolve when through energy medicine we receive the first inkling of potential healing and wholeness inherent in our lives. When, a desire for such healing arises if only for a moment, it reveals the innate yearning of Heart for Heart. It is the supreme motivation for the complete liberation of all beings, which we need to lovingly fuel and expand to the farthest reaches of our existence.

If we do not fuel and expand our motivation, it cannot be sustained. We will forget about it. Seemingly more pressing matters in our everyday lives will interfere, and we will fall back into the belief that we need to struggle in order to survive. There will always be something else that vies for our attention until our desire for healing is completely forgotten and buried under the never-ending routine of our mundane existence.

If we fail to nourish the spark for real truth and freedom, it will certainly die. It will not grow into the all consuming and inner mounting flame of the compassion of a true healer who has experienced and thus acknowledged the ever-present Grace to heal self and others. In this respect, the desire for healing is very much connected to the desire for the freedom of self-realization. At the highest level they are one and the same. Ultimate healing can only happen in ultimate freedom.

If the desire for freedom is continuous, then all the habits and distractions of mind will drop. Think only of freedom and you become freedom because you are what you think.

> *The desire for freedom is the high tide,*
> *which will wipe out the sand castles of doubt. -Papaji*

If we do not nourish, the spontaneous and selfless aspiration to heal, to be free, and complete, more and more obscurations in the form of the ordinary tendencies will sneak back in our mind, until they finally take over and dominate our lives. Whenever the supreme motivation for true healing and freedom is not kept vibrant, the obscurations, like pride, greed, aversion, lust and delusion, will contaminate our aspirations. The desire for self-aggrandizement may replace the wish to heal. Under their sway, our Reiki practice can become very narrow minded and self-serving. It can become an ego game.

We may then have the tendency to style ourselves in the 'big healer', and begin to be very concerned about this new self-image. We may feel urge to pretend to be more than who we are, perceive ourselves as knowing more than we do. We may be tempted to make others believe for example that we have done Reiki for fifteen years, whereas we took our First degree class only a little over four years ago. We may claim to have had experiences that we have only read about in books. Another typical result of ego-based Reiki is that we may be compelled to add accouterments to the basic practice in order to stand out and be special.

Instead of following our deepest aspirations, we may fall prey to the business of marketing our ill begotten specialness.

None of the above is conducive to the purpose of healing. Instead, it only creates confusion in us and others. Inevitably, it stirs up the proliferation of thoughts, concepts and emotions, which actually are the very aspects of our existence, which are at the root of all imbalance and disease. Thoughts and emotions need to be pacified, not stirred up. Therefore, turning Reiki into an ego pursuit is very counterproductive and can only dampen its liberating spirit. Ego centered Reiki is never in alignment with the supreme motivation of ultimate healing.

The Tip

Practice Helps Explore Our Real Motives

How exactly can we nourish and support the motivation for freedom, for healing? First, by strengthening the desire because inevitably we always attract, what we desire most. The challenge is, that most of the time, we are not even aware of the motives of our actions. Very few people are aware of their true motives and so for most they are ill defined.

Quite often the mind subconsciously stays focused on what it resists, and therefore attracts exactly that. For most people, personal motives remain somewhat vague. As a result, they often get exactly what they don't want, or even detest. The reason for all this is lack of focus or awareness of what they really wanted in the first place.

To strengthen the desire for healing, a simple way is to practice the Usui Method of Natural Healing in a consistent manner. It will help us to remain aware of our deepest aspirations and selfless motives. We can acquire a marked sense of accomplishment with the use of Reiki in the same manner that we accomplish ordinary, mundane goals. For example: If we want to become a professional dancer, we have to train to develop both our physical strength and endurance as well as become proficient in the steps and moves. We have to watch a lot of performances in order to imbibe the grace of the experts. If our motivation is to become a pianist, we have to practice the piano and listen to recordings of many great pianists. In fact, if we want to do anything really well, we cannot afford to take it for granted that we already know everything about it or that we have reached the pinnacle of accomplishment. To allow such an attitude, is a sure way to have our motivation wither on the vine. Therefore, in order to become proficient with Reiki, we need to practice a lot of Reiki, and preferably on many different bodies.

All of this is very obvious, but as humans, we often tend to miss the obvious. Our minds are sometimes too clever for our own good, always 'futurizing' and fabricating abstract ideas. We most often don't see the tree because our minds are preoccupied with the concept of 'forest'. We may talk about how great and wonderful Reiki is, but may actually shy away from using the energy in the present moment, because of the possible feelings that might come up. Soon thereafter, if we continually follow the avoidance impulse, we will easily forget about Reiki, and in all likelihood, also forget our motivation for healing, wholeness and freedom, until it pops up as another glimmer of unsustainable hope and short lived enthusiasm at some point in the distant future.

The only chance we will ever have to free ourselves from the pull of this downward spiral into mass un-consciousness is to practice Reiki, provided of course, that Reiki is what we want to do. Once we begin and get into a flow, it becomes effortless. The practice itself and its ensuing benefits become our motivation. Consequently, practice endows us eventually with more and more experience. Experience, in turn, feeds motivation. Motivation then again inspires us to continue practicing, and so forth, creating a sustained upward spiral.

The Heartfelt Desire to Live in the Moment

Selfless motivation is an essential point, because where our motivation directs us, is where our Reiki practice is going to lead us. We want our practice to be expansive, in order for us to grow and become expansive ourselves. However selfless motivation does not infer that we should abandon all self interest for the sake of an abstract and unlivable ideal of altruistic purity. This would be as nonsensical as total selfishness, because such false construed altruistic purity amounts to just another form of denial.

Selfless motivation simply means that it is our heartfelt desire to continuously notice in every moment now, the original, all encompassing goodness, always present in us and in others from beginningless time; noticing goodness for our own sake and for the sake of all sentient beings, wherever they are in this vastly immense universe.

Selfless motivation helps our practice to become all-inclusive and more expansive. It counteracts any tendency toward narrow mindedness. If our sole motivation, for example is self-aggrandizement, only to become rich and famous through Reiki, this idea will seriously restrict the possibilities and impact our practice can have. We would then only do things designed to advance our own agenda. Everything that doesn't would be pushed aside. We need to ask ourselves: Is this worthy conduct for someone who calls him or herself a 'healer'?

And what would the repercussions be of such behavior on our entire outlook on life and the way we practice Reiki? How would it compromise our awareness of the continuous availability of Universal Life Force Energy? These are some of the issues which are important to notice and feel, for they are sure traps which lead one backward into a more solidified identification with ego or a separate sense of 'self', which is the root cause of all suffering.

Since Reiki is in itself limitless, the scope of our motivation needs to match the very limitedness of Universal Life Force Energy. When we want to use Reiki in a meaningful way, the only choice we have, is to do it for the highest good of all concerned. Regular Reiki practice will strongly support such an open attitude, provided we allow ourselves to directly feel and experience the energy, instead of imprisoning it in concepts. If we allow ourselves to feel and savor the energy, we will also automatically feel and express the four immeasurable qualities of love, compassion, joy and equanimity as natural expressions of Reiki for highest good of all concerned.

Dr. Paula Horan has a rich lineage of Reiki Masters traced right back to Dr. Usui, who placed a great importance not only on regular Reiki Practice but also on the importance of the Reiki Attitude. She has been a Traditional Reiki Master for the past 20 years teaching in America, Europe and Asia. Paula introduced Reiki to India in 1989. She is an author of numerous books on alternative healing & non-dual awareness. A long time disciple of Papaji, and for years, a Vajrayana Practitioner, she leads periodic seminars and Jnana Yoga Retreats.

www.paulahoran.com

CHAPTER 17

ThetaHealing®

Shalin Khurana

*"Imagination is everything.
It is the preview of life's coming attractions."- Albert Einstein*

The Essence

Thoughts create everything. Most people spend their time thinking about all the things they *do not* want, and then wonder why the same thing shows up repeatedly in their life. When we give attention to something, the energy flows through us and expands and charges the object of our attention. Focusing on what we do want, rather than what we do not want in our life, is the key to attracting all the best things into one's own life. Our thoughts not only matter, they create matter. Thought is where everything comes from. The universe is made of consciousness - and matter and energy are just two of the forms that consciousness takes. Therefore, in all effect, thoughts create the physical world. And once we comprehend that everything is energy then there is no distinction between matter and energy – and the boundaries of the physical world and the world of our thoughts start to fade away as well.

Beliefs are only thoughts….

Our beliefs are only thoughts. So although wellbeing is abundantly available to us, our mind role playing as the gatekeeper, determines how much of it we experience. Our thoughts and beliefs are the deciding factors to how much we open the gates of abundance. The more positive our beliefs, the gates open wider!

Although negative thoughts seemingly have a lot of power, they are really just thoughts that have been thought about, repeatedly. This then proceeds and takes on the form of reality. Their power is attributed only to the energy we choose to give them. And with *The Law of Attraction* set in motion, these then only contribute to a snowballing effect – of transforming from a purely energy realm into the physical realm. When we repeatedly think certain thoughts, they take the form of beliefs. The Universe then is left with no choice but to deliver to us, what we choose to believe!

However, in the end, beliefs are just thoughts. With some effort we can change them and our lives!

In the wide spectrum of alternate healing modalities, available today, ThetaHealing® stands out as an extremely powerful yet gentle form of "energy" healing. It has the potential to resolve an enormous range of physical, emotional, financial and spiritual issues. Post Theta sessions, one tends to experience enhanced wellbeing, abundance and joy.

The Process

How ThetaHealing® works:

The theta brain wave state has been scientifically verified and measured by electroencephalography (EEG) lab tests. We are in a theta brain state every day; at the moment when we first wake up and just before we fall asleep. It is an extremely powerful brain wave to use for healing and manifesting. Other types of brain wave states are beta (when you are studying or in conversation), alpha (light meditation or taking a bath), and delta (deep sleep).

What makes ThetaHealing® a unique and powerful form of healing is the ability of the practitioner to get into a theta brain wave state (deep meditation), and facilitate a healing from God (Source/Creator) for the recipient. The healer then witnesses the healing. The healer's role is to be a clear channel for the healing from Source. We are all interconnected in a web of consciousness that holds infinite possibilities. ThetaHealing® simply taps into that web for positive transformation and healing for the highest and best.

ThetaHealing® realigns and re-balances your energy field, while also removing energy blocks from traumas, diseases and accidents. These energy blocks can cause physical (including genetic), financial, emotional, mental and/or spiritual issues and challenges. As a result of the ThetaHealing® sessions, harmony and balance is restored, resulting in wellbeing.

Healing occurs on four levels –

- Core: conscious and subconscious
- Genetic: ancestral; DNA
- History: including past life
- Soul

ThetaHealing® is essentially a two-step process –

- Identify the key beliefs, feelings and traumas that are at the root of the problems and issues. These may be experiences from this lifetime, including childhood, genetic history or previous past lives. All of these have created subconscious belief systems and feelings that can still affect the present. ThetaHealing® practitioners are able to identify the subconscious belief systems and feelings causing the problem by using special techniques; asking questions and using intuition.

- Remove or resolve the belief systems and feelings that are the root cause of the issue or problem and replace them with empowering and positive beliefs. By entering a Theta state, practitioners are able to connect to the energy of the Creator of All That Is and request that deeply held subconscious beliefs, feelings, emotions and trauma are instantly removed and resolved. The unconditional love of the Source / Creator has the power to heal any illness and to resolve any situation.

When we receive a ThetaHealing®, we are also helping those around us and the universe, since we are all interconnected at some level. When we heal at a genetic level, we are also healing our ancestors, our relatives, and future generations of our family. Remember, scientists have learned that in quantum physics, the distinction between the past, present and future does not exist as we perceive.

ThetaHealing® is -

- A way to change beliefs that impact the reality we experience.

- A way to heal the energy rifts and blockages that occur due to our thoughts and beliefs.
- Transformation that creates physical, psychological/emotional and spiritual healing.
- Aligned with current understanding of quantum physics and quantum mechanics relating to how and why thought influences matter.

ThetaHealing® facilitates balance and harmony between the conscious and subconscious minds, while infusing a sense of security and wellbeing.

Through the processes of – feeling and belief work – our reality can change and healing can occur in an instant. It can be permanent and lasting. The USP of ThetaHealing® is that we can identify the belief that is causing the issue, pull it, insert a new one that better serves us and we're done! As simple as that!

What it resolves:

ThetaHealing® effectively removes, resolves and clears emotional and physical issues that hold us back in the journey of life. The subconscious holds secrets, past issues, memories that may be invisible to the conscious mind. One can, with fabulous results, cancel, replace or resolve past or current issues and memories and initiate the healing process with ThetaHealing®.

Resolve issues -

- Deep emotional issues, including trauma from abuse
- Physical pain, problems and illnesses
- Fears and phobias
- Subconscious blocks and obstacles
- Bad habits
- Negative feelings
- Anger management
- Grief and bereavement
- Stress, anxiety and depression

- Past life karma
- Soul contracts and agreements
- Releasing energetic cords that no longer serve you

Improve lifestyle -

- Lose weight
- Build confidence and self-esteem
- Attract a compatible, loving soul-mate
- Create wealth and abundance
- Overall health and well being
- Relationships
- Energise and balance Chakras

There are also some other interesting elements that are a part of this modality, which encompass interesting and meaningful exercises, that deal with –

- Manifesting what one truly desires in life, including financial aspects as well as soul mate or twin flame.
- Getting rid of parasites, viruses and bacteria that do not serve any purpose.
- Instilling positive feelings that one may never have fully experienced before.
- This includes feelings of joy, abundance, respect and honour.
- DNA that holds unfavourable cellular memories; scientists used to think of this DNA as junk! Changing DNA is part of what enables one to reach one's full potential.
- Repairing chromosomes that have been damaged by aging. The telomeres (caps) of DNA strands fray from aging and can be energetically repaired.
- Making the transition for those passing (or who have passed on) from this plane to another easier.
- Traumatic foetal memory.

- Broken soul, which for example may happen from chronic and/or severe abuse.
- Ending vows and oaths that no longer serve us.
- Dark night of the soul
- Ending curses and psychic hooks or attacks.
- Releasing etheric cords of attachment that no longer serve a person; this includes unnecessary ones we have as well as ones others have with us.
- Radiation detox
- Releasing traumatic free floating memories resulting from an accident or illness (including during anaesthesia), abuse or drunkenness.
- Gene replacement or repair of defective genes, including ones involved in addictions
- Soul fragments; retrieving pieces of one's own as well as returning ones that we hold, that belong to another person. Our soul fragments (which are part of our essence) also hold our power (or that of others if we have soul fragments of others stuck in our energy field). One way for these fragments to be transferred is during intense verbal or physical exchanges with another person or group.
- Replacing our spirit guides if sometimes we outgrow one of them!
- Connecting with our ancestors' spirits, angels and guardian angels.

The Tip:

As Dr. Michelle L. Casto sums it up beautifully, "The time is now for transformation. It is a new era and we are poised with the opportunity to bring in a new consciousness and co-create a new reality. Why? Because the light within each of us has been turned on, and it's our job to turn that light on brighter and brighter until all false thought forms dissolve in the light of our Truth."

"The message that underlies Healing is simple yet radical: we are already whole….. Underneath our fear and worries, there lies a peaceful core which is unaffected by the many layers of our conditioning. The work of healing is, peeling away the barriers of fear that keep us unaware of our true nature of love, peace and rich interconnection with the web of life. Healing is the re-discovery of who we are and who we always have been. Alternative healing does not always offer a quick fix of a symptom, but it does offer a permanent healing that resonates beyond physical well-being. It creates a total uplift in attitude, enhanced spiritual awareness, and so much more that will change the way you appreciate life every day. Embracing alternative healing by focusing on the cause and trusting the process as it unfolds will be a journey that can be trying or difficult at times, but it will always be extremely rewarding."

You are a powerful, unlimited and eternal soul who is here to enjoy the experience of creativity and contribute to humanity's evolution, by the process of conscious and purposeful co-creation of one's own life and destiny. And ThetaHealing®, having carved out a niche of its own, and by virtue of its purity is equipped with the appropriate set of tools to help you through the process of co-creation.

What is important is that are you willing to step out of your comfort zone, to reach out and embrace the very thing that will empower you?

Shalin Khurana is a spiritual guide, clairvoyant, psychic and an intuitive healing practitioner with an extensive experience in a wide range of healing modalities. She is in an expert in ThetaHealing®, Pranic Healing, Space Healing, Distance healing and is a gifted intuitive – she does aura reading, water reading and land scanning amongst other things. She has been practicing ThetaHealing® since 2004, and is the most sought out practitioner in Delhi with a loyal following of clients among other people. Her sister introduced her to ThetaHealing® and Shalin hasn't looked back ever since, she learned personally from Vianna Stibal – the founder of this healing technique, and is one of the top few practitioners in the world today, and the senior most teacher-practitioner in Delhi.

www.shalinkhurana.wordpress.com

Chapter 18

Aura Healing- The Basis of all Energy Healing

Nishant

The Essence

Scenario 1: Well I met this person the other day and shucks his vibes were so negative. I wanted to run away from him.

Scenario 2: Do you remember that teacher who conducted the meditation the other day. His presence was so peaceful and overwhelming that I almost wanted to cry.

Scenario 3: I visited this resort in the hills of Uttrakhand; it was so peaceful and serene. The moment I entered the place, it was some kind of positive vibes that took over me. It was a warm feeling as if I have come back home. I felt so good and healed.

Well, I am pretty sure that at some moment in our lives we all have been in the above 3 similar scenarios. We might have met a person for the first time and instantly clicked or we might have wanted to run away from that individual and never want to see him again, some places we visit seems to be inviting and have a warm feeling of belongingness whereas some feel cold and uninviting. Every time something like this happens, we are actually unconsciously reacting to some kind of invisible energy which we feel and call it casually as the 'Vibes' of a person or a place. We do not know what is it but we know and feel it as a part of our gut feeling.

But have you ever wondered what exactly are these 'VIBES' that, we casually refer to in our daily conversation?

Some might know about it whereas majority of people do not care. But here's an interesting fact about them:

Holistic Wellness in the New Age 147

These invisible vibes are actually energy emanating from everything in this universe, whether visible or invisible. Spiritual people & Healers know this form of energy as the 'Aura'. Scientist call the same energy as the 'Bio field or the Electromagnetic field'.

It is a measurable field of energy, which not only controls your physical health but also plays a major role in your emotional, mental & spiritual well being. It is now a scientific system of study & research in some of the major institutions worldwide.

Over centuries it has been an intriguing subject of scientific research and spiritual studies. No matter which painting or art form you look at across any tradition around the world, almost every spiritual master or religious deity has been depicted by a halo of light surrounding the head. This was the starting point of research for the people who wanted to know and understand what is the basis of this Halo? Is this something divine & mystical that only a few people possess or something common that is available to everyone?

So with this question in mind, scientists started to research and came up with this interesting fact, which makes absolute sense. As per the theory of Quantum physics: The whole universe (visible & invisible), is made up of virtually the same particles of energy. All Energy vibrates; some at a faster rate while some at a slower rate; this rate is called the frequency. Now scientifically, frequency is the number of vibrations of a particle per second. The unit of measurement of frequency is Hz (Hertz).

So, when we say that the frequency of this object is 10 Hz, it means that the particular object is vibrating at a speed of 10 vibrations per second. That means literally everything that you can see or cannot see is energy and is vibrating at various frequencies. You are energy and so I am, even this book that you are reading or the so-called 'empty space' around you is also energy, which you can't see but you can surely feel it.

Now going back a little to the elementary science we studied in our school time, we know the basic laws of energy like:

> *"Energy can neither be created nor be destroyed*
> *but can only be transformed from one form to another"*

And the famous equation postulated by Einstein i.e., $E=mc^2$ (Where E is Energy which is equal to M = Mass multiplied by C = speed of light in vacuum), which means that Matter and Energy are inter-convertible. Now the famous scientist of the last century also said the same thing as the current findings say, that matter is just condensed form of energy and what is not visible is simply energy flowing freely all around us.

Some of you might be wondering that Why am I telling you all this? What is the use of this piece of information? Hang on with me and you will know why I want you to educate yourself about 'Aura'.

The Process

Our body is made up of atoms and molecules. In each atom we have charged particles called electrons, protons and neutrons which when further expanded are made up of quarks (particles of light) which again on further expansion are made up of strings and super strings and on further expansion its empty space. Yes nothing else but empty space, so in a way all the matter is originating from this empty space of energy, this is called the Nothingness or the zero point energy. Now this theory coincides with the spiritual theory that 'The universe came from nothing and will go back into nothing'. Coincidence, I bet not as it is the real science.

The Aura is actually the result of the electrical impulses generated by the movement of electrons and protons around the nucleus in our cells. According to the famous law of Electromagnetic Induction wherever there is an electric field, an equivalent magnetic field would be induced around that electrical field. For example: You use a particular screwdriver to open and close electrical circuits, over a period of time it gets magnetized and now has the ability to attract small iron fillings. So no wonder, Aura is literally the Electromagnetic field.

We all know how Doctors use ECG (For measuring Cardiac rhythms) and EEG (For measuring Brain signals), uses Electrical signals as an input to test the health level of the human heart & brain respectively. Then how can we not believe in the Electro-magnetic field generated by all other organs in the body?

Till the time your body is ALIVE & PULSATING, it's generating a "MEASURABLE BIOFIELD CALLED THE AURA"

Holistic Wellness in the New Age

But here's the twist now, the Aura is not just limited to your Physical body. It is much more beyond that and encompasses your mental, emotional, spiritual and astral bodies too. These 4 bodies are called the subtle energetic bodies which can be seen only if you train yourself well to operate at a level of energy which is in sync to their own frequency or perhaps use gadgets like RFI Aura Imaging systems or PIP (Poly interference photography).

You can imagine our different bodies by taking the example of an onion. On the outside it looks as one whole but if you remove the covering, you see various layers overlapping onto each other and having a common core. Now take this example to understand the human energetic system. The inner core here will be the soul, the various layers will be the different bodies and the outermost covering will be the aura.

So technically Aura is just a medium to hold everything together as one system! The nature of Aura is to reflect what is happening inside the various energetic layers. So if you are having depressive or negative thoughts about something or you are having some physical health issue, it will all be reflected as an energetic imbalance in your aura.

The Tip

Reading Aura gives you an edge to know what is really happening at the invisible levels of your energetic anatomy. I have experienced it myself in numerous cases that I was able to predict and map out the imbalances up to 3-6 months in advance before they actually came into the physical body as DIS-EASES. Being a clairvoyant gives me an edge to see the aura energies and having an engineering background coupled with my extensive research in the field of energy medicine and aura imaging allows me to validate my knowledge with the use of aura imaging systems. My personal favorite is RFI ™ as it gives you a comprehensive report on what is happening at the various levels of your body, mind and chakras. You can use any or all of the below mentioned methods to check for aura imbalances and then correct them.

- Intuitively through your third eye or sixth sense. (I highly recommend because it is powerful & accurate. Combining my research work & experience I have put together a whole new step-by-step method of activation of third eye and using it to scan & detect energetic imbalances in the aura & chakras)

- Using tools as Dowsing, Lecher Antenna, Universal Scanner, Pendulums etc.
- Energetic Scanning via hands as taught in various modalities
- Using Aura Imaging systems like Kirlian aura imaging system, Poly Interference Photography, Energy Field Imaging or using the most updated and reliable system like RFI™ (Resonant Field Imaging)

Our Energetic body is the Key to Wellness and is the Core from which the physical body derives energy. So to maintain the physical health, we must maintain a strong and vibrant aura. Once you are able to detect the imbalances it's absolutely necessary that you do something to heal it. As the science of aura says, energetic imbalances in the layers beyond the physical body are much easier to heal than the imbalances in the physical body because matter is also energy but at a denser rate of vibration which requires a lot of effort to shift and heal.

Nishant is an IT Engineer by qualification but an Energy Medicine enthusiast by choice. He is passionate about "Integrating Science & Spirituality" and has over 10 years of rich experience in Human Energy Field (Aura) & Spiritual Mediumship. Blessed with unique gifts like Channeling & Mediumship, he has the ability to connect with beings in the higher dimensions and the spirit world for guidance & healing. He has also channeled several books on Shamballa as guided by the Saptarishis. With this Intuitive gift he can also SEE the Invisible energy that surrounds us. He works with the most prominent doctors and scientists around the globe as an expert in the field of Aura, ESP, Psychic & Paranormal phenomenon, Radionics, Consciousness and Energy medicine. As a result of his channeled knowledge, experience & scientific research studies he has developed a method for "Aura Awakening" which empowers people to understand the Human energy system and a step-by-step method to harness our Energy system for Improving & Balancing every aspect of our lives. After all, all energy healing starts with Energy body so it is very crucial to understand the nature of our energy body and its energy system clearly.

www.biofieldglobal.org

CHAPTER 19

Emotional Freedom Technique

Dr. Rangana Rupavi Choudhuri

"I suggest that the body and soul react to each other in sympathy. A change in the state of the soul would necessarily have an effect on the body and vice versa." Aristotle, 400 BC

The Essence

While living in Florida and working for a medical company I was undergoing tremendous stress. Mostly self-inflicted stress, as I had a pattern of wanting to do a good job. This stress resulted in chronic daily migraines, nausea and debilitating pain in my shoulders and back. I was on shock therapy, physiotherapy and a cocktail of medications to narcotize the pain. I came back to the UK and got used to taking the pain medication, until one day I was at my sisters' house and she was running her first seminar on EFT (Emotional Freedom Technique). At the same time I also had an intensely painful migraine and my mother persuaded me to try out EFT or "Tapping" to help with the pain. I was naturally resistant and reluctant to try anything new, particularly a method of alternate therapy I knew nothing about. Being a scientist with a PhD from Oxford University, I was a bit skeptical and quite frankly, I thought the technique was a bit strange. To my surprise, after just 5 minutes of EFT with my mother, my headache completely vanished. However, my pride got in the way and I told my mother that there was still a mild pain remaining. On the inside, I knew that something had shifted that day and I embarked on my own secret exploration of EFT studying with 20 of the 26 EFT masters around the world. Using EFT, my migraines and pain have completely cleared. More importantly, I feel grateful and have deep reverence for my mother and what she taught me on that day in my sister's house.

"EFT is easy, effective, and produces amazing results. I think it should be taught in elementary school." Donna Eden, Author, Energy Medicine expert

Poor health is related to emotional stress and trauma

"Pro-actively clearing daily stresses and past emotional upsets and traumas is the best health insurance. Once we have health we have everything."

Did you know that 85% of illness is stress induced? Chronic as well as unconscious stress upsets the natural balance of the nervous system, disturbing the body's natural ability to maintain and repair itself, making the body vulnerable to the effects of poor diet, environmental toxins and microbes. This breakdown of the body's natural ability may result in disease and illness.

A study by Kaiser Permanente involving over 70,000 individuals showed that childhood emotional trauma was a significant factor in the development of chronic disease later in life, specifically:

- Alcoholism and alcohol abuse
- Depression
- Illicit drug use
- Risk for intimate partner violence
- Smoking
- Suicide attempts
- Multiple sexual partners
- Health-related quality of life issues
    - Liver disease
    - Chronic obstructive pulmonary disease
    - Ischemic heart disease
    - Sexually transmitted diseases

In addition, 70 published studies from the community on nearly 70,000 trauma survivors showed a tenfold increase in depression as well as two studies following 11,000 people for up to 20 years, revealed an increase in depression of up to tenfold. Childhood maltreatment has been shown to result in increased cardiovascular disease in women and depression in both men and women.

Emotional hurts and trauma can vary from person to person. For someone, it may be a parent or teacher saying 'shut up' and for others, it could be verbal or even physical abuse. Trauma is upsetting no matter what the severity.

Negative upsets can be experienced at school, home and workplace in the form of bullying, shouting, angry outbursts, overwhelm and a feeling of being controlled by others. I wonder what hurts you are holding on to? What events have occurred that have caused you emotional pain? What is it that you get stressed about? Clearing past emotional upsets, hurts and traumas and stress using clinically proven techniques like EFT can help.

Emotional stress and upsets can be cleared

Emotional Freedom Techniques, EFT, is now used worldwide by millions and clears emotional stress and upsets.

EFT combines tapping on acupressure points while saying statements out loud. It is clinically proven to lower stress, tension, depression, phobias, fears, past trauma to create health and wellness. The technique is used by Celebrities for overcoming performance anxiety, being able to speak confidently in public and sports performance.

"After 6 sessions of EFT 90% of study participants were free from symptoms of post-traumatic stress disorder." PTSD Study, Dawson Church, 20104

The technique can eliminate the negative charge from past memories and shift limiting thoughts to empowering beliefs, which can create a space for manifesting abundance. Once negativity is cleared, it creates a feeling of wellbeing and calm.

The action of tapping on acupressure points while repeating specific phrases out loud releases stress and emotional traumas. The technique integrates ancient wisdom and the science of acupuncture with modern day psychology without the need for needles. It is one of the few therapies in the world that combines talk and touch.

Negative emotions cause a disruption of the body's energy system. The EFT tapping process re-wires the energy system creating a feeling of peace, calm and letting go. In many cases, after EFT, people experience a shift in thinking that is more empowering.

The Process

"EFT is a simple, powerful process that can profoundly influence gene activity, health and behaviour." Bruce Lipton, Author of The Biology of Belief

EFT is a popular alternative therapy modality that combines tapping on acupressure points on the body with saying specific statements out loud. It combines ancient eastern medicine with modern psychology and has been clinically proven to relieve stress, anxiety, tension, pain, fears, trauma, depression and past negativity.

Emotional Freedom Techniques, EFT, is now used worldwide by millions and clears emotional stress and upsets. It is easy to learn and create stress relief in seconds. You can learn EFT "Tapping" as part of a self-help personal development program or to get professionally qualified.

EFT for a range of challenges

Extensive application of Energy Psychology treatments like Emotional Freedom Techniques has shown impressive improvements in a wide variety of issues, including those listed below.

Personal performance

- Abundance
- Weight loss
- Business and career goals
- Self realisation/spiritual growth

Emotional challenges

- Children's behaviour
- Relationship issues

- Anger management
- Depression
- Insomnia
- Severe trauma (PTSD)
- Addictions
- Sexual abuse
- Phobias

Physical diseases

- Allergies
- Migraines
- Pain management
- Chronic fatigue syndrome
- Multiple chemical sensitivities
- Hypertension
- Fibromyalgia
- Cancerous cells
- Muscular dystrophy
- Parkinson's disease
- Cystic fibrosis

Other

- Animal healing
- Surrogate applications

EFT for stress relief

Stress, particularly emotionally related stress, is considered to be the silent killer in the western world and fast spreading to the east. A recent report indicated that those suffering from emotional stress had a much higher chance of cardiac challenges. The Medical Journal JAMA reports:

"Stress can cause a heart attack, sudden cardiac death, heart failure, or arrhythmias (abnormal heart rhythms) in persons who may not even know they have heart disease. Individuals with congestive heart failure, coronary heart disease, known arrhythmias, or other heart or blood vessel diseases should avoid emotional stress whenever possible and learn to manage the effects of stress."

Stress can cause an increase in the stress hormone 'cortisol' which can cause havoc with the body's circulatory, hormonal, immune and digestive systems. For example, Irritable Bowel Syndrome (IBS), a disorder of the digestive system, is now known to be caused due to stress.

The good news is that studies have shown, a regular practice of exercises: breathing, physical exercise, meditations and emotional release can reduce cortisol and stress levels resulting in a feeling of calm and well-being. In particular, EFT has been clinically shown to reduce stress as well as stress hormones like cortisol. A recent clinical study in War Veterans has shown EFT to be effective in reducing extreme stress know as Post Traumatic Stress Disorder (PTSD).

EFT points for stress relief

In the event you suddenly get stressed or overwhelmed with emotions just tap under the eye, collarbone and under the arm. This is known as the Triple point calmer or Anxiety stopper.

Next steps

1. Use the EFT sequence in this chapter as part of a daily routine to lower stress.
2. Attend EFT Training to learn the technique to clear past emotional hurts, cravings, physical tension, negativity, limiting thoughts and disempowering mental patterns as part of a personal development program.
3. Consider learning the technique to become a practitioner to work with others as a profession. Helping others is a rewarding profession and contributes to increasing health, happiness and confidence. Our EFT programs can be found on http://vitalitylivingcollege.info/bookme/

4. Book a customised session with a certified EFT practitioner by e-mailing india@vitalitylivingcollege.info

The Technique

Clear stress and upsets with EFT

"EFT produces great healing benefit." Deepak Chopra MD, Author, and, Mind, Body and Spirit Expert

The pace of life is becoming increasingly hectic, and with demands made on us from numerous places, it can be difficult to allow yourself the time to focus on yourself and your wellbeing.

This can lead to a life that is unhappy and stressful with very little excitement or sense of self worth.

Given the choice, most people would live a life that has reduced stress, increased self-belief, free from past upsets and with a positive outlook.

So I am including the step-by-step instructions below on how to use EFT as part of a daily stress-bust and healthy wellness routine:

1. **Identify the problem by asking yourself**
   - What am I stressed about? What is upsetting me? Who is upsetting me?
   - How does that make me feel? How does that really make me feel?
   - Where in the body do I feel this stress or upset? What kind of a sensation is it? How does that make me feel?

2. **Measure the problem from 1 to 10 by asking**
   - On a scale of 1 to 10, how high is this stress where 10 is a very high stress and 1 is no stress at all?
   - On a scale of 1 to 10, how high is this emotional upset where 10 is really upset and 1 is not upset at all?
   - On a scale of 1 to 10, how high is this negative feeling where 10 is really high and 1 is not high at all?

3. **Start with tapping on the side of the hand**

    - Tap with the fingers of one hand on the karate chop of the other hand (side of the hand below the little finger) and say the following three times with feeling:

    - "Even though I… (Name problem with specific information of what happened, who did what as well as the negative feeling and number), I deeply and completely accept myself."

    - For example: "Even though I am really stressed because I have too much work and it makes me feel anxious and it's a 10/10, I deeply and completely accept myself."

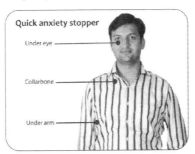

4. **Tap each point 7 times as you say a phrase from the problem**

    Repeat key phrases out loud from the problem, for example the emotion of specifics about the problem, while tapping on the points shown below.

    - Eyebrow – at the beginning of the eyebrow just above the nose

    - Side of eye – on the bone bordering the outside corner of the eye

    - Under eye – on the bone just under the eye

    - Under nose – between the bottom of the nose and the upper lip

    - Chin – midway between the point of the chin and the middle of the lower lip

    - Collarbone – at the junction where the breastbone, collarbone and first rib meet

    - Under arm – under the arm about 10cm from the armpit

- Thumb – on the outside of the thumb, level with the base of the nail
- Index finger – on the side of the index finger closest to the thumb, level with the base of the nail (miss this point out if pregnant)
- Middle finger – in the same place on the middle finger
- Little finger – in the same place on the little or baby finger
- Karate chop (side of the hand) – on the edge of the hand

5. **Final clearing. On the Karate Chop say the starting set-up phrase again (name the original problem again).**

   "Even though I… (Name problem), I deeply and completely accept myself."

6. Relax. Take a gentle breath in and out and take a sip of water. It is very important to drink water to flush out any toxins that get released. 70% of our bodies are composed of water – drinking water is vital to our health and vitality.

7. Testing the results. Measure the problem again from 1 to 10. Notice how the problem and original emotion feels different. If there is an emotional charge left, repeat the tapping process again till you feel better.

For more information you can download a free booklet - http://vitalitylivingcollege.info/free-resources/

Matrix Reimprinting – the latest advancement of EFT

Although EFT is widely available with thousands of testimonials and accolades, most people are not aware of the more advanced forms of EFT, which can allow for instantaneous healing. Matrix Reimprinting with EFT is an example of a powerful advancement of EFT.

Matrix Reimprinting combines inner child healing with EFT and quantum physics to re-program the body and mind in conjunction with the spirit. The process culminates in a deep healing heart meditation while simultaneously programming the neurological system for health and abundance.

The technique literally re-imprints our limiting experiences creating harmony, balance and empowerment. This process is excellent for being at peace with any kind of trauma, powerlessness or helplessness.

For example:

- Job loss or being put down at work
- Relationship break-up or divorce
- Accident like fractures, car accidents, injuries
- Bullying, made to feel small or weak
- Over-worked mom or employee
- Coping with loss, grief or sadness
- Fighting in the home or at work
- Financial worry
- Illness, health issue
- Physical pain or tension
- Verbal, physical or sexual abuse

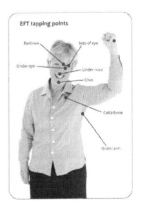

The beauty of Matrix work is that it makes a connection with the inner child who felt powerless and helpless and that can also get frozen in time. This inner child is known as the ECHO in Matrix Re-imprinting. The ECHO becomes the client, enabling the child to claim their power back. It is a very gentle, powerful and potent technique.

Case studies with EFT

Dr Rajesh CM heals his back pain completely after attending EFT Training and now routinely helps his patients heal from body pain with results in only a single sitting.

"After attending EFT Training with Vitality Living College I became even more powerful and effective in my private practice. I now have 5 – 6 patients daily and every patient is satisfied through EFT. For any kind of pain, for example in the knee, back or head I am getting good results. The best part is, in a single sitting my patients get more than 70% and sometimes 100% relief. In my own case before attending EFT Training I used to have severe back pain and through attending the EFT Training session it has gone completely." Dr Rajesh CM, Navi Mumbai, India

Sejal Mehta, a very accomplished trainer and therapist, resolved her ongoing Edema and Fibromyalgia, after only 2 days of EFT Training.

This is what she had to say "… the last 2 days of attending EFT has brought huge physiological, temperamental and attitudinal changes in my life. I have become not only sympathetic but also more empathetic. My edema and fibromyalgia (debilitating pain that can takes years to treat) of 7-8 months has disappeared miraculously and after months I have slept so peacefully" Sejal Mehta, Mumbai, India

After EFT Training Daisy helps her son overcome his learning difficulties and it has brought them closer together

Working mom Daisy Anand learnt EFT to become professionally qualified and one day she noticed her son's grades had dropped and the teacher called her in and explained to her, that her son's behavior had become aggressive and was experiencing learning difficulties. Instead of pushing EFT onto her son she started to use it in front of him on herself and explained to her son, it was helping her to feel calm and relaxed. Her son became curious and allowed his mom to use EFT with him. Through EFT they uncovered an incident where the teacher inappropriately insulted her son and they used EFT to vent out all the pent up anger and frustration. Daisy shares "After EFT he was better able to concentrate and we no longer even remember that teacher. I even saw him use EFT on his own before a cricket match! Using EFT has brought us closer together and be ourselves with each other." Davinder (Daisy) Kaur Anand, Mumbai, India

Business owner and working mum Emma Voss gives up her Chocolate cravings after Day 1 of EFT Training.

"Just a quick email to thank you for a fantastic day. I learnt so much and feel very positive. Still no galaxy (a Chocolate bar) and I feel in CONTROL of that. I don't even want a hot chocolate, which is what I normally go for if I'm trying to not to have a bar of chocolate. I have come home and done all the work I have been putting off, with regards my website and I did not even think about it. I am so happy that after just 1 day of EFT training I feel so good. I feel in control and feel better!!"

Emma from the UK returned for EFT Training in 2012 and gave up her biscuits cravings. She came back on Training in 2013 when she shared that she was slimmer and could fit into the little black dress, she always wanted to

University Counsellor Mallika overcomes all her food allergies during Matrix Reimprinting

During the Matrix Reimprinting training in Delhi, University Counsellor, Mallika Ramachandran, had a long list of food allergies and she wanted to clear these during the training sessions. She had a range of different food allergies and was asked to pick only one allergy to work with. 'I chose to work with my mushroom allergy and used the process taught during the seminar in the practice session. After the session, I went home and insisted that my husband take me out to dinner and that too, only to one particular restaurant. I chose the Taj Palace, mainly because I'd often seen my husband order the mushroom cappuccino there. And I had always noticed the look on his face as he told me how Yummy it was! So, having just gotten rid of my allergy, I now wanted to try it. As we sat down, I told him that I wanted the mushroom cappuccino. My husband did not think that I should try this, especially at night, and attempted to talk me out of it. I disagreed and told him that was what I wanted. Soon, the waiter stepped in and told us that it was on the house so we should go ahead and try it. We asked him to get one but he added that we could each have one. Yet, my husband, assuming that I couldn't have it, told him that one was enough. The soup finally came and it was placed in front of me. The waiter and my husband watched me as I smelt it.... felt okay.... then took a small sip...

and still felt okay… then took a deep breath and finally put a spoonful into my mouth! Hhmmmmm…. It was heaven! Now I know what I was missing on while my husband was able to have it all these years… I have now been eating mushroom and fish and all the things I previously had allergies to. Thank you EFT. Thank you Rangana' Mallika Ramachandran, Delhi, India

Apoorvaa Pandit cures her Thyroid after learning EFT & Matrix Reimprinting

Highly skilled Facilitator & Therapist Apoorva Pandit cures her Thyroid after learning EFT, " .. *as suggested by Dr Rangana Rupavi Choudhuri, I started tapping – starting from surface issues, persisting through all what came up. After some weeks, I noticed that the symptoms of Thyroid had come down. A medical examination confirmed that I was free*". Appoorva Pandit Delhi, India

Testimonials

"I feel more confident, I have learnt more and I trust that EFT is something that works." Margaret Bradley, Virtual Assistant

"Confidence to heal myself. I feel full of vitality and love." Kate Rees, Bookkeeper

"That all things are possible. Even my shoulder is feeling better." Stephen Parrott, Instructor

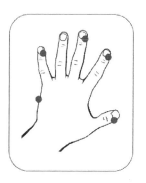

"Although some of the issues raised were very profound, the atmosphere and space felt safe." Linda Munster, Nutritionist

"Cleared all my emotional blockages" Iva West, Utility Warehouse

"A renewed enthusiasm with EFT and renewed confidence in its efficiency." Franki Gifts, Complementary therapist

"I appreciated the time the trainer took to 'help' everyone whilst making a learning experience for everyone else." Dani Diosi, EFT Practitioner & Hypnotherapist for conception, birth and pregnancy

"Now that I have learnt EFT and become a Practitioner with Vitality Living College I am getting more clients and earning a living." Jayant Pawar, Wellness coach

References

1. Psychological Stress and the Human Immune System: A Meta-Analytic Study of 30 Years of Inquiry. Segerstrom Suzanne, Miller Gregory. Psychological Bulletin, Jul 2004.
2. Trauma in the Addiction Family. Claudia Black, Dec 2010. www.addictioninfamily.com.
3. Childhood Maltreatment as a Risk Factor for Adult Cardiovascular Disease and Depression. Batten Sonja, Aslan Mihaela, Maciejewski Paul and Mazure Carolyn, Journal of Clinical Psychiatry, Feb 2004.
4. Molecules of Emotion, Candace Pert PhD (Simon & Schuster 1997; ISBN 0-684-84634-9).:
5. Quantum Healing, Dr Deepak Chopra (Bantam Books 1992; ISBN 90-215-8874-9).
6. The Biology of Belief: Unleashing the Power of Consciousness, Matter and Miracles, Bruce Lipton PhD (Hay House, 2008; ISBN 978-1401923112).
7. Psychological Trauma in Veterans Using EFT: A Randomized Controlled Trial. Dawson Church, Crystal Hawk, Audrey Books, Oliver Toukolehto, MariaWren, Ingrid Dinter, Phyllis Stein. Presented at the Society of Behavioral Medicine, Seattle, Washington, April 7-10, 2010.
8. Heal your emotions to heal your life, Dr Rangana Rupavi Choudhuri, (PhD) Aparajita Publishing, 2010-2015

Rangana Rupavi Choudhuri (PhD) is the Founder & CEO of Vitality Living College® and delivers trainings and seminars around the world. She is an international author, dynamic speaker and heart centered mind-body expert. She is totally passionate about motivating people – about boosting their confidence and helping them to achieve their true potential.

Dr Choudhuri's clear and proven coaching style has encouraged audiences around the world to move out of their comfort zones – inspiring them to meet and exceed their personal and professional goals, over and over again.

For information about our Free Seminars EFT, NLP, Breakthrough Coaching®, Hypnosis, Timeline Technology and Matrix Reimprinting Courses please visit http://vitalitylivingcollege.info/bookme/

Rangana Rupavi Choudhuri (PhD) & Vitality Living College 2010 - 2015

www.vitalitylivingcollege.info

CHAPTER 20

Serenity Surrender (SS)

Minal Arora

Once I was sitting quietly in my patio on a nice windy summer evening when I suddenly had some revelations about some aspects of human life I was introspecting. It was a conversation in my head with the source itself and here it goes!

When did I first decide to come to this planet?

When your eternal soul got entangled in the web of karma, so entangled that it was unable to understand how to resolve itself, it needed a mirror. This is when it was drawn to experience this physical plane.

What's so special about the physical plane?

It is the plane of duality. It gives you mirrors. It shows you what you carry within through your family, your relationships, your life situations and your experience with them. It makes you experience love when you carry love within and blame when you carry blame within. You cannot escape or run away from self for wherever you go, your karma follows!

But beware, it isn't a punishment system, it's a feedback system the voice said.

So what's so special about family?

Family is the set of constant mirrors that one manifests which one must face. They show you different aspects of yourself in so many different ways. Through a spouse comes your relationship of love with yourself, through a child comes your relationship of nurturing yourself, through a parent comes your relationship with accepting your creation and so much more with each of them.

So does that mean I must always stay with my family and each member always?

Well, each relationship in one's life is a mirror to some aspect within. When one's relationship with loving one's self changes, it will also change what is reflected through the mirrors of outside relationships. With every change within, each past / every block / every unresolved memory that one has ever experienced in loving one's self through a friend / family member or through a difficult life situation will be surfaced. The reason isn't to hinder progress but rather to facilitate it through the learning one has already imbibed. It's only when that learning doesn't resonate with one's current awareness or wisdom do they experience conflicts. When conflicts arise, they bring discomfort in the form of pain, hurt, anger, blame and misery. In that moment one either raises his/her wisdom higher by imbibing a new learning or stays with the old pattern and resists the change. Depending on how much resistance is imposed, the intensity of pain or suffering will be experienced.

Have I chosen my family / my work / my life situations?

You have chosen everything my dear, I heard being said. Every situation good or bad, every happiness & misery, every right or wrong, you have chosen everything that you are experiencing. Each choice is made by your soul believing the experience through that choice will give you maximum growth.

There are two parts of you, one that you understand as your mind (conscious mind) and one that you understand as your sub-conscious mind. The understanding of the conscious mind is what is in your awareness, weather good or bad; you believe it's you. For example I am strong, I failed, I am rich, I like mangoes etc. The sub-conscious mind however is a projection of that part of you that either you are unaware of or in non-acceptance of. For example, I feel fear, I think I may not succeed, I don't feel right, I want to become a rich man etc. The sub-conscious carries the soul's perception of self. If it believes "Money gets me love", which comes from a past life where when you loved someone and couldn't marry because you didn't have money, in this lifetime, no matter how much money you have, this belief at a deeper level will keep you in the insecurity of money only to ensure that love is not abandoned or lost. What blood is to the body, love is to the soul.

Have women chosen to be raped? Have people chosen to die of hunger? Did that guy who was reported to be killed yesterday choose to die?

To understand the reasons for why such grave experiences come to soul, you must understand it through an example. Imagine you are a theatre artist and you are chosen for a play. You are ambitious and this seems like an opportunity to prove your skills. You are called backstage and given a choice of 2 different characters in the play. One of them has to keep standing all through the 3 hrs and deliver a lot of dialogues while the other is also the lead role but he has to sit on a chair and not say too much. Which one will you choose?

Maybe the first one, I said in my head almost instantly.

Why? , the voice asked me

Since I am ambitious and I want to grow, it makes more sense to choose the role which gives me maximum exposure & hence opportunity to prove my skills and grow. More learning, more growth I said.

That's it. That's exactly what the soul is doing. Difficult lifetimes offer an opportunity for higher growth. This is what you all believe at a deeper level.

So, is this understanding right? Is struggling with life a good thing?

No, I wouldn't say you were created to struggle. This is your own belief system that has developed through several experiences spread over eternity. You were created to just flow effortlessly. Once things didn't happen as per what you believed was right, you lost trust in the natural flow & started to put effort to have things your way. When you did get things and attributed it to the struggle you did and there began a vicious cycle. Had you just trusted the flow and when things didn't seem right, would have trusted a bigger picture unfolding, life would have been effortless. Struggle is a choice your souls made.

Does that mean we should stop doing any action?

No, effortlessness isn't to be confused with non-action. Action done being a channel of the universe doesn't seem like effort. When your input is required somewhere, the opportunity is presented in the most effortless way and doing the respective action almost happens without you feeling like a doer. Since you didn't plan or intend for the action, there are no expectations from the result and the highest order prevails. This sort of action brings your unconditional input to the universe.

Does that mean if I go out of my way to help someone, it isn't really required?

The way you are a spark of the creator, so is everyone. If someone's journey will need your contribution, it will come your way in a time & place where you will be able to make that contribution in the most effortless way. Everything will fall into place giving you a feeling as if there was a plan. While if you are thinking about someone, worrying over their circumstances or pitying them, then realize that in those moments, you are forgetting that they are sparks of the same creator too. If they need help, they will be able to attract it from the universe. Your concern for them is again mirroring some weakness / insecurity about yourself through them. For example, what if I become like them, what if I lose all my money like them, maybe he is feeling very lonely etc. These are all emotions that bother you or raise your own fears which are why you attracted them in their lives. It's a way to show you how you are not present to negativities within yourself. That is the real reason for their presence in your life.

As long as you are accepting the spark of love that you are, without any effort, you will be able to help so many others in realizing their own inherent power. You will move & inspire them. That is what will bring real growth to this universe.

So what to do when we feel like a victim? When we experience pain and misery?

- Bring awareness to self. The moment we drop any outward action i.e. the blame, the pity, the anger and realize we are attracting it, it initiates the process of that energy dissolving itself.

- Bring complete acceptance of your reality. We usually only accept partial realities, because it's difficult to face our mistakes, our guilt. Non-acceptance of this reality only prolongs the process of resolving the root cause of the misery. Forgive yourself consciously for your contribution or lack of it to the situation and accept everything unreasonably.

- Stop justifying your truth at the cost of others. Stop telling yourself but what happened was really wrong, or what so and so did was wrong, or what so and so happened is why all of it happened. Realize you ATTRACTED all of that you call wrong because at some level you only lack understanding of that aspect which is in conflict. By justifying the existence of this conflict, you will only energize it.

- Empower yourself by knowing you created this pain, this blame, this anger and it has arisen out of a conflict within. If you are its creator, you can destroy it too.

- Create intent to learn the lesson that misery brings through that conflict in the highest and best way.

- Heal the reason for why the conflict exists by taking guidance from the creator. As long as you stay focused inwardly, you can heal it at the deepest level and resolve it forever.

- The healing part of this is done through the beautiful modality of "Serenity Surrender" or SS, which I have talked about later. This sort of healing will do two things. It will resolve that conflict at the soul level forever hence stopping itself to attract it again and it will expand the conscious awareness of your soul so that it does not create further karma based on the conflicted understanding.

Do our relationships last forever?

Yes they do but not necessarily in the way we perceive them. They transform, they evolve as we evolve. If A and B were married 20 years ago, they have served each other as a mirror for that time. When their relationship would have begun, in most cases, they would have started by seeing the love that they carry for themselves through the other and hence experienced love for them. When love is experienced by a soul, it will also surface its lack of understanding of love, the rejection it felt through love, the betrayal it felt through love, the suffering that love brought and the unforgiveness for self above all. All of this will allow the distortions of love to be dissolved and hence a deeper understanding of love shall emerge. All of this comes up not to bother one but to free one's perceptive experience of love from anything that isn't the highest understanding of it. Now if A's soul believes love is betrayal and unforgiveness, it will manifest / attract it through a life situation / relationship / person. It won't be easy to face and accept the betrayal as one's own choice. There will be a need to disown it, to blame, to justify it was never my fault but all of this will never even begin the healing process because one will be defying the basic principal of the 'law of attraction' which works all the time that we are the soul magnets and we attract everything BUT from the sub-conscious level. We may or may not carry, a memory of our deserving of something we detest now and yet, it's there, deep within.

If A is able to stay focused inwardly, he/she will be able to heal his/her relationship with B, because B was only a mirror to what A carried within. BUT, their relationship will also transcend to a new level now. If B is able to make the same journey inwardly and both meet at a point of self-love and compassion, they will stay in compassion and in a mutually agreeable relationship forever. However if A makes it and B doesn't, then A will be facilitated out of the situation and in spite of B's need to hold-on to A, the universe will resolve it for the one who is able to forgive oneself.

It's also possible that B was always there, it is just A who couldn't see it. In which case, they will meet where they will share mutual love & growth.

In either case, the relationship MUST go through a transformation because one learns deeper about loving one's self as we move forward. What A could see through B, 20 yrs. back, was what A could understand about loving self then. In 20 yrs. both have learnt deeper about loving themselves and hence what they see through each other is only a deeper understanding of loving self. If the relationship seems less loving or sour now, it only means at a deeper level, they have not been able to establish a higher understanding of love for self through each other. The deeper you go, the more intense it gets and hence the gravest mistakes / lacks that the souls believe as a part of them will also surface. This only facilitates further depth to self-realization.

The need of A to hold-on to B or B to hold-on to A...the need for A to stick to the relationship 20 yrs. back or B for the same is only non-acceptance of themselves in this present moment. It is bound to give misery.

Love never meant possessing or holding-on. Love only meant allowing self and the other to be. It also means if the one you love has a role to play in your journey and you have in theirs, it will be facilitated lovingly so. If not, realize that you are only limiting your experience of love within. Realize when you are being guided to rise above your fears and find yourself through other means. Love isn't and cannot be forced. If one loves self, they will experience love from everyone around naturally and effortlessly so.

What is fear?

Fear is the need to believe in the presence of an outcome in the future of a situation / relationship or behavior, which will bring misery. Fear itself means that you are energizing that outcome which didn't even exist before the fear arose. It could be coming from some unresolved past in which this situation expected to come in the future did arise and gave misery & hence the belief system from then onwards, believes in the respective outcome & the misery tagged along with it.

From the soul's perspective, the fear arose because it wanted to go. You, instead of realizing that it wants to go, started believing in it. It then gets heavier & more energized and settles down back again. It slowly grows big enough to be mirrored through your physical reality or what you feared will happen. You then justify that you knew it was going to happen and that's why you feared it, but that isn't true. You feared it & chose fear over faith, which is why it became a part of your reality because it was made to believe it's significant enough by none other than yourself.

What do we need to do when we fear?

Stay with faith & heal the fear. Follow the 6 steps I gave you (written above). Do them and then you will be ready to heal that fear. It will dissolve forever. If done pro-actively, on the first sign of the fear, many grave life situations can be avoided. Remember, the soul was never meant to suffer. Suffering is a choice it makes; only when it doesn't believe in its ability to resolve its conflicts otherwise.

Finally...

Finally, if you want the mirror to show you differently, the only way is to change yourself within. Life is about moving forward only and in complete trust that whatever is needed for your growth, will flow to you, effortlessly so. Holding-on to any person / relationship or life situation only brings misery. Letting go in compassion, trust and surrender expands the love we carry within and our experience of love too.

Forgiveness for self and others is the key. Life is an experience. It grows and changes mirrors. Accept change. Accept the flow.

This conversation was elaborate & profound. This was just after I found my connection with the source through "Serenity Surrender" or SS. I didn't even know my potential to receive such profound knowledge.

Serenity Surrender (SS), I realized is the most amazing way to connect with the divinity in each of us. It has been brought to this planet by Shivi Dua, who is an inspiration for all those who get touched by her. She started her journey of healing out of her need to be able to help her daughter who was diagnosed with asthma at the age of 3. Starting with Reiki in year 2000, as she progressed inwardly through healing herself & others, she found her connection with the creator. Through this connection, she was revealed deep knowledge about her soul's journey & life. She started using this knowledge via her healings to help others and in year 2010, she was guided to pass on this knowledge to others on a journey to realize self. The name itself suggests arriving at serenity within through practicing surrender. SS has been helping many souls to grow in their understanding of self empowerment by the way of transforming themselves at both the conscious & sub-conscious level ever since.

Here is an excerpt from Shivi's book "Let the power be with you" that published in Speaking Tree, Times of India in Oct 2009.

"Everything that we think about receives energy through our thought. When we accept our power, we also learn to send our power packets to the all that give us happiness. We stop sending them to those that upset us because we don't want to energize them and increase their role in our lives.

At times, when we are praying, we might be asking the Creator to help us forgive those who have done us wrong, while at other times; we might be busy condemning the person for doing the same. Brooding over the past in this manner will give rise to anger and possibly, revenge. In our ignorance, we are sending our power packets to the wrong that we experienced, the person we believe wronged us and to the emotions of anger and revenge. These will then easily negate those we sent during our prayer for forgiveness. Later, we might even find it convenient to blame the Creator for not answering our prayers.

Accepting the past and whatever unpleasant may have taken place helps us to integrate it in us. Reminding ourselves that the other person in question is entitled to his own way of looking at things; handling his life helps us accept whatever happened between him and us in a neutral manner and in moving on. Only then we can continue to create positive vibrations to 'forgive and forget' though it really should be 'accept and forgive'. Accept them as they are and forgiveness follows naturally. Trying to forget only makes us remember it again some other time. Accepting it actually frees us of the burden.

It was about four months since we had moved to Chandigarh, when one morning on her way to school, the bus my daughter was travelling in met with an accident. A truck hit the bus and a windowpane broke and fell on my daughter's hands, leaving her with cuts and scratches. While narrating the incident, she also told me that all the children in the bus were concerned about her. She said despite the blood and the pain, she felt good. She recollected earlier incidents in other places we moved to where it was through some sort of suffering that she made friends in the new place. She finally said: "I knew something like this will happen and I will make friends here also." Needless to say, I pointed out to her that it was this belief of hers that was creating this misery for her time and again and that she deserved to make friends wherever she went easily and effortlessly ... All you have to do is to believe in your power to create your life afresh and send the right power packets out to the Universe."

This book is now an integral part of the Serenity Surrender healing modality. It is a beautiful and simple way to understand how to live a life of awareness & feel empowered each moment.

SS is a channel by the way of which it becomes possible for each to see their life, situations, relationships & concerns from a higher perspective. When we look at our lives from the limited understanding of our physical reality, we tend to blame, get angry or feel victimized. This is because in that moment, what we can see, hear & feel from the physical life situation & people, takes prominence. We fail to see how we have attracted the respective relationship or situation. Over our journey right from the creation of the soul, we have judged ourselves, punished ourselves and believed in experiencing evolution through struggle & misery. All of this happened because from the moment of our creation as a soul, we have perceived ourselves as other than the creator. We developed an identity, which was other than what we implicitly were. This need for identity gave us the need to attract various experiences, by the way of which we sought who we are. Having chased who we are, we many times identified ourselves as different people in different roles and each role we played at each stage, only brought us closer to believing that we are bigger than that role. Whenever we got stuck in the role than looking at ourselves as the one who's playing it, we got trapped in it till we realized our power over that role, the power of having chosen it.

SS happened to me at a time when I needed these answers. I guess I attracted it and it was the universe's way of telling me that I am guided & supported in so many ways. I say it happened to me because I look at it as a phenomenon, which transformed my being deep down to the cell level. As we transform our understanding of self, by the way of healing the SS way, we eventually bring a change in our DNA, thus defying any rules of horoscope; destiny or genetics that were meant to imply on us and give us a certain way of life.

All of us have desires we would like to manifest. All of us also have undesirable situations, which we'd rather do without. Whatever we desire & our soul desires it too, we have it in this moment. Whatever we don't have in this moment & yet we desire it, simply conveys that we have reasons within our sub-conscious for why we can't have it. It could be a fear of losing something else or a lack of understanding growth through it or simple lack of deserving. The way the conscious mind can carry unresolved experiences which were 20 years back, the sub-conscious can go back 20,000 years. Today, what we experience as ourselves, internally / within or externally through relationships, money, work, responses, society etc., all of it is the cumulative understanding of who we are as per our combined consciousness. The sub-conscious carries memories and learning from past lives too, which it has held on for further learning.

We need to be able to know what's in store with my sub-conscious mind and learn what is due to feel whole & complete in this moment. Else, that unresolved past that hasn't "passed", interferes and distorts our present. This is what Serenity

Surrender gave me...the ability to know what it is that I am still holding on. It taught me how to overcome hurdles experienced by my soul.

To understand how SS works, I will explain how it contributes to one's journey. This will make it simpler and inspire those who have at the soul level already chosen it as a path of self-discovery.

The conceptual base for growing through SS is that we all are a spark of the Creator, of pure unconditional love. As we start to understand our journey by traversing backwards from now, everything that we are other than pure unconditional love is only a perception of who we are rather than what we really are.

When in this moment, we are faced with a difficult life situation or relationship or person, it means that we have encountered a deep energetic block in the understanding of self at the sub-conscious level. Imagine a ball of light, which is throwing its light to the surroundings. Suddenly, within the ball, there is a block / obstruction to the spread of light. Something like a dark patch is created inside the ball. The flow of light through it seemed to get blocked. Wouldn't the projected area, wherever externally it was throwing its light, seem to create darkness now? Isn't absence of light only what we know as darkness? Yes indeed it is. That ball of light is us while that distortion in our flow of light is projected as a difficult situation / person or relationship in our life. While this happens, also notice that within the ball, all the light is now falling on the dark patch. If that process is allowed and we start recognizing the power of the light that we are, we can focus on the reason the dark patch exists, heal that energetic blockage and restore the flow of light.

To heal an energetic blockage coming from sub-conscious beliefs, here are a few things that need to be understood first. Let me share a few examples of such blockages and what was revealed during SS Healing Sessions to help my clients overcome their concerns. This will allow a deeper understanding of the modality.

Case Study 1

- **Symptoms / Concern**

    Client was a woman named Radhika (name changed), 35 years old, healthy, married & had 2 kids. Her concern was double edged. One was that she since the last 2 years was having a relationship with another man (name given is Shekhar) outside her marriage. That guy was also married and had a happy family. Both of them felt very connected at a deeper level. She felt she was cheating her husband by holding on to this guy but she couldn't let him go either. She justified her stand by telling me that her husband (name given is John) had a relationship with a colleague a few years ago and ever since that was revealed, although she forgave him, but something between them had changed. Her second concern was the lack of love & passion between her & her husband. Through this emotional & mental tug of war, she was also feeling confused, torn & lost. She needed guidance to what was the right thing for her to do.

    Now as these kinds of cases come in, the first thing that I intend to make people understand is that something of this intensity, could potentially have a lot of past associated with it. The depth of the problem can tell you the depth of unresolved memories or understanding at the soul or sub-conscious level. It is a journey & although the changes at the sub-conscious level happen instantly, in some cases it might take 3-4 sessions also to see the affects in the physical reality. In one's thoughts & emotions though, mostly instant changes are reported.

- **Therapy -**

    In the first SS Session, I connected with the Creator & asked for her karmic links from her past with Shekhar. A past life of hers was revealed where she is a young lady in her early twenties. She was wearing some ethnic dressing of some Asian civilization. Shekhar is a man who's with her. Both of them must be in their mid twenties. They seem to be very scared and it seemed as if it's evening time, and they are hiding in a quite lonely place. As I progressed in the story, I saw that a few people who seemed to belong to the lady's tribe / village manage to find them & drag the guy with them. The woman was screaming & shouting but they didn't listen. She follows them to a place where there are more people of the same village / tribe. They are angry that she had chosen to run away with a guy from a different / rather enemy tribe and hence they were looking for them. They eventually kill him and she then commits suicide after him, in grief & unforgiveness for self.

This lifetime indicated that she carried extreme guilt for Shekhar's death, for being responsible for his loss of life because of her tribe, intense need to be with him while strong fear that the society (tribe in that life) won't allow it to happen. In this life hence she had manifested him in a position where all of these beliefs of the soul manifested and since they are in a relationship other than marriage, she fears she will never be able to be with him in a legitimate relationship.

Using SS, I healed this past life in her sub-conscious, which meant I made her sub-conscious see that past life from a higher perspective. Through doing that her grief, sorrow & guilt for shekhar's death dissolved and her soul understood that the adverse situation that both of them faced with each other was only meant to be that way since they chose it to see their fears of being with each other & society and be able to rise above them.

While I was experiencing her past life, she felt slight pain in her chest area, which also went away as I healed the life. The pain was a sign of her grief and sadness upon shekhar's death, which she experienced in her emotions and hence body at that time.

She felt lighter after the session and her anxiety over her relationship with Shekhar reduced from a scale of 9/10 to 7/10.

Slowly, in a few more sessions, we went beyond this past life to trace their journey together. It's not only past lives having unresolved karma but sometimes we carry deep karmic roots from beyond earth times also. The soul has lived eternally and possibly many of us have lived before earth too, in other planes. I realized that even before she came to the earth, she had distorted her understanding of the masculine aspect and hence had experienced pain or suffering through her masculine counterparts. I worked through these beliefs in her sub-conscious to bring a conceptual understanding of what her masculine energy means to her and how only suffering through it was not the only one.

It emerged as a pattern that Shekhar and Radhika couldn't be happily together in several lifetimes. In one lifetime, both she and Shekhar were friends. They were both men. They were young. They used to steal things and rob people in that time. They did it more for fun, than any limitations. One day, they planned to rob a house. As they entered, the owner was a very beautiful young lady and there was a 2-3 years young baby playing there. Radhika (a man in that life) was extremely drawn towards the mother of the baby. He found her extremely attractive. Shekhar resisted but Radhika made a move towards the young lady. Since they were robbers and were armed, she got defensive and ran. It didn't seem like either of them meant any harm to her but she got more scared than expected, maybe due to her own fears. She instantly ran towards the stairs and in the anxiety fell off the stairs and died. All of it was very instant and what happened made Radhika extremely shameful for that child & the young lady. He didn't mean to take things to that level but he couldn't ignore the fact that the young boy had lost his mother.

That young baby is John (her husband) in her current life. When I revealed this life to her, she shared that indeed her sexual relationship with her husband isn't good. She felt as if she's punishing herself by sleeping with him. She also recalled that she had an extremely volatile relationship with his mother and she unnecessarily blamed her to have separated her from her son. The dots started connecting.

From this recent lifetime, her soul was carrying extreme guilt & sense of responsibility for John and the need to provide for him & care for him for a lifetime because she carried the shame for having deprived him of his mother & shelter. Then she mentioned that for many years her husband didn't earn well and she used to work and take care of the entire family. This was another validation that she was indeed carrying this past.

When I asked her about Shekhar's stand on her marriage, she says he believes my husband is a nice man and I must stay with him & care for him. That also reflected that somewhere deep inside, their souls were in acceptance that they can't be together and yet the unresolved karma with each other drew them closer to each other too.

As we resolved more & more of her past, her belief system at the sub-conscious level altered. The way we do what we believe in our mind, our life is created by what our soul believes in to be its reality. As the belief system of the soul is altered, its need for misery, suffering, pain and failure can also be resolved and one can move forward & evolve only through love.

She noticed that her emotions for Shekhar were changing. He anyways was less involved with her than the way she was. He was clear that his family is a priority to him. She started feeling greater acceptance for her husband. She complained that he never expressed his love for her, which started to change. They started spending more time together and discussing their differences. She then did the 3 Day SS Basic workshop with me to learn more about her soul journey and to learn to heal her own sub-conscious. She also wanted to heal her husband out of his concerns so that both of them could mutually grow together. Today she leads a happy life. I believe Shekhar & Radhika are still friends but she got over the intense desire to spend her life with him & is now in acceptance of her current reality.

She particularly mentioned that her way of looking at life had changed post the workshop & now when she saw someone better or worse than her, she didn't judge them or herself and still feel love & compassion for them. How beautiful does that sound?

I particularly chose this case study, not because I want to say when you are married then staying in the marriage is the only way to be. Had my client's soul been with John only to see through her karma with him & there was no further scope of mutual growth, these healings could have also facilitated them to part ways effortlessly, without having to blame or fight with each other.

Healing through SS facilitates the soul to move forward in the direction that is the best for the soul in question, without having to deal with suffering on the way.

Case Study 2

- **Concern / Symptoms**

    Bella (name changed) had Auto-Immune Disorder when she came to me. She was already on allopathic medication & treatment and she had been also helped by a holistic healer friend to overcome her fear of death. When she came to me, her primary two concerns were

    The symptoms of the disease were there and she obviously wanted to overcome her disorder

    She had lost her hair due to the disease. She had developed this whole complex about her looks because of the loss of hair. This troubled her even more than her disease. She had stopped working and stopped facing people completely only because she feared what will they think of her when they see her without her hair. The doctors said she will slowly grow her hair but she couldn't trust them. Something inside told her as if she was meant to lose that hair.

    She had an old friend whom she liked and they were planning to take their relationship forward. The guy lived in another country and was due to arrive in 5 weeks. She was very anxious as to what will he think of her when he sees her minus the hair. This guy had been very supportive of her emotionally throughout her treatment and she knew he wouldn't logically feel anything of the sort but her fear wouldn't let her believe this.

- **Therapy –**

    I first discussed Bella's opinion on self & beauty. I realized she had a lot of judgment about her looks and thought she was a tall, young good looking & fit woman to look at, she carried too much insecurity. She would diet, she would exercise like a freak, she would weigh herself every day and she would make sure when she stepped out of the house; she was looking perfect each time.

    It isn't a bad thing to take care of one's body but when we are too focused on the body, somewhere we may also be using it to stay in aversion of the soul. One's beauty is a projection of how they feel within.

As I connected with her energies and then the creator, I was guided to a past life of hers. This time the guidance was more feelings & thoughts based.

I saw her as a young lady who has a slightly dark complexion. She is smart, confident and happy. She meets a guy whom she is attracted to. The guy doesn't give any indications of the kind but he's nice to her. In her heart she falls for him. They are good friends and they share a lot of their life with each other. Once, while Bella crosses his room, she hears him talking to another woman who's also his friend. It seemed like the other woman confronted about his emotions for Bella and he says something to the effect that "She's a good friend but I don't love her. She's a little dark & ugly for what I want as my companion". Bella overheard this conversation and her heartbreaks. She cries and cries for days, looking at herself in the mirror. She is unable to get over the fact that he called her ugly.

She lost all her confidence then and pretty much spends her life alone. She is never able to bring her to the understanding that she is worthy of love. She starts to believe her life and her ugliness is a punishment she must endure.

She marries a much older guy upon the suggestion of her parents who are old and want her to just get married before they die. She doesn't care about whom she's marrying and after marriage, even the old man makes her realize that she isn't good looking enough. She further falls into depression and pretty much wastes away her life in the grief.

While dying through a disease in that life, she realizes that she pretty much wasted her life and got into a self-destructive pattern. This was exactly what she was doing now. Autoimmune disorder at the sub-conscious level means the soul is in a self-destructive trap. It's destroying itself and only through that destruction does it believe it can move forward. This is what her soul did when she destroyed her dreams, her life only to believe she could have move forward only this way. This guy in this past life was the guy she liked in the current life so she also carried a fear of being rejected by him on account of her looks.

I healed this past life of hers for her judgment of her looks, her need to believe that only if she is good looking can she get love and her need to destroy self. She also carried the fear of rejection from her friend.

Soon after, I directly asked for her specific concern of her hair. Why did she attract the hair-loss and how will she start growing them again.

There was another past life. This time it was just one scene in which Bella was a boy who promised her deity whom she worshipped in a past life that when she will get something she desired, she would get her head shaven. However she didn't keep that promise then. Now in this life, she feels that losing her hair is the only way to punish herself so that her desires will start getting fulfilled again or so that "God" will start listening to her. So her sub-conscious believes losing the hair is the only way to move forward.

I healed her guilt and shame for breaking her promise to her deity. Her sub-conscious was given a higher perspective of her evolution & the role her body plays in it.

We healed 5-6 times over gaps of a week each between two sessions. When her friend came in 5 weeks, he was completely supportive of her and stood by her. Her hair had started growing and in-spite of her medical reports marginally changing, her body symptoms like headaches, feeling lost, lack of confidence, hot flushes etc. vanished. She even joined office in 3 months time.

These were 2 case studies, just to give an idea of all that goes on within our sub-conscious and what can be done to resolve it.

Serenity Surrender (SS) is a revolutionary methodology to be able to not only know & understand our soul's eternal journey but to bring it to learn its lessons faster & free this moment of suffering. A believer or a non-believer is only a choice but by virtue of being in a human existence, and yet, we all go through conflicts between our conscious & sub-conscious, we all have un-fulfilled desires or fear of losing what we have, we all have attachments & dependencies and we all wish to move forward to a state of peace & joy.

The typical concerns that can be resolved using SS are in the areas of:
- Relationship Concerns
- Fear & Phobias
- Blocks in growth / work / money
- Physical Ailments of any kind
- Depression
- Anxiety & Stress
- Marriage Related Concerns
- Lawsuits / Manifested Fights / Conflicts
- Getting rid of external negative energies
- Finding a soul mate
- Deeper into self (spiritual journey)

There are two ways of seeking help using SS.

You can opt for private sessions. SS is a New Age modality specifically channeled for souls who have chosen to expedite their journey and face self at a deeper level. A typical SS session lasts anywhere between 1-1.5 hrs. SS is a fairly simple & extremely effective technique that does NOT involve hypnosis of any kind.

You can attend the 3 Day SS Basic Workshop. The SS Basic workshop enables one to learn the SS way of healing for self & others. Post the 3-day workshop, you will be able to experience and heal your own past, including past lives.

The SS Workshop is a transformatory experience and one attracts it only when they are ready for their life's perspective to completely change & align itself to their highest best. The 3 day session includes theoretical understanding of a soul's journey, how creation ever began, how we perceived ourselves to become who we are today, how the conscious & sub-conscious operate & communicate, karma, past lives, how our past impacts our present, what do relationships mean to the soul, concepts like marriage &

money, how to receive guidance from the creator (pure unconditional love) and how to heal past life karmic memories to instantly transform in this moment.

It also includes practical healing sessions done in pairs, for self & group healings provided to all participants by the trainer. Ideally everyone gets what he or she comes for and more from the workshop. They go back home feeling empowered having found their divine connection through which they can instantly shift their negative thoughts, emotions & relationships and change their life on a daily basis. It makes them more complete within & they are able to free themselves of everything which isn't helping them in being happy & blissful now.

The process enhances a deeper connection with self. Let's endeavor to become the limitless pool of love that is hidden within our perception of ourselves.

Minal Arora is an IT Geek transformed into a spiritual healer & mentor. Her 12 years of chasing software programs & logics started looking less interesting as she saw an opportunity of inward growth. Starting her spiritual journey by becoming a Past Life Regression therapist, she soon discovered that growing within self is the only way to help others too. As she realized the need for self-healing at a deep level, she got drawn to finding a way and miraculously met Shivi Dua, who guided her to the Serenity Surrender way of life. She found a mentor & a friend in Shivi who has been her source of inspiration ever since. She is also the author of "Maaya- A Tryst with Self".

www.pastlifeconnection.com

CHAPTER 21

Beyond Self-Sabotage[1]

Archna Mohan

Just a couple of days ago, I had accompanied a friend to the local hospital for his regular check-up. As I waited for him in the café, I gazed out of the big glass window from which I could see a vast expanse of woods. The sight of the woods, in autumn, was heavenly. I have been to these woods many times, as this is my favorite dog-walking route. I looked at the people around me in the café – some, who like me, were there accompanying a patient, some who probably worked in the hospital, and some would have been patients, waiting for their appointment. Like me, some were admiring the view outside, some were just engaged in their own thoughts and some (presumably staff) were busy discussing their work. I wondered how many of these people have ever walked in woods just to get out of their daily routine.

Do they know how deep these woods are? Have they ever paused to observe the beautiful trees, flowers or the birds, which come every season? I was not judging them; rather the question was to me too. Why, after having lived there for nearly eight years, I never visited the woods? Why did I start going out in woods almost every day since last 2 years only? I love fitness and have been going to a gym regularly since a long time. And then I bought a puppy. I needed to take her out for walks. At first it was a chore for me as I never saw how walking in nature would be fun. Looking back, the root for this belief emanates from my own belief system as growing up; I was not used to see women of my age taking their dogs out for a walk. After sometime, I started enjoying my chore. Once I became aware of the trees, the greenery, the birds, the nature, it no longer remained a chore. So what changed; my awareness of the surrounding or

---

[1] Special thanks to my friend and colleague JP Sears for this term, which I gratefully acknowledge.

my spiritual awareness? Once that changed, I started enjoying my walks; rather looked forward to it. Every day was a new revelation – the trees, the woods, the greenery tells you so many things. I started learning so many things and till date I am learning something new each day.

The walls around us

Sitting in the café, I realized the walls that I had built around me – the walls that had to be dismantled for me to realize the mere presence of woods near me. As human being, we build walls around us to make us feel 'safe' and 'secure'. The walls provide us comfort that nothing will change around us, that there will not be any new challenge to face that my environment will continue to remain the same.

In the past couple of years, I have worked extensively on myself and with my clients on various issues that confront us. Each of us is unique. We face challenges or environment that may be similar, yet everyone deals with it uniquely. I will demonstrate this using my own example. Being the youngest of four siblings, I was born – and grew up – in the shadows of my siblings. Perhaps the very first experience learnt was to get myself noticed among the siblings. I was friendly little girl, talkative and easy-to-get-along-with. However, in school or among relatives I always found myself being compared with my own siblings or a cousin or a friend – (unfortunately) someone who was smarter than me. It was a constant pressure to perform, to prove myself better than the others, to excel and to keep raising the bar higher. I was not up to this challenge. I found an 'easier' way out. I self-accepted that I am a mediocre and that nothing is great about me. So rather than matching the (ever-rising) expectations of people around me, I learnt the best way to deal with this was to believe that I was 'non-special'. This belief served me well and made me feel safe and secure.

A few years back, I had a client who used to harm herself. She was in a relationship with a married person and had drugs related issues. Working with her, I gathered that her parents had migrated to the USA from India. As with first generation immigrants, the parents worked very hard to provide good living conditions to their kids. At same time they wanted to ensure that the kids carry all the values (read belief system) from the culture that they have immigrated from. As someone who has made a change from one environment to another, I do not want to let-go of my belief system, and at the same time 'enforce' it on people around me. As a child, adhering to two-belief system (one abstract, which is 'loosely' followed within the confines of my home; the other, more defined, to which I am exposed to most of my conscious life) is a difficult task. So long as a child is dependent on parents they do things to 'please' their parents, but deep inside, they do not feel connected to those acts. As humans, we are born to express ourselves. When this opportunity is denied to us – either due to circumstances or environment - we are unable to contain this need (to express) within ourselves and, in some cases, start abusing ourselves. The root of my client's abuse lay in her desire to be heard, to be recognized as a person and to feel worthy in her own eyes.

The walls around us are everywhere. They are expressed in our common parlance:

- "I can never lose weight, I am fat."
- "I am not beautiful."
- "I am not worthy."
- "I will never be rich."
- "I am not talented."
- "I am never heard."
- "I may not speak."

These are just some examples. There are many such 'walls' that are deeply embedded within us. We build them, and with each adverse event, the walls get strengthened, and finally we believe them to be true!

Self-Sabotage

As a child, we experience events that lead us to firm beliefs (walls). Some beliefs are inherited – the parents pass them to their children; some are based on the societal norms (do's and don'ts), and some are even related to past-life experiences. The belief system that we are born with (past-life experience), coupled with those we have inherited and those we are expected to 'conform to' sometimes inhibits our need to express differently. We are expected to be 'polite' to people who may have harmed us; we are expected to 'pay attention' to someone who we find boring... and the list goes on. Our inability to conform instills 'shame' in us. We are shamed for non-conformity; we feel shameful for being what we are. And the shame in us, results in self-sabotage.

So what is shame and how does it affect our self-belief and feeds self-sabotage?

As a coach, I come face-to-face with shame with almost all my clients. Once I realized the impact of shame on my clients, I took time to study it deeply.

Another client, in her 20's, came to me complaining of some physical issues. She suffered from severe lower back pains, had irritating skin and was in depression. After my first consultation I could sense that the root of her problems lay somewhere else. I started working with her nutrition and exercise, knowing fully well that she was suffering from some type of shame. As a Coach you don't want to confront her – you need to gain your client's confidence before you start. It is you – as a coach – who needs to listen, not the other way round!

As a child (aged 9) she was in love with a boy. When this came to the knowledge of her parents, she was severely punished and deported to stay with a relative, far away from her home. This led my client to 'believe' that she is not loved, not worthy of being loved and that being in love is not good. She felt betrayed by her parents. It was 'shameful' being a kind of girl none can be proud of. This shame in her led her to believe further that she was not worthy of anything good happening in her life, and if someone is being good to her, then the person has some ulterior motive. As a result of her belief, my client lost trust in people. The pain in her lower back was the manifestation of an event when she was sexually abused while being 'deported'.

In 'shame' my client tried her very best to please her parents, to make them love her. When she failed, she tried 'self abuse'. She learnt the hard way that she can 'control' her parents by harming herself! When I met her she was in her 20's with some physical issues, her low back pain was severe, some skin disorder and deeply in depression. She had an inner child of 8 year old. She was fearful of outer world and it was difficult for her to trust any man – even her husband.

When I asked her to write down everything she believed in, below is what she came back with:

"I am not worthy enough to be loved."
"My parents are perfect people, I betrayed them."
"All men are dishonest."
"I will die one day in depression."
"I believe art is the best form of presentation."

It took my client a good few months to come up with her beliefs. To me, it was the first break-through. My next line of work was how to make her being loved again. When I asked her this question, she laughed for good few minutes and said it was impossible. Her belief that she is not loved was so deeply rooted in her that she was fearful to address it and move to a strange zone which was not familiar to her. The shame in her was giving her comfort.

> *"You, yourself, as much as anybody in the entire universe, deserve your love and affection."* - Buddha

I asked my client to answer some questions honestly. They were:

1. What are your beliefs about people?
2. Why do you fear people?
3. What is the worst thing that can happen when meeting people?
4. Are my beliefs in this area improving the quality of my life?

For someone, who is stuck in similar situation, it helps to realize whether their beliefs are helping them move in their journey. Once they realize that the belief is not serving them, they let it go.

In her beliefs, my client had written something that caught my eye: "I believe Art is the best form of presentation". I was curious what she means. Like me, she loved to draw. I introduce her to Mandala making and every week, I'd ask her to make a new Mandala for me. Her Mandala started speaking in depth of what her self-sabotage belief was. Mandala also helped her relax. There was a noticeable difference in the way she walked and breathed. Her shoulder muscles start relaxing - a tight shoulder is indication of holding anger and closeness of your heart chakra.

Healing is a slow process. Getting rid of your beliefs – some that you have been carrying for a very, very long time – is not easy. Your beliefs – good or bad – give a meaning to your life, your actions and your thoughts. Getting rid of them is like 'reset' button on your life. As a coach, my aim is to help you identify your beliefs, help you evaluate them for alignment to your goals, and, if found unfit, help you replace them one by one. My clients slowly started working on her self- sabotage and belief. Today she is a proud woman, full of self-confidence, brimming with life and an example to others.

So what works for you if you want to get out of the self-sabotage?

The first is being aware of your beliefs. Most of the times, we do not realize the existence of beliefs that we carry. In the above case, I asked my client to write down what she feels in front of a person or strangers, and if she could notice a pattern of fear or anger in her feelings. I, then, encouraged her to work on these issues during her "quiet time" by trying to address them with love and compassion.

The second is taking responsibility of your own life and actions. It is important to create some values in your life. It can be as simple as waking up early, doing something that helps you to grow as person, or getting to discover nature. Values help in grounding and it provides a sense of belonging.

What other says often upsets people. We need to remember that we all carry our own perceptions and if someone does not fit in our paradigm, we react by denouncing them, making them feel down or shaming them. You can change or mould only *your* perception; it is hard to change others.

If someone criticize you with the intention of shaming you for things in past while you are trying to heal, you need to see that person with empathy. The other person's belief to feel strong or loved comes from shaming others but they themselves are lost souls.

As a kid, we all are born beautiful and worthy. However, instead of building upon this beautiful fact, most of the time what we experience is totally opposite of it.

Let me give you another example – one from my own life.

As a kid, I wanted to write and do theatre as these activities made me happy. When I was growing up, writing and acting were never appreciated as 'serious' professions to pursue. Given my fondness for writing and acting, I remember being punished, as I was too busy preparing for my school's annual function drama or writing stories at the back of my mathematics book. One of my teachers called me STUPID and said I would never pass from school. As a kid, I was shattered and shame engulfed me. I remember getting fever every now and then, and did not enjoy the school. My body was showing all the signs of something, which I believed was not right. Eventually, my creativity took a back seat and I start preparing for my exams. I passed with distinction but for a very long time, I thought I am not talented or smart. My belief was so strong that instead of applying for an admission in a good college (where I could have got admission), I ended up applying at colleges, which did not have good standing.

My belief about me being stupid and untalented continued to grow stronger with everything I did. If you have one belief, you start creating many 'sub beliefs' to support that belief. I enrolled for computer programming course. I excelled in the examinations, but I thought (believed) it was my luck that the questions were too easy. By the time I married, the self-criticism and my self-sabotage were deeply rooted in me. I did not feel like being loved or like deserving love. And I received exactly the same response from people around me – about being unworthy and unloved. My 'shame' that I am not worth anything made me feel I was not attractive too. Instead of talking about my vulnerability with my close ones, I moved towards food. Eating is your best companion when you are suffering from shame, depressed or loneliness. Food never talks back to you; it does not criticize or judge you. They help you forget your worries. No wonder, very soon I was overweight. As my belief got stronger every day, I stopped caring about myself. In order to earn respect and love from others, I became very giving and tried hard to please people.

One belief gives rise to more beliefs in time. If the first belief is positive, the subsequent beliefs (or the sub-beliefs) too are positive and help you find the purpose in your life. However, if the first belief is self-negating, then that, combined with other sub-beliefs makes you sink in them making you a prisoner within your own body with shame and guilt.

When you are shaming yourself you always have three persons around you - one who shames you, second who is a witness and the third who shows empathy.

Depending on the level of your shame, at times, you have to wait for long for the third person to come to your life.

When the third person came to my life, my self-sabotage and limited belief started getting weak. I started noticing the deterioration of my body, which was getting weaker day by day. I seriously questioned to myself:

1. Why do I need other people's approval to feel worthy?
2. My beliefs are not giving me happiness; it is worth to feed it?
3. Do I need to create something else to feel grounded and supported?
4. I need help.
5. I need to create new belief for myself.

How do you approach your deep-seated belief? To change your belief that is not serving your purpose, at first you need to be aware of them, to identify those belief that are prompting you on a course of self-sabotage. Then you need to identify how they are harming you and finally acknowledge how deep rooted they are in your system. The deeper their roots are, the harder it would take to uproot them. More depth needs more patience, more love and more time. You need to express your emotions behind the belief leading to self-sabotage - the anger, sadness, tears, love, gratitude, forgiveness and compassion towards your own self. These all are part of it.

My belief that I am a good writer came true when people started following my writing. And it was not easy. Expressing yourself, after years of silence was the first step towards it. I started writing for myself. Then I started sharing it. After sometime, I started receiving positive comments on my writing (with a fair share of negative comments too, which I chose to disregard!). This gave me courage to open a hitherto unknown door of my belief, to see a vast field of lavender – the color of enlightenment.

I distinctly remember my first workshop in the UK. I was stricken by a firm belief that I am not a native English speaker and hence, conducting a two-hour workshop for native English people was scary. It took a lot of effort to counter this belief. Add to it, a deep-rooted belief of being stupid and unworthy! To counter this negative belief, I had a positive belief that I know what I want to convey to my audience, and I am good at it. I address that fear by my opening my workshop with my admission about my strong Indian accent and poor vocabulary. I asked my audience to interrupt me, if they did not understand what I was saying. At the end of two hours, I was the one most (pleasantly) surprised that no one had interrupted my talk once, for not following what I wanted to convey!

My next desire, stemming from my penchant on writing was to publish my own book. My first little tiny book "A Pearl for this Day" was published on Amazon as an e-book in 2013. It was not a best seller. Nor did it get nominated for any prize! But it did not make me unhappy. I was taking one baby step at a time. The fact that I published a book germinated another belief in me on my ability to write. And now, I am working on a major book on the value of Chakra system. I have achieved this by looking deeply inside me, my belief system, my perceptions and the rules, which I created for myself based on my fear and shame. Once I decided not to adhere to those rules, the beliefs and the perceptions, every obstacle started disappearing from my mind, making way for new, positive thoughts and perceptions. As an astute farmer, we need to keep an eye on our garden to see that weeds do not spoil the beautiful lavender field.

I mostly work with women clients. One day I got a call from a man who sought my help. As an ex-personal trainer, I had worked with lots of men. However, as a life coach this would have been my first experience. The person had been following my writing for a long time and decided that I could help him. He desperately needed my help but I was not sure whether I would be able to understand his spiritual and emotional self to help him. My belief or self-limitation told me that being a woman, I was an excellent coach for the client of the same sex, but may not be able to appreciate the spiritual needs of a person from opposite sex. The more I thought about it, the more I could discern the fallacy in my argument. And then I thought if nothing else, it would help me to understand two men in my life – my growing son and my grown-up husband! I decided to accept the challenge and signed up my new client.

My first meeting with him went very well. My new client was a successful businessman who came to me seeking help for constipation and recurring knee problem. As with any other client, I could see that his ailments were symptomatic

Holistic Wellness in the New Age

of deep-rooted issues. And, it took him longer to open up, to admit his issues. In our society it is okay for a woman (weaker sex!) to ask for help, to cry and to talk about her weakness. For man, it's a different set of rules altogether.

The male child is bred to be strong, to protect the weaker sex. He is taught to resolve his issues on his own, without seeking help from any one else. He is expected to hide his emotions – *"don't cry like girls!"* this *'manliness'* results in a man hiding his emotions and his expressions deep in his body. As they do not get expressed; they accumulate in your body, in your mind. As a result most men suffer from ailments such as diabetes, heart issues, stiffness around neck and shoulders.

After some session, I gained my client's confidence to explore his issues. He came from a family where his father was very strict and disciplinarian. His mother loved kids, but would never go against her husband. During childhood, my client loved to sing. His singing was never appreciated in the family (remember *manliness*?) and was discouraged. The discouragement made my client believe that singing would be a curse to his family. He became quite, went to a prestigious school and university, now owns his own business. He was successful in every sense – a provider, a good son to his parents, a loving father to his children and a good husband. Yet, in one of the sessions, he mentioned he saw himself as a failure and that that nobody listened to him except his daughter.

I asked my client to define success and failure and this is what he came up with:

- Having enough money in bank is must.
- You should be a perfect example for your family as a good provider.
- Your own sacrifice counts for family prosperity and happiness.
- Failure is not achieving any of these.

When we discussed happiness, what surprised him most that he was making everyone around him happy, but at a cost; in return he was making himself unhappy. A common belief that most of us carry from childhood is that someone else is responsible for our happiness.

My client was very attached to his daughter as she was inclined towards singing. In his daughter he found his long-suppressed desire to sing. He made her believe that she was a good singer and that she should pursue singing with all intent. There was nothing wrong in his encouragement; through this he was indirectly fulfilling his own unfulfilled desire. He might achieve some happiness but his own desire to sing would not be completely fulfilled.

The next task that I had for him was to focus on happiness: If he could reverse his childhood what was one thing that would he like to do? What is one act or thought which would bring greatest happiness to him? And which belief does he consider to be like a prison to him.

His belief that he will be unfaithful or disrespectful to his parents was for the first time challenged when he decided to sing again. He enrolled at a local singing class. He wanted to give his parents and family a surprise on Mother's day by singing for them. By enrolling for the singing lessons, he replaced his old belief with a new belief, that which was positive and served him happiness. His belief that singing will upset his parents was gone too. His physical body started showing a sign of improvement. Knee is where we store our chronic fear. Once my client started releasing his anger, sadness and explored his talent he could notice a definite improvement in his knee problem.

Most people can bring drastic change in their quality of life by identifying the top five or ten of their limiting beliefs and changing them. Each belief has power to create unhappiness or joy in your life. And as every belief has sub beliefs within it, so if you have a belief you are not worthy, will create more sub beliefs on various aspect of self-loath. And on the contrary, a good positive belief spawns many sub-beliefs to support the positive belief. On a subconscious level, every belief has a secondary benefit. A secondary benefit means that while something causes pain or discomfort on one level but it may provide pleasure on another level. This is the reason why we protect our beliefs, even after being aware that they are not helping us. We create justifications for our beliefs. For example, a client, who was unhappy with her job and yet she was fearful of changing her job. Her secondary belief was even if she changed her job, the new job would be like the current one. This secondary belief provided her the 'comfort' to stay in her current job.

> *"When patterns are broken, new world emerges."* - Tuli Kupferberg

We create meaning in whatever we do. And this meaning is deeply connected to our emotions. Hence, our emotions are in alignment to the meaning that we have created. If you create a meaning on your unworthiness, it is very likely that you will experience emotions that are negative. I come across people who are angry with someone and they believe it is the person who has made them angry. In reality, that anger must have been carried inside since some time and the person who they are blaming may no longer be present. This is the emotion that they are carrying. You are the cause of any emotions that you carry. If you understand this, then you will understand your own power to stop it any time you want.

> *"Let go of all that is no longer serving you and realize that an infinite power lies in your present moment".* Mateo Tabatabai

We make our own rules for success, happiness, health, in short everything that matters to us. I often get clients who say they would be happy after losing 'x' amount of weight and then their relationship would also improve. So losing weight becomes a belief, on the success of which rests the key to their happiness. Like a pot of gold at the end of a rainbow! There are some for whom earning a certain amount of money is believed to make them happy or winning a lottery! The truth is it never does. We create our belief in future merely to provide ourselves comfort in the present. So we do NOT take care of the present – to improve our living conditions, and chase a rainbow in the future for the mythical pot of gold! In addition, the rules that we create – the beliefs – are usually, not practical or worth and hence destined to fail. The failure, in turn spawns another belief about our unworthiness. This cycle goes on and one till one day we just give up hope or seek help to change ourselves.

As we think of the same thoughts and entertain the same beliefs, we experience the same outcome. You need to create awareness of your beliefs to be able to challenge them and attempt to change them.

> *"Lets us not look back in anger or forward in fear, but around in awareness."*

We stop living in present and worry about the future. Are we aware that today was the future of yesterday for which we had worried?

Being aware of your belief requires a quite time. Sometime people find it hard to be quiet. Having a quiet time does not always mean meditating. There are many activities that can calm you like making Mandala, which is a art created through energy and the colors represent your state of mind, or gardening, walking in nature, making something from Lego or going for a ceramic class, anything that will teach you how to live in this present moment.

Being aware of present brings quality to the normal thing you do. If you have prepared dinner, present in a way to make it special; if you're spending time at home, dress up as if you were going out; just making an effort to do something great by being in present and being aware of it. When did you last sit down with your child and listened to their stories – just you and your child, no TV at the background. When did you listen attentively to someone – without your mind 'judging his or her motive'? Being in present one hundred percent creates new meanings and beliefs to your own world.

Getting under the root of any belief is like digging deeper and deeper in earth till you find the water. It is painful and sometime it is very scary too. It is like invading in a strange zone where nothing is familiar. Like an invader, you have to be ruthless; you need to crush your old beliefs that are no longer serving you.

If we wish our lives to be different in the future it is necessary to change our belief today. This, in turn, changes our thinking and emotions, and finally our lives. And it does not end there; it also impacts others around you.

If the belief is good it starts spreading the emotions of happiness, positive energy radiates outward. Our physical body shows the sign of health.

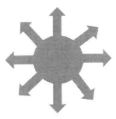

If the belief is negative it brings back hatred, jealous, envy, worthlessness and it affects our physical body because energy gets trapped inside.

Self-sabotage arises from our beliefs. When our belief – and myriad sub-beliefs reach a stage that overpowers us, we move to self-sabotage. It is the ultimate form of expression for the one practicing it – a cry for help, for recognition, for acknowledgement.

When I was approached to write for this book, before writing, a thousand thoughts crossed my mind and worried me – who will read this book, how will it be received, will it be good enough….And the thoughts went on and on. As I became aware of the beliefs, I calmed myself and started writing –one thought at a time. Very soon that thought spawned the other, then the other and the result is what you are reading now.

You were born to write your own play. You are the director of your play and it is you who has to decide what type of play you want to create and watch. I bet we all like to watch something meaningful and which has got purpose. Look at your life and the potential that you hold inside. It is our false beliefs that because of some event in our childhood we have left the true essence of life. We are born perfect. Why doubt that perfectness now? During consultation I always ask all my clients "What do you want to leave behind as your legacy?"

Give a good thought on this and when you will get the answer, you will know which belief has to be replaced by others. Do not be a prisoner in your body or within the false walls that you have created. Go out and take a stroll in woods that you have been watching for so long from your windows. It is yours and it is waiting for you.

Archna Mohan is a holistic life style coach, REPs qualified level-3 personal trainer and a nutritional advisor. She is passionate about what she does and it shows in the way she works and the way she lives her life. She moved to UK, from India, ten years back. With her hard work and dedication, she has made her name in the fitness industry not only in UK but all over the world. For over a decade, Archna has been implementing programs developed as specific solutions for the struggles that so many women face. She helps women around the world to find the time and motivation to exercise, to end the vicious cycle of dieting, improve their health and energy, or just improve their daily functional activity levels. She understands the issues of women over 40 because she is one of them.

www.archnamohan.co.uk

CHAPTER 22

Fitness: The Challenge Within

Tarini Khetarpal

To exercise, to eat right. What is the Big Challenge?

Why do we gain weight? Why do I fall sick?

Where do I find a solution? Should I go to a Gym or should I first visit a dietician?

Better still, let me join a slimming class

All tried and tested solutions, proven testimonials by housewives and celebrities. Before and after photographs. Logical conclusion "surely these instant solutions will work for me!"

Sorry to disappoint you but you are wrong, wrong, wrong!

Today there are various solutions towards weight loss and attaining a fit body. However all these strategies for weight loss lack in one important element-dealing with the battle of the mind, which is essentially the most important battle.

Come to think of it...

If one could control one's cravings towards chocolate

cake (or any other craving for that matter)...

If one could remain enthusiastic towards exercising

on a daily basis...

If one could follow the healthy diet chart

without any cheating...

...Would one need to shop around for finding an external agency to help us win the battle of weight loss?

It is here that the role of NLP comes in.

What is NLP?

'NLP' stands for Neuro Linguistic Programming. 'Neuro' refers to the way we experience the world through our senses; linguistic refers to the way we use language to make sense of the world, capture and conceptualize our experiences and then communicate that experience to others; and programming addresses the way we code (mentally represent) our experience and adopt various behavioral patterns of response.

In short, NIP is a powerful mechanism involving the programming of our mind. It can impact you both professionally and personally. It is applicable to all spheres of one's life-be it weight loss, overall health, business management psychology and all forms of personal development.

NLP can help you with:

- It can remove the mental barriers blocking you from reaching your goals and set new higher expectations from yourself.
- Replace negative behaviors and habits with positive ones.
- Transform the way you go about everyday tasks.
- Better understand you own motivations, needs and behaviors to have the greatest impact in your life.

NLP helps you understand your current mind as each person has their own unique map of the world. It helps you unlock the subconscious beliefs, limitations and filters that you have created and stored in your mind.

Be it with respect to fitness or your ability to lose weight.

NLP will help you change your mental perception

NIP will help you understand that emotion which drives you to eat more and exercise less. It will help you to come up with alternative solutions towards satisfying that emotion. Find alternate mental and emotional states that lead you to overcome eating disorders, exercising less, staying depressed and being lethargic.

We humans represent the world to ourselves with our senses

- Visual (What we see)
- Auditory (What we hear)
- Olfactory (What we smell)
- Gustatory (Taste)
- Kinesthetic (Our Emotions)

It is possible to enhance or depress the qualities or attributes of the representations you make by using your five senses and their sub modalities. NLP can help you frame a picture of your favorite physical activity in your mind. It could be going to the movies, dining at your favorite restaurant, your favorite food or being with your best friend. The technique will help you visualize your mental picture in color and with intensity.

It will help you to evoke a positive response to it.

NLP can also make you visualize another picture in black and white and make you take notice of your response. The technique can change your sub modalities by bringing closer or pushing certain images further away from yourself, in doing so the technique can help you to love something or in turn detest some other thing. NLP can help you to stop procrastinating and to act on what is good for you. The interesting thing to note here is that once you understand that you create your internal world, you realize you can change it.

Here is a Technique You Want to Try

The Swish Technique

- If you eat food which is not good for you and you want to change this habit, you should try this technique
- Shut your eyes and imagine yourself eating hot chocolate fudge ice-cream. Now think of a healthy food item which you'd rather have instead. Perhaps…I'd rather have a bowl of yoghurt instead of chocolate.

Holistic Wellness in the New Age

- Shut your eyes and now imagine a picture of eating yoghurt. Mentally picture how you feel the positive emotion whilst eating healthier food. Visualize this new picture as big, bright and close to you…
- Next gradually shrink this yoghurt eating and feeling picture, making it smaller and dimmer. Gradually push it into the right hand corner of your brain.
- Open your eyes.
- Bring back the Hot Chocolate eating picture (your craving) in your mind.
- Make it bright, big and close to you as possible. Remember, you still have on the right hand corner the dim yoghurt eating picture.
- Say 'SWISH!' and expand the small picture into a big one such that it covers the chocolate eating picture. Feel the positive emotion that you would feel of eating a healthier food. Open your eyes.
- Do the Swish 10-12 times. Each time Swish it faster and faster.
- Open your eyes.

Result: You would have either forgotten about your craving or would have the 2nd picture in your mind. Practice the Swish technique on yourself on a daily basis. The more you do it on yourself, the more the success shall be of this technique. The Swish technique is also equally successful in curing you of your bad habits be it biting nails or to attain one's ideal body image.

Tarini Khetarpal is a Certified NLP Master Practitioner from the NLP Academy. She has learnt NLP from the pioneer of NLP himself, Mr. John Grinder in London. She has been in the field of training for 5 years and has conducted 800 + training programs on various avenues. In addition she is a certified and licensed 'Heal Your Life' Workshop leader, certified by Hay House, USA and has also conducted programs based on Louise Hay's philosophy.

t.khetarpal@gmail.com

CHAPTER 23

The Four Pillars of Health

Nandini Gulati

In the winter of 2003, a few months after my father's death, I was visiting my cousin in Paris and one evening he took me out for dinner to a special place. It was a Lebanese restaurant where a "coffee reader" of considerable repute was available a couple of times a week. A coffee reader makes you drink a sip of dense black coffee and then "reads" the trails and marks left behind in your cup to reveal some insights about your life. They also answer your questions about your life much like a palm reader or a tarot reader does.

Due to the difficult emotional period I was going through following my father's sudden passing away, my cousin wanted me to meet the coffee reader and find some solace in his insights and predictions. Although, skeptical of occult sciences, I was open to the idea. I suppose when your heart is broken due to the loss of a loved one, you become more open and vulnerable. I was looking for any fragments of hope and reassurance that I could find amidst the complete disorientation and confusion I was feeling as a result of my father's unexpected demise.

I can recall clearly the words of the coffee reader (as translated from French by my cousin) as if it was yesterday, "Your heart and head are not connected." I remember asking my cousin and my best friend who accompanied me, "What does this mean? What does it feel like to have a connected heart and mind?" I really was innocent in my cluelessness; I could not fathom what it even meant to have a disconnected heart and mind, let alone to experience a connectedness.

Switching to what was happening with my body and my health. I was overweight ever since I stopped playing basketball after college. It was slow to build up at first but when I moved to the US, I ballooned to a gigantic 95 kilos! In 2007, I

Holistic Wellness in the New Age

was diagnosed with high blood pressure and put on medication and soon after diagnosed with Rheumatoid Arthritis, a chronic autoimmune and degenerative disease. My journey of re-connecting my head and heart or mind and body had begun.

In 2009, after further deterioration of my hypertension, I was taking 3 medications a day to control it and suffering from various side effects. In addition, I was on multiple medicines for Rheumatoid Arthritis. My health future looked bleak. I felt depressed and could not see any hope on the horizon. Following the crash of the economy that year, I lost major projects as a corporate trainer and circumstances led me to focus on myself and my failing health. At that time, I sent out a heartfelt intention to the Universe asking to learn more about connecting better with my body and to heal from my various ailments.

To cut a long story short, in my search for healing, the Universe conspired to send me various books, videos, healing techniques and teachers. Collectively, they led me to a path where I found the clues to put together the puzzle of traversing the journey to connect my head to my heart.

I released 25 kilos effortlessly and more miraculously, this time I managed to keep it off! I completely recovered from hypertension and no longer take any medications to control it. The four pillars of health are my offering to those searching for answers to their own health challenges.

First Pillar

The first and foremost pillar is food. No one taught me at school or at home what exactly was the natural diet of our species. In fact my natural abhorrence of milk, for example was overridden by adding sugar and other chemical additives to make it more palatable. Animals and their products were regularly served on the table and belonging to a Punjabi family that was a treat we all looked forward to.

During my quest for healing in my early 40's, I came across the work of Dr. Colin Campbell, author of "The China Study", a seminal work about the effects of nutrition in a large population and the harmful effects of meat, dairy and processed and refined foods.

Soon after I met Dr. Nandita Shah of SHARAN who has been working in the area of preventing and reversing lifestyle diseases like diabetes, hypertension, heart disease and even cancers and auto-immune issues through educating people about food that supports health and how to prepare it. After attending her one-day seminar entitled Peas vs. Pills, I finally understood the real meaning of our natural diet and how to eat to prevent disease and maximize the natural healing powers of our body.

There are many medical doctors in the US practicing and teaching the health benefits of a "Whole, Plant-based Diet" to cure a myriad of diseases. Some of these, whose books, websites and videos have inspired me, are: Dr. Joel Fuhrman, Dr. John McDougall, Dr. Neal Barnard and Dr. Caldwell Esselstyn among others.

Adopting this abundant and wholesome diet into my life has been one of the most rewarding and centering decisions of my life. I have not only improved my health on all fronts but also feel good that I am doing the best for the environment by eating lower on the food chain. It has also awakened compassion within me and I am at peace that no animals are harmed in order to feed me. It is a clean and wholesome feeling from inside that always leaves me at a loss for words when I try to explain it.

Finally, I experienced a connection and oneness with my body with this single most important change in a way that shifted and evolved my life in many positive ways. I understood the meaning of the Hindi saying from our *shastras* – "*Jaisa ann, vaisa mann*" or "Like food, like mind" or the more famous English phrase, "You are what you eat."

Adopting a plant based, whole food diet is an affirmative, sustainable and tangible action for everything I believe in – compassion for all beings on the planet, healthy living and minimizing my carbon footprint by inculcating eco-friendly habits. And I get to live and practice my beliefs 3 times a day with my fork. Lucky me!

Second Pillar

As you would easily guess, the second pillar of health is about activity and movement, also called exercise. I prefer to use the first two words as "exercise" often has negative and effortful connotations for many. Before I began my own journey of self-healing, I was extremely sedentary and the excruciating pain of rheumatoid arthritis made me even more lethargic.

One day I was sitting on a park bench after another failed attempt to stir up enough energy to go for a walk. I watched as two little birds flitted back and forth from a tree to the ground immersed in incessant chatter. They seemed to be really busy organizing things for their day. I wondered where the birds got all the energy as I felt drained and spent. (This was before I adopted a whole plant-based diet.) Looking up, I saw in the distance a really old woman, bent over in half, walking at a snail's pace. Within me a tiny voice said, "If she can do it so can I. If the birds can do it and the old woman, I can try it too."

Every morning, a battle of sorts went on in my mind about whether or not to get up from the comfort of the bed. My lazy side always won this battle. I thought what is the minimum I can commit to doing, bare minimum at which I really cannot fail. And all I could come up with was to wear my shoes. And so I began wearing my walking shoes first thing in the morning and standing up. I was open to the possibility that my shoes may want to take me somewhere. What I realized was that once I was out and moving, my body wanted to move more and the mind took a backseat. Slowly, I made daily walking a regular habit.

In the middle of my weight release journey, I discover the whole plant based diet and 3 months after I went on it, I had so much surplus energy that I started jogging. I had never been interested in jogging ever as it always seemed too effortful to me. But after the new way of eating, I was like a child who could not walk but had to skip or run!

The self-motivating strategy to get into the routine of moving more is to start with some minimal activity and make it a daily habit in your lifestyle. Even now when the old inner resistance comes up, I fool my mind by saying, just 10 minutes, just one round of the park. And once I am down there my body decides when to stop walking.

Take up any activity on a daily basis. It does not have to be the gym if you don't like the gym and it does not have to be early morning if you are a night person. Make it any time of day and any type of activity that fits into your lifestyle. You can play with the kids, climb stairs, park a little further, put on a piece of music and dance to it in the privacy of your room, walk in the mall – absolutely anything as long as you move a little more than usual. You will find that the more you move, the more you would want to move. This is the secret of adding more physical activity into your daily routine.

Third Pillar

Positive, wholesome thoughts are the third pillar. Ultimately, the control center to change our lifestyle is in the head. Unless we change our thinking, we can't really hope to change much in our lives.

For years, I did not like what I saw in the mirror. I disowned the person looking back at me, as she did not meet my ideal image of what I thought I "should" look like. I just rejected everything from my neck downwards refusing to really acknowledge it as my body. This is perhaps what was at the crux of the disconnectedness I felt between my heart and head.

The sub-conscious communication I was giving myself was that I would love myself after I looked like what I wanted to look like. In other words meet some idealized slim and sexy version of myself. And this was clearly not happening for over 20 years! Finally, I realized if I had to shift my relationship with my body, I had to start loving it exactly as it was. Right here. Right now. Not in the future. Not when it looked like this or that but exactly as it was right now.

This was a revelation and I began to be aware of my self-talk or the words I was saying to myself in my head. I realized that I was judgmental and unkind in the way I spoke to myself. So, I cleaned up my act and started talking to myself as I would to a beloved friend. The conversation inside my head changed my relationship with my body and I became aware of the times my body was communicating back with me too to guide and support me. I developed a new respect and love for my body and its infinite and divine intelligence.

I started getting clues, signals and messages that taught me when to eat and when to stop and what my body was asking for in terms of nutrition at any given time. Before putting just about anything in my mouth, I started checking in with my body first and this was a crucial practice which helped me to get to my goals of weight release.

Fourth Pillar

The final pillar is one of habits - the childhood, family and social conditioning that we get set into without questioning. These habits stem from the beliefs we carry around all our lives. We may have inherited these from our family and friends or picked them from our doctor or read it in books and papers or simply followed the societal norms. Sometimes, we just call it our personality and refuse to budge or change anything saying, "I am like this only." This is all inner resistance to change, our invisible dragons that we are meant to slay in our journey to evolution and self-awareness.

More often than not, we are not even sure why we are doing it, but we are doing it e.g. Drinking milk – we do it because everybody does it and the prevailing paradigm is that it is good for health and the best source of calcium. As if God put the cow on Earth to provide calcium for humans. How come no other animal on the planet needs cow's milk for its calcium needs? Say an elephant, a horse or a deer? Once I started questioning the established paradigms and norms, my body started revealing the reality and truth of the moment and my true education began.

I realized that the body never lies and is always in the present moment. The mind lies constantly and its predominant nature is fear, doubt and judgment. However, if we can love our minds with understanding, we can access the wisdom of our bodies. Our bodies have the capacity to guide us home about our health and physical wellbeing. We don't really need any external expert to do this for us. In fact the entire healing system of "Natural Hygiene" or "Naturopathy" is based on the self-healing capacity of the body. All we have to do to heal ourselves is to get out of our own way and let the body do what it knows to do best which is to maintain a state of health.

Incorrect beliefs about what is the right food to eat are very strong and hard to release. Then there are unhealthy and addictive habits like smoking, drinking, chewing *gutka*, which we may have picked along the way and now we are hooked to them. Seeming less harmful but being equally addictive and harmful to our health is addiction to tea, sugar and fast foods like pizza and burgers or processed foods like fried *namkeens*, chips, commercially sold *mithais*, packaged noodles and biscuits etc.

Not doing some form of physical exercise is also a habit that is difficult to break and so are mental addictions like playing the victim and blaming everyone else for everything that goes wrong in our lives.

In my 12-week program, designed to help people adopt healthier and more wholesome lifestyles, we explore all the four pillars. Health is not just about food or just about exercise or just about spirituality or just about having a few good habits; it is multi-dimensional and permeates every aspect of our existence. Becoming aware of all these four aspects brought me back to wholeness and helped me integrate my disjointed heart, body, mind and soul.

I am eternally grateful to the many teachers that have guided and inspired me on this journey to live a more connected and abundant life. I wish you the very best of health and much happiness.

Nandini Gulati is a Holistic Health Coach. She offers many programs to help people lead healthier and integrated lifestyles. The programs range from one time consulting, healthy cooking classes to a 12-week customized health-coaching program. She is affiliated with Dr. Nandita Shah of SHARAN who is working in the area of preventing and reversing lifestyle diseases like diabetes, high blood pressure, high cholesterol, heart disease, asthma, allergies, thyroid and many other lifestyle related health issues. SHARAN organizes one-week retreats and even a 3-week retreat once a year, which is successful in reversing many illnesses just within 21 days!

www.nandinigulati.com

CHAPTER 24

Program your mind to a slim body

Preeti Subberwal

Growing at an annual rate of more than 10% for the past five years, the market for weight-loss products – methodologies and procedures, diets, drugs, supplements, services, devices, accessories and cosmetics in 2014 is projected to reach close to $600 billion. In spite of all these developments in weight-loss industry, obesity is constantly on increase.

So why don't most people lose the desired weight even though they have tried over and over?

This question has been bothering so many of us for so many years. Most people make the decision to exercise and eat right but some challenge comes up that sabotages their weight loss plans and they give up. However we know of other people who one day determined to lose weight and became healthier than anyone ever imagined. If we understand the crucial distinction that makes the difference between these different set of people, we can be a part of the ones who get the desired results.

Why Diets don't work?

Extensive studies show that around 95 per cent of all people who lose weight through dieting alone subsequently put it back on again. Most of the diets rely solely on restriction of food intake and no way teach people to eat healthily, nor help them to modify their lifestyle. So, once you are off the diet, you return to your old eating habits and start piling your weight back on. Moreover fad diets and unnatural calorie restriction actually causes your body to store fat more effectively, and create cravings for high-calorie foods thus drive you to bingeing no matter how strong your self-control is.

Weight Loss, a quite complex issue!

The process of weight loss is complicated and challenging because it is not just about shedding pounds, it is about the awareness of how do you sense food cravings. And it is a commitment towards personal change, which is always insight-out.

As obesity is not simply a function of laziness, emotional instability, poor eating habits, lack of exercise or any other factor, there are several different areas that probably need addressing for each individual regarding weight loss. And there may be lots of different types of temptations and issues that can come to light when weight problem is properly dealt with. Perhaps you need to sit down with someone close to you and discuss all the issues surrounding your current situation such as what you have tried in the past, what succeeded and what was difficult for you.

Is your behavior under your control?

The problem is that we believe we have more control over our behavior than we really do. Stress, anxiety and addiction can limit the conscious control you have over your choices. What drives your behavior is not logic but brain biochemistry, habits and addiction, states of consciousness and the people in your environment. We are emotional beings with the ability to rationalize and not rational beings with emotions. If we are stressed, depressed or addicted, no matter how good the advice we are given, chances are that we will not be able to act on it.

Why are you not thin yet?

There can be any of these patterns that may be responsible for your inability to lose weight till now.

Pattern one: Obsessive Dieting (Are you a Yo-Yo Dieter?)

Pattern two: Emotional Eating (Are you a Comfort eater or the Depressed Overeater?)

Pattern three: Faulty Programming (Are you unable to visualize yourself thin?)

May be you have other problematic patterns like speed eating and eating quickly can delay the onset of 'fullness'. A lot of us were brought up not to leave food on our plates and you may not be able to resign the clean plate club.

Fitness starts in your head

Our body is the result of the choices we make. You don't have right to complain about your body if you are not willing to change. You must make health and vitality a must and choose to eat right, exercise regularly and treat your body with respect. You don't have to be more fit than anyone else. You just have to be fit than you ever thought you could be. **Fitness is not 50% exercise and 50 % diet but it is a 100% commitment to diet and exercise.** It is rightly said that food is the most abused anxiety drug and exercise is the most underutilized anti-depressant.

Enough of all such excuses!

- No time
- Too busy
- May be tomorrow
- Not enough motivation
- I love food
- No willpower
- I hate exercise
- Too tired
- Too hard

If working out is important for you, find a way, if not, you find an excuse.

So are you ready to do something different?

Now just imagine if salads could be more appealing than ice creams and exercise could be something to enjoy. How much sense of control you could have felt?

Using mind programming techniques and models, you can change your habits so that you can lose weight easily and effectively. Our brain works on pain-pleasure principle. And you can utilize this principle for your benefit instead of being a victim to this principle. You can program your mind to associate enough pain for overeating and eating junk and immense pleasure for eating health and exercising.

Weight loss through mind programming aims to help you to achieve permanent weight loss by breaking the patterns and habits of poor or over eating and take control of your hunger and weight. Taking a psychological approach can help you deal with the hidden patterns behind poor eating and over-eating as they occur deep in your unconscious mind. Such an approach can be helpful in the following areas:

- Build up and maintain your motivation to lose weight
- Prevent you from over eating
- Motivate you to exercise
- Help you make the right choices about the food you eat.
- May even train you to eat slower
- Deal with any issues you may have with regard to losing weight
- Control your cravings
- Overcome anxiety, depression and mood swings
- Learn to be completely satisfied with smaller portions of food
- Eliminate emotional baggage and control emotional eating

Motivate yourself to create the body you desire.

Muscle weighs much more than fat but it is much better to look at. You don't have to be great to start, but you have to start to be great. Some statements that you can use to charge yourself up:

- I have reached the threshold, I must lose weight now.
- I must take complete responsibility for creating the desired body.
- I believe in my ability to get in shape.
- My past failures in losing weight don't bother me anymore.

- Metabolism is not something constant, and I can easily increase my metabolism.

Get clarity about what you really want and use the power of goal setting

- What is your goal for your health?
- What is most important to you? (Your longevity, your energy, your shape, avoiding disease, being healthy enough to enjoy your children or grandchildren?)
- Be clear why it is compelling for you - Why are you absolutely committed to create a light and healthy body?
- When you set a goal for yourself, it is important to understand exactly what actions are necessary for you to achieve your goal.
- Visualize your desired body to direct yourself to your result.

Get rid of your food compulsions and choose to eat healthily

What are some of the behaviors that keep you from doing that that you currently engage in?

Every action begins with an emotion. For example, if you have a habit of over-eating, there is an emotion and a chain of behaviors that lead you to overeat.

Because the location of hunger is usually experienced between the centers of the chest to just below the bellybutton – in the exact places that we tend to generate our emotional feelings. Hunger is not an emotion, but it does tend to occur in the places that we feel our emotions. No wonder then that some people get it so confused.

When you eat right you feel right. Junk food that you crave for a few moments is far insignificant than the body you wanted for years. The junk food that looks good out there looks bad when it is stored as fat on your body. Keep reminding yourself that it is just food, it cannot control you, and it doesn't have any magical power.

**Make Exercise a pleasure, not just a chore.
Get the urge to move every day!**

What do you hate more – a 30 minute workout or those 30 extra pounds?

30 minute of being uncomfortable with exercise is much better than being uncomfortable for life.

Believe it or not exercise is not the 8-letter version of work. It can be fun. A great workout helps you detoxify yourself mentally and physically. Let exercise be your stress reliever and not the food! Losing weight means you look good in clothes, exercising means you can look good even without clothes. Complaining won't burn calories, only exercising will. Workout as if your life depends on it and it certainly does. For every minute, thinking about whether you should workout or not, you could be working out. The more you sweat during the workout, the less you cry on the scale. So blast that music and work it out!

Affirmations for making you enjoy your workout:

- You see a sweat, I see a glow.
- I don't have the time to work out, I make time.
- On good days, I work out, on bad days, I work out harder.
- I wear black when I work out; it's like funeral of my fat.

Commit to yourself:

- I will take the required action
- I will eat healthy food
- I will drink lots of water
- I will exercise regularly
- I will get enough sleep

I Will See The Desired Results

Preeti Subberwal is the Founding Director of Thoughtful Engagement, a firm that facilitates quick and sustainable change and transformation in individuals and organizations through powerful and innovative programs. As a Transformational Coach and a Facilitator, she is passionately committed to deliver personal and professional development workshops, seminars and coaching programs that empower the participants to attain their next level of success, fulfillment and self-mastery. She is a Certified Master of Spirit Life Coach, Certified Life Coach, Licensed NLP Master Practitioner and Theta Healing Practitioner. She believes in the holistic approach to wellbeing and leadership that promotes mind, body and spirit unification.

www.thoughtfulengagement.com

CHAPTER 25

Allowing the Magic to unfold: Access Consciousness

Seema Sharma

The Essence

Do you remember the unfettered, unbridled bundle of energy you were as a child?

Everything was bright and shiny; the sound of your giggles and laughter reverberated everywhere you went...

Whatever you did, you did for the joy of it and nothing else mattered! What happened to that?

When did you learn to be serious?

When did you learn that laughing heartily was ridiculous?

When did you learn to be realistic and put aside all those dreams you thought were so within your reach?

Who sold you the lie that life was a struggle?

Who made you believe that you were limited by this reality?

Whose reality did you entrain to?

Whose limitations did you buy as real and solid and then built your reality around that?

These are some of the questions I have been pondering on and strangely just asking these questions, leaves me feeling lighter and expansive. The invisible weight on my shoulders lifts and I feel connected with the Universe and the magic of possibilities.

Holistic Wellness in the New Age

All our gurus and scriptures tell us that we are infinite beings with infinite capabilities, yet for all practical purposes, we believe our limitations are more real than our potential, and create a life based on limitations rather than possibilities. I wonder why that is so.

Elephants that are huge and powerful animals are made to wear a metal anklet when they are a baby, which hurts them if they try to pull on the rope attaching it to the pole it is tethered to. They get entrained to this pain and even as adult powerful animals believe they cannot pull on the flimsy chain tethered to a small wooden pole even though they are capable of pulling away an entire tree.

Interestingly and sadly so, we humans are disempowered too by similar beliefs which are untrue yet we believe those to be the truth. How many of us would like to create and have a better life, a better job, better finances, better relationships, but are held back by seeming limitations of background, religion, gender, finances, pedigree, education, language, credentials etc.?

How many of us stop dreaming about a better life as we grow up, as the limitations that we think we have seemed to loom large in front of us? What if all those limitations that we bought from our parents as the ultimate truth for us, were just beliefs that could be changed? What would happen if we began to question those beliefs that we bought as true for us? What if the beliefs that worked for our parents did not really work for us? What would it take for us to begin to question those beliefs and change what does not ring true for us?

Access Consciousness

I have always been a seeker all my life. The search for answers to basic questions about life, about suffering, about pain, misery and sadness continued to bother me and I attended seminars, classes, read books looking for solutions and solace. I enjoyed learning Reiki, Quantum Touch, EFT, Pranic healing, Theta healing etc. As I look back, starting from Bhakti marg each one of the teachings I came across offered a special nugget that was just right for me at that time of my life, the search continued and my life continued to heal itself just like Louise Hay says - You can heal your life, and indeed you can!

Access Consciousness entered my life like a fresh breeze of ease. Like most of the people who will pick this book, I have been a seeker, looking for ways to ease pain and suffering for self and others. Access is a large toolbox with tools to deal with just about everything. There are verbal processes, bodywork, and tools that can be used to shift and change anything that you would like to change. Having used these tools for the last almost a year and a half, I now feel empowered and at ease with most things in life. There have been other modalities that I have studied and applied over the years that have contributed greatly as well, and Access has given the key to areas of my life that I had made peace with, having concluded that those areas were immutable and hence could not be changed.

Do you remember the exuberance you had as a child, when no pain or suffering lasted for more than 10 seconds and you were happily skipping about seeing rainbows and joy oozed out of your being? Remember that questioning spirit you had? And no question was too silly, you could ask ten question in a row of how, when, why, what about everything you came across?

Where is that spirit of question now? Did it get smothered when the parents and teachers told you that your questions were too silly? Or did you perceive the sadness and defeat your questions invoked in them and therefore you suppressed the urge to ask questions about changing stuff and started mimicking their way of maintaining the status quo? Did they say you wasted too much time asking questions when you should be learning the answers in your text books that you found too boring? When did that boisterous spirit of knowing that you could change everything and that everything was mutable got smothered? When did you decide that by aligning and agreeing with "this is how things are in our family" you could help create peace in your world? Or did you choose the other way round of resisting and reacting to "this is how things are in our family" as your way of creating peace and change in your world?

Has any of that worked for you? If yes, please don't read further. If not, please continue.

Being in the Question

One of the biggest takeaways from Access Consciousness for me has been – to stay in the spirit of being in the question. Growing up, becoming serious about life, meant I had to give up that boisterous questioning spirit in favor of seeking the theory- of- the- correct- way- of- living- life. Somewhere I also began to suppress my own knowing about what was right for me, in favor of seeking answers from the adults who had more experience and therefore knew better than me. I thought I could create a nice life for myself learning from other people's lives, trying to come to conclusions about what worked in other people's lives and could therefore work in my life as well.

Unfortunately, this trying to live by proxy hasn't worked very well for me. Somewhere along the line, I gave up being me in favor of trying to become what worked for other people rather than myself. As we start to live from conclusions, we begin to shut off the magic of the Universe and limit the possibilities of change showing up in our lives. Access encouraged me to start asking questions, and the best thing was I did not have to have the answers! It was a bit confusing as first and the habit of staying in conclusions or finding conclusions is so ingrained that it doesn't come naturally to me to ask questions.

So what happens when I remember to ask questions? Magic shows up, synchronicities happen! It can't be that easy now, can it? Well how can that be? Indeed how can that be? Well, the way to go about it is that you ask a question and then get out of the way, yes, get out of your own way! What happens when we ask a question to the Universe is that it starts the quantum entanglements in favor of our question. Everything is interconnected, and in response to our question, the Universe begins to rearrange itself to offer the most creative and best ways to bring to us what we asked for. There are no co-incidences indeed; it is all coming to us through our own creations. But when we ask a question and come to a conclusion, we limit the Universe and shut down the myriad pathways that opened up. It's like planting a seed one moment, and pulling it out the next to see if it has grown yet.

On the other hand when we ask a question without coming to a conclusion and stay out of being vested in the outcome, the Universe gets to work for us and opens up quantum entanglements so that the energy that matches the energy of our request, brings together more such energies and new pathways get created and the people or circumstances required for the fulfillment of our desire come to us without too much effort on our part. It still requires some 'doing' but this 'doing' happens with ease, without the 'struggle' part.

Making a demand of the Universe

Sometimes I ask the Universe to show me magic, show me the gifts that I have that I haven't acknowledged. And magic gets created in so many ways. Money flows in unexpected. In sessions with people, the contribution they were looking for appears effortlessly, there is no hard work required, and it is a seamless match of demand and supply, simultaneous gifting and receiving for both.

The Process

Access Consciousness Bars

We have learned a lot of concepts through the Law of Attraction, Jerry and Esther Hicks (and now Esther) talk a lot about Ask and its Given, and so many beautiful ways of allowing the Universe to gift to us. With Access, using all of these concepts has become easier and effortless. 'Access Bars' is a therapy that makes 'receiving' from the Universe easier, each Bars session helps to release limiting beliefs that do not allow us to receive freely.

The Bars is a hands-on process that requires gentle touching of 32 points on the head, the worst that can happen after a Bars session is that you feel as if you had a good head massage, and the best your whole life could change. The Bars are designed to open you up to receiving from the Universe, that too without much effort on your part. You just need to lie down and allow the practitioner to touch some points on your head. How does it get any better than this? There are Bars points for money, control, creativity, time, hopes, body, etc. and when the practitioner touches these points gently, limiting beliefs, thoughts, emotions related to that area get released in the form of electromagnetic charge resulting in greater peace and ease in these areas.

Personally for me just this one process itself has brought in so much ease within my life that I can hardly recognize myself. Each Bars session brings in more peace and more ease, the stress melts away as if by magic. I feel so liberated and light now. There were some incidents from the past that I was holding on to, and those incidents defined my story and as Eckhart Tolle would call it – when the "Pain Body" surfaced, those incidents and the charge of trauma, pain, sadness, victimization etc. would rear its head and I would recreate the trauma and add charge to it to feed the "Pain Body" and quite surprisingly now, there is no charge on any of those incidents and no need, and no desire to feed the "Pain Body" as well. This has been a huge contribution not just to my life but to the lives of my immediate family as well, since my energy affects not just myself but all of them too.

Verbal Processing

While giving a bars session to one of my clients, I sensed the bars for money to be running with a lot of intensity, and asked if the client would like some verbal processes to facilitate more change in the money area. He agreed and we ran some verbal processes after which he relaxed so much that he slept through the rest of the session. Much to my delight, the next day he shared that he experienced a financial breakthrough in a case that he was following up for the past six months.

Verbal processing is a unique way of changing energy around things we wish to change. When we talk about an issue that we wish to address, there's an energy that comes up and around the subject. This energy is the solid wall that gets in the way of our changing the things that we wish to change. This energy could come from either aligning or agreeing with others, or resisting or reacting to them; instead of choosing from the space of being ourselves. It could also be the limitations that other people think are real and solid for them but not necessarily true for us. Access has a clearing statement that clears up the energy that gets in the way of this change. The verbal processing brings up this charge of limitations and shifts the energy thereby making it possible for change to happen with ease.

The Technique:

I would like to introduce some tools for you to use in everyday life. One of the tools that I use most of the time is – HDIGABTT. Its not Greek speak, it stands for How Does It Get Any Better Than This – use it for when things are going great so you get more of the good stuff, and use it when things are not going great to come to something better. An example of this which is often shared during Access seminars is – a lady learned this tool and on her way home, she found a Dime on the pavement, she picked it up and said, how does it get any better than this? Went a bit further and found $10 on the floor, and gleefully asked, how does it get any better than this? She took a cab home and found a diamond bracelet and what did she say – it doesn't get any better than this! This illustrates the way what we say affects the vibration we are in, which affects how the Universe responds to us. The energy of "how does it get any better than this?" is expansive and full of possibilities, whereas the energy of "it doesn't get any better than this!" is that of closure and conclusions and there's no room left for further possibilities to show up.

I have been using this tool along with "What else is possible?" for every situation that I find sticky and it works like a charm every time. Have you ever noticed how we are conditioned to look at and prepare for everything that can go wrong, do we ever spend time looking at what could go right? Or if we share our plans with others they tell us to stop daydreaming and come back to the reality of how things are supposed to be difficult by default. How often do we come to conclusions about things we can't change and give up on things we would like to be or have? What if instead of giving up we could just ask this one question (even if we don't have the answers right away) - 'What else is possible that I haven't even considered'? This opens up possibilities that we haven't even conceived of! It's like opening doors, windows and balconies in a corridor that earlier had solid walls with just one door at either end, so now we can see and explore options from a fresh perspective rather than looking at things the way everyone else does from the limited perspective.

Likewise there are a lot of tools that Access offers to bring ease into everyday life. What would it take for you to play with some of these tools and create a life with ease and joy?

Another thought that I would like to leave you with is – Is this a benevolent, abundant Universe or a Universe of lack and scarcity? What happens when we allow Nature to be, does it thrive? What would happen if we get out of our conclusions, limitations and control over our lives and our future? Would we allow the magic of the Universe into our lives? Could we???

Seema Sharma is a certified Access Consciousness Bars Facilitator; a Marketing and Corporate Communications professional, she always had an active interest in Energy healing techniques. She practices healing modalities including Reiki, Quantum Touch, Pranic Healing, Theta Healing, Aura Reading, Past Life Regression, EFT and Ho'oponopono among others.

seemasharma.accessconsciousness.com

The Body Approch

CHAPTER 26

Ozone – Nature's Detox Doctor & Healing Superhero

Dr. Paula Horan

The Essence

Have you ever noticed how a shower takes away all of your tiredness as it removes the sweat and dirt, and makes you feel refreshed and rejuvenated? It is the first thing you need to relax after a hard day at work. In a similar way, cleansing our system of toxins or pollutants internally is all we need to help our body maintain a robust mechanism.

Ozone is the element that is nature's gift to us for cleansing and energizing internally. It is revolutionizing medicine when it comes to healing and rejuvenation and its applications and benefits are evolving as we make progress in our understanding of it. However despite its proven benefits for over a century and the fact that it has no side effects, ozone treatment has not yet entered the mainstream of alternative healing.

As a result of general lack of knowledge regarding ozone and lack of access to ozone clinics, millions of people are either unaware or cannot avail of its benefits. It is my deep aspiration to spread knowledge and awareness about this wonderful element which can help us maintain our well being in the midst of our environmentally challenged lives, where we need to be constantly attentive to an ever increasing army of free radicals, heavy metals, pollutants, not to mention the mental and emotional toxicity that we gather everyday.

My own experience with Ozone tells me that it is by far the best and simplest method for detoxifying the body, which is a basic requirement for any kind of healing, be it for an acute or chronic ailment. And here I will present a basic idea of what Ozone is, how it works, its healing properties, applications and how you can combine it with other modes of treatment for faster healing and recovery.

It will surprise many people that Ozone and its healing properties were discovered more than 150 years ago. We all know that Ozone plays an important role in our atmosphere's composition as it protects life forms on earth from harmful radiation of the Sun. Few are aware however of Ozone's important effects on our body. Ozone is actually the most powerful regulator of our immune system. It is the main component in the redox system, which maintains a perfect balance between oxygenation and oxidation (between energizing our cells and burning up old dead, weak or damaged cells). It thus acts as a natural cleanser that keeps your system free of germs, viruses, fungi and pollutants, and it boosts your metabolism and increases the oxygen content of your cells which is all you need to become free from any diseases.

Medical doctors learn briefly about the redox system, but the medical texts themselves basically misguide young medical students as they focus only on the dangers of oxidation and not so much on the positive aspects and even the essential nature of it. All free radicals are thought of as bad (which most are) but little or nothing is mentioned of the good free radical: the extra O1 in triatomic oxygen or ozone, and how it can actually discern the difference between healthy and weak cells and will only oxidize weak or damaged cells (contrary to chemo therapy which is a free radical that attacks and burns up even healthy cells).

The Process

What is Ozone and how does it work?

Ozone is a naturally occurring form of elemental oxygen, which is essential in maintaining homeostasis or natural balance on the planet.

Ozone is tri atomic oxygen, which means it has three atoms of oxygen temporarily held together. Because only two oxygen atoms can bond with each other, the third atom remains free to attach with any other atom. Oxygen being a beneficial element, the third atom becomes a positive free radical and this is what makes it a powerful oxidant. Thus ozone oxidizes any negative free radical i.e. pollutants and effectively burns them up.

Holistic Wellness in the New Age

Ozone in the atmosphere does the same thing on a macro level, neutralizing the pollutants in the air and in the water, in the same way our body does on a micro level by oxidizing the toxins in our body.

It has been determined by scientists at Scripps Institute, La Jolla, California that the human body itself produces certain amounts of Ozone to oxidize its own pollutants. This happens during the process when antibodies also known as immuno-globulins fight off bacteria and kills them. However if there is any disturbance in the number or efficiency of antibodies it is certain that the body's capacity to produce its own ozone is affected, which is the case with most people having severe or complicated health problems.

The following statement from Tom Harrelson elucidates the connection between ozone and the cleansing of toxins in our body: *"Since body is mostly water, and ozone is primarily used throughout the world to eliminate any chemicals or pathogens in the water supply, than it stands to reason that ozone will also do the same for water in your body, to clean and heal itself more efficiently."*

If you look at the industrial uses of Ozone you can easily draw parallels to the kinds of benefits it can offer our body, which is no less complicated than a giant industrial plant with all its various systems serving different functions.

Ozone and Healing:

Ozone therapy can truly be called a futuristic as well as holistic healing method because it does not foster the divisive approach of modern medicine that approaches every disease state as a battle to be conquered, leaning on the fight and kill idea. Rather ozone therapy works by changing the very ground on which this so called battle of body v/s pathogens happens.

And that ground is that of toxic waste, in the absence of which the battle ends and we regain our well being. The popularly accepted idea that the cause of disease is a germ or bacteria or virus is the result of the skewed perspective and manipulation of scientific studies done by ignorant scientists who were only looking at the subject from an isolated view.

Pathogens are always present in the body, which has sufficient mechanisms to keep their activity in check and maintain our health. However, the real cause of disease is the filthy pile of toxic waste which when not eliminated becomes a veritable breeding ground for pathogens. As any game is a numbers game, the antibodies lose out to the fast increasing pathogens, which accumulate in a body overloaded with toxins and we fall sick.

However in truth, it is not the disease itself that is the real threat, it is our body's unhealthy environment, which fosters disease that is the real cause of concern. If the toxic waste can be eliminated harmlessly, our body's well being can be assured. And nothing works better than ozone in this case.

Ozone acts as a panacea, as it frees our system from its toxic waste without any harm, enabling healing to happen naturally as the body gains control over its various systems. If applied in the right way, Ozone therapy can eliminate the need for many expensive and complicated treatments and minimize the time of recovery.

We need to regularly detoxify our body; it is a need of the hour with ever increasing pollution and adulteration in our food and the chemical attack through many other products, if we do so we can give our body the clean environment it needs to stay healthy.

Instead of purchasing innumerable drugs to cure the countless ailments we face, we should rather shift our focus towards good nourishment and detoxification, which can fortify our body against any impending danger. Such is the efficacy of this approach that you can live fearlessly despite the threat of so often health hazards highlighted by the media and medical fraternity.

The Benefits of Ozone

In the same way you need a diamond to cut a diamond; free radicals can only be hunted by another free radical. While pollutants are negative free radicals, ozone acts as a positive free radical and thus it kills or disables the negative free radical without causing any harm to the healthy cells.

The negative free radicals are responsible for causing degeneration, aging and morbid conditions like cancer. Ozone with its O1 free radical only eliminates the diseased cell and does no harm to the healthy cells, how this happens has been explained in detail in my book, 'Heal Yourself with Oxygen', but for a simplistic understanding I will explain how it works.

What happens is that the harmful free radicals have a positive electronic charge and the ozone free radical or O1 has a negative electronic charge and as we know opposites attract. The negative charge of the ozone attracts the pilfering toxic waste carrying the positive charge and neutralizes it and carries it out of the body. The antioxidants contained in all the healthy cells are actually helping the process of oxidation. And all the healthy cells are bypassed when the O1 seeks its pairing and thus the healthy cells remain unaffected.

Unlike chemotherapy where healthy cells are also destroyed and the body is weakened, ozone therapy does no harm to the healthy cells and rejuvenates the body besides cleansing it. Considering this benefit, ozone therapy should be the primary method for treating not just cancer but many other ailments.

It is important to know that, oxidation is a very key process of the body without which the toxic waste cannot be neutralized and flushed out. The body has its own mechanism for oxidation to occur; however ozone also acts very much in the same manner as an external catalyst and boosts the process. When a person is suffering from severe disease and has high levels of toxic waste in the body, we need vigorous oxidation and the way to do this is to give an external catalyst to the system like ozone.

Thus if the process of oxidation in the body can be boosted and regulated, any disease can be easily controlled. Some key benefits of Ozone are that –

- It disinfects the blood by destroying bacteria, viruses and fungi and by oxidizing chemicals and heavy metals.
- It improves circulation by breaking down the clumping and rouleaux formation of red blood cells.
- It stimulates the antioxidant system and it is a metabolic regulator.
- It has marked effect on cellular metabolism.
- It corrects intra cellular hypoxia (poor oxygenation) by regulating the mitochondria respiratory chain
- It activates the nutritional exchange in the cell.
- Stimulates and modulates the immune system.

A detailed explanation of how these benefits actually take place is given in the book. And readers can find in depth information on various internal physical processes and how they parallel the way ozone purifies the oceans, lakes and streams of the planet when it blends with the H20 in the clouds and rains down as hydrogen peroxide.

The Spiritual Aspect of Detoxification

In my own experience, all suffering is a wakeup call to see where we are out of balance in life. Serious ailments that shock us out of our slumber, give us an opportunity to finally tune in with awareness, to listen to the body/mind and integrate the different aspects of our life that we have been out of touch with.

For the mind it is awareness and observation which fosters growth and for the body it is the cellular metabolism which is the key to well being. Both must be tended to. Cells are the primary unit of the body, and thus if your body is healthy on a cellular level you experience wellbeing. Cells thrive on two main ingredients, water and oxygen and thus if we supply our body with sufficient water and take in good amounts of oxygen, we can support our body in maintaining its systems without any malfunction or disturbance.

Health and wellbeing are required by everyone, no matter what our focus in life is. However for those who wish to wake up and are working toward their spiritual evolution, they especially need regular detoxification to ensure that their efforts are not dampened by a lack of cellular well being.

This is the very reason why fasting has been practiced by seekers in all traditions, as it is a natural way of detoxification. With today's lifestyle however, unless you do periodic retreats, you cannot avoid day-to-day activities, which need your time and energy. In such a condition, long fasting is neither feasible nor advisable. It is for this situation that Ozone therapy can be used to obtain the similar benefits.

The state of our body and mind is not different and each affects the other; they truly are one continuum. Thus, if your body is full of toxins and waste, it will hamper your experience of the movement of finer energies in your body and your awareness will be affected as a result. Only an efficient vehicle can sustain you for a long journey and your physical wellbeing is the first and foremost condition for developing your spiritual practice.

Many pollutants also directly affect our thoughts and emotions and conditions like bipolar disorder, depression, fatigue, lack of interest, confusion etc. are caused by the presence of many of these harmful toxins in our blood.

This statement by Dr. Kurt Donsbach illustrates how mind's activity is related to the oxygen activity in the body; he says, *"Negative Mental attitudes can become a major factor in oxygen depletion. Think for a moment perhaps you remember the last time you felt depressed. Were you breathing in a shallow fashion? In addition, the very thought patterns that are associated with negativity and depression produce toxins in the body that increase the need for detoxifying oxygen."*

To include certain practices for our wellbeing and to follow them with discipline is a very small effort to make in order to gain health and longevity. Relying on drugs and taking an approach that deals with symptoms and not with the actual causal factor of disease, only leads us to suffering both financially and physically.

It is high time that we shift gears and adopt this simple and very basic therapy in our life and minimize the environmental impact on our body. When we ascertain our well being in a holistic way such as with the use of therapeutic ozone, we also contribute to the wellness of the earth and its ecosystem because we are the part of that same ecosystem and we are interconnected to all the various streams of life forms and life-elements of the earth.

The Myths about Ozone

Like any other alternative healing method, Ozone also has many misconceptions and myths surrounding its applications and benefits. It is important that people become aware of the true facts about Ozone therapy so that they can dispel their doubts and make the prudent decision to incorporate Ozone in their treatment.

A general myth about Ozone is that it is a toxic gas. The media, because of its ignorance of the whole story, propagates that high Ozone count in the atmosphere can cause allergies and irritation. However the truth is that Ozone is present along with pollutants to oxidize and thus burn them up. It is the burned up residue of pollutants until dispersed that remain in the atmosphere, which causes irritation to our lungs.

The fact is, in today's heavily polluted atmosphere, the ozone amount is low compared to the smog, which means the process of oxidation is never complete. Thus the burned pollutants are not able to fully disperse, which is what causes the actual problem to the lungs. In the same way if we breathe ozone directly, because we have so many toxins in our lungs, the ozone will immediately burn them up and we end up coughing from the left over residue that has just been oxidized. Thus ozone itself is not the culprit. If the air we breathed was pure we could theoretically breathe ozone without a problem.

The ratio of Ozone to pollutants in smog is 1:3 i.e. pollutants are three times greater in quantity compared to ozone, however Ozone is often illustrated as the main component of smog and the highly harmful chemical pollutants are often not mentioned. This has created a gross misunderstanding about ozone and an understandable apprehension in people about Ozone and its application in therapy.

If only the media were to act responsibly and do serious research and people could become more aware about the essential role ozone plays in both the health of the planet as well as the human body, Ozone would not be looked upon as a toxic or dangerous substance.

Another myth about Ozone is that it is very unsafe to use in therapy. It is true that when taken directly into the lungs continuously, it can be harmful for the reasons listed above, however when breathed through oil (turpene) it can also heal tuberculosis. When used in the right concentration, Ozone is very beneficial. It is an obvious fact that any substance when used in extreme quantities will be harmful, (you can drown from drinking too much water), and so Ozone is not an exception to that.

Ozone's benefits are extensive in the various medical applications, which have been used on millions of people in Russia, Germany and Cuba. Industrial use of Ozone is well established and many people are using ozonators in their homes as well. When applied with the right guidance, Ozone therapy can work wonders for your body.

In a study done by the German Ozone Society in 1980, 644 therapists gave Ozone infusions to over 3,84, 775 people and only 0.007 percent reported side effects which were also only due to improper administration of the infusion. None of the side effects were serious or fatal, which is nothing compared to the thousands of annual deaths reported in America due to the side effects of dangerous prescription drugs.

In reality Ozone is a much safer therapeutic tool compared to what most allopathic treatment has to offer. People should be encouraged to work with alternative therapists to study about Ozone therapy and make a confident choice of using it for regular detoxification.

The Tip:

Applications of Ozone

The applications of Ozone are as varied as its benefits. Ozone therapy can be used for almost any ailment from malaria to cancer, allergies, infections, arthritis, diabetes, migraine etc. and even in diseases like HIV or AIDS.

Ozone therapy can also be used for Hair treatment, Eye Rejuvenation, Skin treatment etc. Besides an infusion of Ozonized saline for degenerative diseases, you can also drink freshly Ozonized Water, use Ozonized Oil for Massage and take Ozone steam bath and Vaginal Insufflation.

The book 'Heal Yourself with Oxygen' illustrates in great detail the various applications of Ozone mentioned here. Another area where Ozone treatment is making headway is dentistry. Ozone helps to stop the seeping of blood and thus it is very useful in dental surgeries. More important, it fully sterilizes the tooth in a way no other chemical compound can, giving the tooth a better chance to heal and not become decayed under the new filling. The upcoming edition of the book covers an entire chapter only on the application of ozone in dentistry.

It covers a new form of dentistry (Minimally Invasive Dentistry) which avoids high speed drills entirely that destroy the enamel on your teeth, which in turn, allows decay to seep in within a very short time. Also Biomimetic Dentistry - the science of rebuilding overly treated teeth without having to use crowns and effectively destroy the whole tooth is discussed. This is vital information not only for dentists but also for patients. It is my wish to inform more and more dentists across the world so that they become aware of the new art and science of dentistry which has been around for over thirty years but is still only practiced by about 5% of dentists worldwide due to simple ignorance and the greed of certain industries.

Many amazing experiences have been recorded with Ozone treatment for ailments like cancer, AIDS, Depression, Infertility, Alcoholism, Paralysis, Skin disease, Ulcers and many other problems. Ozone is also used in veterinary treatments as well.

Just like turmeric, basil, honey or any other natural element Ozone is nature's gift for healing. In the same way we use these ingredients everyday in our home remedies, ozone can be integrated into our daily detox program. All we need is awareness about Ozone and the initiative to take action.

In combination with Ozone Therapy, I find that pulsed electromagnetic frequency therapy is very beneficial, because it increases the blood circulation, which then helps carry the toxins out of the body which ozone effectively neutralizes. I personally use the Swiss IMRS machine, which I even carry on my long tours to overcome jet lag quickly (as it recharges the brain as well) and keep myself energized during hectic schedules.

The IMRS machine increases our blood circulation through simulation of the Earth's natural magnetic frequency. It is a technology that was developed after the first Russian who went into space for two weeks came back with strong effects of aging. They eventually discovered it was due to a lack of the earth's electromagnetic energy that he was so depleted. Today, the earth's precious frequency is also depleted due to a number of factors, so even if you walk a lot, you still don't receive the same effect our ancestors once did. Simply lying down on the IMRS mat and soaking in the energy has an amazing effect.

Along with the blood circulation, it boosts the metabolism. It also has varied frequency settings for different ailments and different times of the day. I recently used it to heal a broken toe very quickly. There are many PEMF devices available; however the IMRS is the most comprehensive in terms of "bells and whistles". It can actually measure your heart rate and adjust the frequency to your need at the moment. This has complemented my self-healing practice (Reiki and diet) so well that I have seen some wonderful results in my own energy and stamina.

Normally, a person with an acute ailment can feel the difference very clearly while lying on the mat, whereas with a healthy person, the energy is so subtle it is barely palpable during the treatment. However the relaxation and rejuvenation one feels after a PEMF Treatment is testimony to its effect.

It is important to realize that blood circulation is the most important process of our body. We breathe to provide oxygen to our cells and blood is the carrier of this oxygen. If blood circulation is poor it can lead to many health problems and any healing will not be fully effective if our blood circulation is not at its best. Healthy blood circulation is very crucial to detoxification and can positively affect the detoxification process and reduce the healing time.

Thus, I strongly recommend that people follow a protocol, which includes ways to detoxify and simultaneously boost the circulation. This includes drinking at least three liters of water every day, which improves the viscosity of the blood, doing physical exercise to boost metabolism and making your heart stronger, and to do IMRS therapy on a regular basis.

Many healing results have been experienced by people using PEMF therapy for a number of different physical issues; similar to the way Ozone acts as a panacea for healing. I believe that the combined effect of Ozone and PEMF can do wonders for any patient.

It is essential to remember, we don't need to wait to be sick to avail ourselves of these benefits. In today's world, we need to do regular detoxification with these therapies. Life is always a challenge as we learn and grow. If we are physically and emotionally in good shape, it makes the journey so much easier. Today, ignoring health is like attempting slow suicide, as our bodies are constantly overloaded with toxins even for those with the best diets and exercise schedules. Why wait for a life threatening disease to knock and give you a wakeup call? Make a commitment now to do at least twice a year major cleanouts as well as some form of daily detox.

It is my wish that through what is shared here, the message regarding the significance of Ozone and its role in detoxification and healing be noticed by many. Humanity needs healthy people with open minds, and both need constant care and periodic cleansing to foster a flushing out of the inner dross, in form of both matter and energy.

Dr. Paula (Laxmi) Horan is known worldwide for her numerous books, seminars and retreats on alternative and complimentary therapies, authentic forms of vibrational medicine, integrative body/mind therapeutics and ground-breaking approaches to spirituality and non - dual awareness.

An American Psychologist born in Boston, she lived her childhood years in Italy and Germany. Completing her undergraduate studies in sociology and English literature in Britain, she completed both her MA (focusing on dance therapy) and her Ph.D in psychology at San Diego, California.

From 1992 through 1997, she spent much of her time with her spiritual master Shri H.W.L Poonjaji in India, who gave her the name Laxmi. Shri Poonjaji or 'Papaji', as he was affectionately called, was a self realized being who left his body in September 1997. Quickened by his presence, Paula shifted her focus from self-improvement to the self-inquiry that awakens the quiet stillness of awakened presence.

Another factor in Paula's life that inspired her to become an avid researcher on detoxification and rejuvenation therapies is her personal success in treating both a breast and ovarian tumors with a raw food diet and Reiki. Fifteen years ago she also became acquainted with the therapeutic effects and astonishing benefits of oxygen in its tri-atomic form, ozone, in regard to healing degenerative diseases and also as a restorative rejuvenation therapy. Her knowledge and personal experience in this field has put her at the forefront of longevity treatments and for sustaining peak health in an increasingly challenged environment.

Paula's seminars and retreats on an expansive range of wellness subjects and on non-dual awareness are whole-heartedly received, due to her unique ability to communicate complicated concepts in a simple and easy manner. She is well known for her warmth, for her inspirational teaching style and her enduring smile, indicative of the joy she finds in sharing her knowledge—which enliven and motivate her students to manifest the richness inherent in their lives. Her first book, Empowerment through Reiki has been translated into 20 languages. It was followed by Abundance Through Reiki, Core Empowerment, Reiki – 108 Questions and Answers: Your Dependable Guide For A Lifetime of Reiki Practice, The Ultimate Reiki Touch, The Nine Principles of Self-Healing and Heal Yourself With Oxygen. Her eighth book called Fierce Innocence was out in 2011.

www.paulahoran.com

CHAPTER 27

PEMF – The Fifth Element of Health

Bryant Meyers

The Essence

Pulsed electro-magnetic fields (PEMFs) are an essential element of health. This is why we are calling it "the 5th element of health." Most people are familiar with food, water, and oxygen being essential. Sunlight is also essential.

We now know that there is a fifth element that is equally, if not more important, than some of those others. In fact you can live longer without food and sunlight than you can without the pulsed electro-magnetic fields of the earth. The good news is there are devices now available that actually simulate the earth-based frequencies and can actually charge up all 100 trillion of your cells. This is why we call PEMF a "whole body battery charger."

The Energetic Universe We Live In

Quantum Mechanics predicts that each cubic centimeter of space has at least 10^{52} ergs or energy, which is more then a trillion-trillion nuclear explosions, or a one followed by twenty-four zeros. (1,000,000,000,000,000,000,000,000) An amount of energy like that can drive our galaxy, and its one hundred-billion stars, for a million years! There is that much energy in every little cubic centimeter.

The solar wind is a relentless storm of energy emitted from the sun that race through space at fast and wildly fluctuating speeds of 200-700 km/second. This is actually what creates the Aurora Borealis or "Northern Lights." The Dynamo Theory explains that the magnetic field of the earth is dynamic and changing, not static, and these pulsing flows of energy create an enormous pulsing electro-magnetic field throughout space. Modern cosmology-models predict our visible universe is only 4% of the total energy of the universe, with the remaining being mysterious dark matter and dark energy.

Here on earth, we are in the relentless storm of energy emitted from the sun, along with lightening strikes (several million per day) with roughly 400,000 thunderstorms. These lightning strikes "ring" the metaphorical bell of the earth's ionosphere cavity creating the Schumann waves, a fundamental earth-based pulsed electro-magnetic field of 7.83 Hz (along with higher harmonics mainly in the 0-30Hz range).

The Body Electric

The human body is primarily an energy, or electrical being, and is secondarily chemical. Conventional and alternative medicine proves this. The ancients called this energy "Qi," "Chi," and "Prana." Acupuncture and much of the ancient Eastern Chinese and Japanese therapies are based on an understanding of the energy fields of the body. The Indian system of the chakras and the nadis also understand this idea.

Modern terms for this energy include "Life-force," "Aura," "L-field," "SOEF," "Biophotonics," "Orgone," "The Body Electric" and "Corona Discharge". Here in the West it is becoming overwhelmingly evident, thanks to modern technology, that yes, we are energetic. Conventional MRI's, cat scans, EEG's EKG's EMG's NCV's and other new technologies are showing us that we are primarily energetic.

As far back as 2750 BC electric eels were used by Egyptians to treat headaches and various mental illness. Reportedly Cleopatra slept on and wore a lodestone to keep her skin youthful, and magnets have long been used in China with the ancient art of acupuncture. The ancient Greeks understood this and Plato and Aristotle wrote extensively that many things cannot be identified with, or explained in terms of, [the] physical body.

Today, "Energy Medicine" is a new field of alternative medicine that uses energy instead of chemistry to heal, these include the following: Pulsed Electro-Magnetic Fields, RIFE machines, Radionnics, Zappers, Scenars, Cold Lasers, Infrared Therapy, Ionic Footbaths, Biofeedback defices, Multiwave Oscillators,

Gas Plasma, Scalar Energy Devices, Activated Air, Whole Body Vibration and more.

Yuri Gagarin's Historic Flight

The Russians won the space race with Yuri Gagarin's historic flight around the earth, however he came back in bad shape. When he arrived back on earth he had depression, bone loss, muscle degeneration (had to be carried out on a stretcher) decreased metabolism, and impaired perception. He was only away from the earths pulsed-magnetic fields for a one hour, 48 minute flight around the earth!

Since that historic flight, "Zero Field Studies" (experiments done in chambers made of Mu Steel which blocks all magnetic fields of the earth) have confirmed that if living cells do not receive the pulsed magnetic fields of the earth they die within hours. We now use pulsed-magnetic generators in every space suit and in every space station because we have to! It is an essential element.

Earth-based PEMF's are required elements of health. You can live longer without food, water and sleep then you can live without pulsating electro-magnetic fields. Yuri Gagarin's historic 108-minute trip was the first evidence that PEMF's are critical for life, without them we die, and with not enough we get SICK!

Why Don't We Get Heart Cancer?

Why don't we get heart cancer? Think about that for a minute. One interesting theory is the heart is the most electrical organ. Heart cells have a voltage of 120 millivolts (mV) and in some cases slightly higher. This is almost twice the voltage of some of the other cells in the average person. PEMF acts as a whole-body battery charger by recharging EACH of the 100 trillions cells in the body. Though we can not charge the cells as high as the heart, we can raise the voltage of the cells in our body up 70mV, and even 100 mV or more in the case of high-end athletes. In most people you can get 70-90mV.

PEMF acts like a spark, ignition, or impulse that keeps the cells charged at an ideal voltage. Just like a car, the human body needs fuel, oxygen and ignition – a spark-plug. Within the human body that spark is pulsed magnetic fields. All metabolic processes are driven by this cellular charge: ATP production, oxygen and nutrient absorption, waste removal, defense and reproduction (ATP or adenosine triphosphate is the mainly currency of energy in the body).

According to Nobel Prize Laureate, Dr. Otto Warburg, cells maintain a voltage across their membrane, which is analogous to the voltage of a battery. He found that healthy cells have a measureable voltage from 70-100 millivolts, with the heart cells having the highest (upwards to 110 millivolts).

Dr. Warburg found that due to the constant stress of modern life along with a toxic environment and the aging process, cellular voltage drops. A sick cell looses energy and there is not enough ATP. People with chronic illnesses and chronic fatigue unilaterally had a diminished cellular voltage (30-50 millivolts). Cancer patients displayed the lowest voltage at less than 15-20 millivolts. Cancer cells only have a voltage of 15-20mV and are in anaerobic respiration (creating ATP without oxygen) and need ten times more energy from the environment.

PEMF therapy enhances and improves the uptake, binding and absorption of oxygen, allows nutrients to be assimilated and delivered better. Earth-based PEMF also enhances your water-based blood and lymph so it has an ideal pH, voltage, lower surface tension (viscosity), which enhances microcirculation so that essential minerals, vitamins, amino acids, fatty acids, nutrients, water and oxygen are delivered to cells, and absorbed by the cells. This gives cells all they need to create energy, mainly in the form of ATP and the cellular voltage across the cell membrane.

NOW you can see why earth-based PEMF is literally a whole body battery recharger, capable of energizing and "charging-up" your 100 trillion cells with energy and life!

The 2-Fold Problem – Not enough of the Good and Too Much of the Bad

But there is a problem when it comes to the earth's natural geomagnetic field and Schumann resonances. The problem is two-fold: first we are simply not getting enough of the good earth PEMF and magnetism due to a decline in the earth's magnetic field and the growing trend of people spending time indoors in shielded structures (that partially block the earth's fields). The second problem is the increasing exposure to unhealthy electrosmog from cell phones, power lines, cellphone towers, cordless phones, TV, computers, microwaves, hair dryers, Wi-Fi, Bluetooth, etc. To put it simply, we are getting not enough of the GOOD (earth PEMFs) and we are getting too much of the BAD (electrosmog, negative

EMFs). We are unplugged from nature and plugged into artificial energies from our modern world. To be healthy we need to reverse this trend and plug into nature and unplug as much as possible from unhealthy electrosmog.

Remember that natural earth geomagnetic and Schumann frequencies are essential, just like food, water and oxygen. We just are not getting enough exposure to the life nurturing and life enhancing pulsed magnetic energy of the earth. But fortunately, like nutrient deficiencies, you CAN and SHOULD supplement your day with an 8-minute session on an earth-based PEMF device.

While we can always go outside and lay on the earth to get these frequencies, over the past 300 years the earths magnetic field has declined 50% and Many theorize that we are in the process of a pole reversal over the next couple thousand years so the earth's magnetic field and the essential PEMFs of the earth is most likely going to continue.

The other problem is the average person stays inside 90% of the day. On top of that, we live and work in concrete structures; we drive in metal cars, and wear rubber soles as we walk on concrete. There are some Japanese researchers that call Fibromyalgia: "Magnetic Deficiency Syndrome."

Besides not getting enough of the "good" earth PEMFs, we are getting too much unhealthy PEMF's "electro smog"; from power lines, computers, cell phones, digital clocks, microwaves, T.V.'s, and hair dryers. These unhealthy PEMF's cause a "sub-molecular electronic disturbance." This phrase was coined by a former Nobel Prize winner to describe these unhealthy energies that bombard us on a daily basis.

Because of this two-fold problem, it is going to become increasingly important to supplement with a good earth-based PEMF device. And if you are still a little skeptical, consider that PEMF therapy is one of the most well researched forms of natural healing.

The Process

Many of the initial studies have been carried out in Russia and Eastern Europe, but more and more research is now taking place in the United States. PEMF is a non-contact, non-invasive, non-pharmacological and effective treatment for many conditions. Worldwide more than 2,000 double blind studies have demonstrated that PEMF therapy is a safe and effective treatment for a variety of conditions, as well as to promote and maintain general cellular health and function.

PEMF therapy has been used extensively for decades for many health issues, and results can be seen in animals as well as humans. The National Institutes of Health have made PEMF therapy a priority for research. In fact, the FDA has already approved many PEMF devices, some specifically to fuse broken bones, wound healing, pain and tissue swelling, and also to treat depression. Most therapeutic PEMF devices are considered safe by various standards and organizations.

Just to be clear, PEMF therapy or any energy medicine device for that matter does not heal or cure disease. What it's really doing is jump-starting our body's own natural healing process. The body is self-healing, self-regulating and self-regenerating. It has the natural ability to heal when given the proper energy and elements needed for sustaining life (more on the five essential elements in the next chapter). In light of this, let's look at the many "benefits" that PEMF therapy provides.

Top 8 Benefits PEMF therapies will give YOU.

(These benefits will allow you to experience a super-radiant and healthy life!)

1. **Stronger Bones**

    One of the first discoveries with PEMF therapy was the effect it had on healing and strengthening bones. A low frequency sawtooth PEMF signal has been shown to stimulate the osteoblast cells in the bones to produce bone matter.

2. **Endorphins and Pain Relief**

    It's been proven that earth's PEMF is essential to creating endorphins (the bodies natural "opiates") and additional endorphin synthesis can be promoted by PEMF therapy. This is one of the reasons why PEMF helps immediately with symptomatic pain relief. Also PEMF generates microcurrents to run through the neural pathways, which reduces the signal needed to create the feeling or sensation of pain. Less signal = Less pain perception. So PEMF not only helps to increase endorphins but it also directly decreases the triggering of the pain response.

3. **Better Sleep and HGH secretion**

   Pulsing magnetic fields (especially the Schumann and geomagnetic frequency) stimulate the production of Melatonin in the pineal gland. Melatonin is one of the most important hormones for sleep and anti-aging. A good PEMF therapy system has a biorhythm clock which can directly improve sleep by entraining the mind to the delta and theta frequencies (.5-7hz).

4. **More Energy ATP**

   At the most fundamental level, your body, organs, tissues and cells need energy to heal, period! No matter what your problem, disease, condition, or current state of health, if you give your body and cells more energy, YOU WILL get better and feel more vitality. We already discussed how PEMF therapy improves cellular voltage and ATP production, but it bears repeating.

5. **Better Oxygenation and Circulation**

   The primary function of the circulatory system is to deliver oxygen and nutrients TO THE CELLS and remove waste products FROM THE CELLS, to the organs of elimination. The cardiovascular and respiratory systems are intimately intertwined. Better respiration and circulation results in optimal ATP and energy production. Research shows that pulsed magnetic therapy enhances the cardiovascular and respiratory system in delivering oxygen to the cells and removing carbon dioxide and waste products.

6. **Improved Immunity**

   And there is direct research that PEMF improves immunity. Lymphocytes are important immune cells that protect our body from unwanted invaders. They have been found to proliferate in vitro in response to weak pulsing magnetic fields, thus improving overall immunity.

7. **Relaxation & Stress Reduction**

   One of the great benefits of PEMF therapy is that it assists the body in relaxation, repair, and healing. It will shift your body into a more parasympathetic mode if you are overstressed. It will energize, invigorate, and stimulate your body for optimal performance.

8. **Nerves and Tissue Regeneration**

   One important peer reviewed study showed that pulsed magnetic fields promote the growth of damaged nerves after traumatic injury. PEMF therapy helps to promote the binding of nerve growth factor of the receptor proteins on the surface of nerve cells, which facilitates regeneration.

The Technique- The PEMF Solution

The solution is earth-based PEMF devices. The iMRS made by Swiss Bionic Solutions is the only PEMF devices that actually duplicate nature, both in intensity and frequency. It does this with a saw-tooth waveform which delivers bunches of the frequencies from 0-30Hz simultaneously. In eight minutes twice per day all the bodies trillions of cells will be fully recharged and oxygenated. With a total of just sixteen minutes per day, the iMRS full-body matt gives the human body the energetic equivalent of walking barefoot in nature for 2-4 hours!

The applicator pad and probe uses the NASA-proven square wave that helps to break-up cycles of pain and allows the body to perform its own healing work. Additionally the iMRS is the only device that utilizes a biorhythm clock to ensure the body receives energizing frequencies in the early part of the day, and relaxing and sleep frequencies in the evening.

By using an earth-based PEMF system like the iMRS made by Swiss Bionic Solutions, you give your body a safe and concentrated dose of natural earth frequencies, which is the solution to the two-fold problem of the decline of the earth's magnetic fields and the rise of unhealthy electrosmog. Plus, PEMF therapy provides dozens of additional benefits such as more energy, better sleep, pain reduction, healing and regeneration, better oxygenation and much more!

Bryant Meyers, BS MA Physics, is a former physics professor, TV show host, and leading expert in the field of energy medicine and PEMF therapy. For over eighteen years, he has researched, tested, tried, and investigated well over $500,000 worth of energy medicine and frequency devices, studying with many of the world's experts. During the past six years he has dedicated his life and research to PEMF (Pulsed Electromagnetic Field) therapy, which he feels is the crown jewel of energy medicine. He has also helped and personally assisted thousands of people in this exciting new field. Bryant currently lives in Sarasota, Florida, near the beautiful Siesta Key Beach.

www.pemfbook.com

CHAPTER 28

From the Desk of Hermina

Hermina Danniel

The most frequently asked questions concerning magnetic resonance stimulation.

Our journey will guide us through many published observations as well as my own experience with PULSED MAGNETIC FIELD THERAPY (iMRS) and its users which I was privileged to witness over a period of 15 years+

What does this stimulation do?

The primary feature of this treatment method is the resonance effect of pulsating Electro-magnetic fields in the body. Vibrations or frequencies corresponding with the frequencies of our own cells are transmitted as purposeful information to unhealthy or energy deprived cells which function has been restricted and disturbed. In other words, magnetic resonance stimulation increases the body's cell potential due to higher oxygen supply and accelerates the function of ion pumps due to increased ATP (adenosine tri-phosphate - energy or fuel for the cell)..

What does resonance mean?

Resonance is the principle of using precisely those oscillations with which a cell

in the body or the entire organism oscillates independently. So naturally the original fundamental oscillation is amplified. The cell membrane oscillates at a certain frequency and at a certain amplitude. Unhealthy cells have the same frequency, however a different amplitude because of weaker oscillation. At precisely this point the resonance phenomenon of the magnetic field stimulation comes into effect because the amplitude of the oscillation can be reinforced by resonance.

What do I feel during therapy?

Although magnetic fields cannot be felt with our senses, some users perceive a certain sensation during this treatment. The most common observation is a slight feeling of heat on the parts being treated. This is a slight temperature increase due to improved circulation in the skin or the muscles. Tingling of the hands and feet is one of the sensations reported commonly. The occurrence of a slight increase in heartbeat is very rare and usually contributed to some anxiety and fear of what is going on. Preferably, one should perceive that 'warm fuzzy' feeling caused by deep relaxation due to a balanced autonomic nervous system.

Summary:	40-50% of the patients initially feel nothing during the first treatment
	40% feel pleasant warmth
	10% feel tingling or other sensations
	70-75% feel a loosening of the back muscles following treatment

Are there any side effects or can I do too much therapy?

Clinical studies on more than 200,000 patients have shown no side-effects detrimental to health due to magnetic resonance stimulation.

15 to 20% of users experience a first reaction similar to a spa reaction.

It may also be considered a 'healing reaction' which can occur by slightly increased pain. Usually these people are sensitive to magnetic fields in general, also to weather changes.

On the average the duration of first reactions is between two and four weeks.

To experience it as a single event is not uncommon either. It is important that users are informed ahead of time not to be discouraged to continue the treatment simply out of fear.

More water intake can help in case of adverse reaction or reducing time or intensities at the beginning of treatment.

THERE IS NO OVERSTIMULATION POSSIBLE. Needless to say, staying within the recommended intensities should be stressed to achieve optimal results.

The user, however, needs to be informed that the whole body application should not exceed one hour during one day. (Recommendation by the World Health Organization)

How do I know that it helps me?

'Simply lay on it for at least four weeks and allow yourself to enter the high success rate statistics which is available. Trust your body's ability to regulate itself when given the right tool', could be one answer to this question.

29 years of scientific research on magnetic resonance stimulation, and over 6500 scientific publications have already proven the medical effect of pulsating electromagnetic fields. Double blind studies and clinical observations can claim a higher success rate using this treatment method than can many drugs.

How can the effect of magnetic resonance stimulation be verified?

- The most valuable verification is the user's personal perception before and after
- MRS application.
- Clinical documented case histories
- Dark field microscopy and thermography before and after treatment
- Observation of daily life activity (improved energy and stamina)
- Mobility test - finger-floor distance test - muscle measurement test

How long does it take for the magnetic field to act?

The onset of effect varies from person to person. It is determined by the body's reactivity and various influences. High doses of medication, internal scar tissue, dehydration or the body's acidity level may also play a role, needless to say, smoking.

A young person will react more quickly than an older person. In addition, the type of complaint and its cause need to be taken into consideration, as well as the duration and the damage, which has already occurred in the body.

In treatment of pain, relief occurs on the average after four to eight weeks. If this is not the case, above mentioned influences may have to be examined.

Important: Magnetic resonance stimulation is a regulatory procedure in accordance with the body's own reactivity. The longer a painful condition has already existed, the longer it will take to improve. However, the immediate effect as explained prior is occurring during the first and all applications even though the user is not aware of it. Numerous testimonials share unexpected and sudden wonderful 'side effects' while applying the MRS regularly.

What can be done if the effect does not last?

Variations in success of the treatment are observed in patients with chronic complaints. This situation could be re-examined by adjusting the dose or by adding additional remedies. For instance vitamins or herbal supplements.

In many cases, a declining effect is due to careless use with a treatment time that is too short or not continuing over a longer period of time. Sometimes because of the euphoria about the initial success, users forget to consistently maintain their changes of a better lifestyle or diet. Even magnetic resonance stimulation cannot help undo the negative effects of continued poor habits. (Never forget to exercise and to walk: 'These boots are made for walking'! -Nancy Sinatra)

What is the actual role of the Chinese Organ Clock?

According to the Chinese Organ Clock, organs have their peak function at different times within 24 hours. Every two hours a different organ becomes very active energetically for approximately two hours. It is not necessary for us to apply the MRS at a certain organ time. Thanks to innovative technology the MRS 2000 and iMRS use these biological daily rhythms in all its time settings.

Why does the polarity change from North to South?

The polarity of a magnetic field plays a crucial role and changes every two minutes. Different structures in the human and animal body have a certain polarity preference. Applying magnetic resonance stimulation, organs are treated according to their preference.

For instance:

North pole flow seems to have a positive effect on pain, swelling, acidification of tissue, sleep disorders and agitation. South pole flow should result in improved metabolism, better circulation, faster wound healing and general regeneration of the body.

Why is this treatment method not recommended by doctors?

Energy medicine is not part of the regular university medical curriculum.

Many patients ask their physicians about their opinion regarding magnetic resonance stimulation only to find out that they have never heard of it.

Nevertheless, many MDs have taken time by now to study this treatment method, especially in Europe, and are incorporating it as supportive measure into their own treatments. In addition several European Universities offer lectures relative to magnetic field stimulation and have provided their own double blind studies of which many have been published.

The Biggest Misconception About The MRS 2000/iMRS

The term 'magnetic resonance stimulation' may suggest to potential users that there must be magnets placed in our whole body applicator. Some may even search for them, while in fact, we are only creating an electro magnetic field within the same frequency range of mother earth and the frequencies of our cells.

Static magnets are not able to achieve a resonance effect. Neither should the MRS stimulation be compared with other so-called 'Magnetic Field Therapies' which operate with much higher frequencies.

Pulsed Magnetic Resonance Stimulation is altogether different and scientifically proven most effective.

Hermina Danneil is a PEMF Expert for low frequency MRS devices with fourteen years theoretical and practical experience. She is fluent in German and English. Hermina has served as an International Promoter for over twenty years, exchanging cultural, educational, economical and medical programs between the US and Germany. In this capacity, she received numerous international awards.

Hermina obtained her diploma in energy medicine (pulsed magnetic field therapy) and ten individual MRS certificates during a four and half year educational period in Europe under the guidance of renowned MRS scientists and doctors:

- Dr. med. Christian Thuile (Internationale Aerztegesellschaft fuer Emergiemedizin)
- Dr.med.Rolf-Rainer Krapf, (IMA International Medical Academy, Germany)
- Dr.med. Hartmut Aufschlag, (Radiology)
- Dr.med. Juergen Schmitt (Orthopedics)
- Dr.med. Martin Gschwender (General Practitioner & Chinese Medicine)
- Prof. Frank Daudert (Onkology)
- Dr. med. Wilfried Heltzel (Orthopedics)
- Dr. med. Walter Glueck (MD, Diploma in Homeopathy, Acupuncture and Chiropractic)

Hermina introduced pulsed magnetic field therapy (MRS 2000/iMRS) to the US, with Dr. Joel P. Carmichael, DC, DACBSP, in the year 2006. Dr. Carmichael has since become the author of the book "Magnetic Resonance Stimulation-Using the Field to Maximize Your Health". In a mutual effort, Dr. Carmichael and Hermina in cooperation with Wolfgang Jaksch, CEO Swiss Bionic Solutions (Switzerland), initiated the groundwork for and the understanding of pulsed magnetic resonance stimulation.

Hermina developed a passion to teach on both sides of the Atlantic. Via email service, workshops and private training, she assisted (and still does) MRS users and associates in the US, Canada, UK, Belgium, Germany, Switzerland, India and Australia.

www.pemfassistance.com

CHAPTER 29

The Art of Acupuncture

Dr. Ravi K. Tuli

The Essence

In a battle that happened 50 centuries ago, an arrow hit a warrior in his leg. As the arrow was removed and the wound was being attended to, it was noticed that his frozen shoulder got healed this attracted the attention of his physicians to the relationship between the point punctured and the disease it cured in a distant part of the body.

Chinese monarchy patronized the system of acupuncture. Over the years a cause and effect relationship was worked out by the physicians of the era between the point punctured and the disease it cured. All such points were charted out on the human body. The joining together of these points termed acupuncture points, with similar physiological and therapeutic properties led to the development of what is now known as the system of acupuncture meridians of channels.

The word "Acupuncture" is derived from Latin words "acus" and "punctate", meaning a "needle" and to penetrate respectively. It is recorded to be nearly 5000 years old system of Traditional Chinese Medicine (T.C.M.) in which hair fine sterile needles are inserted at acupuncture points on the skin to rectify the flow of life-force energy (chi) and restore the yin yang balance or the homoeostasis. This phenomenon augments the body's own inherent natural healing energy that cures most of the acute chronic and even conventionally incurable diseases.

In well-trained and experienced hands acupuncture is a complete system of health by itself. Its efficacy improves tremendously when a qualified physician dedicated to acupuncture practices it. It is best used in the cure of commonly incurable diseases like migraine, insomnia, mental disorders, sinusitis, asthma, indigestion arthritis and spondylitis, etc. It may be unbelievable but it's true that acupuncture cures the incurables in expert hands.

Acupuncture is highly effective at all the levels of health:

- **Promotion of health** i.e. to improve the health of the healthy; many sportsmen are using acupuncture during their training to enhance their performance.
- **Prevention of sickness:** The ancient Chinese paid their physician as long as they were healthy, and stopped his dues when they fell sick!
- **Early diagnosis and cure:** Traditional observation of the pulse or tongue helped to diagnose sickness well before it manifested physically, enabling an early cure.
- **Supplementing acupuncture** with the knowledge and diagnostics of modern medicine helps to cure any sickness much quicker, thereby minimizing/eliminating the adverse effects of prolonged sickness or medication.
- **Disability limitations:** Timely diagnosis and effective cures limits the after effects or residual disability of sickness.
- **Rehabilitations:** Acupuncture has been found to be excellent in the relief of most of the chronic incurable diseases and restoration of the individual to a state of positive health.

Usually Acupuncture cures acute ailments almost instantly, and chronic ailments faster than any other system usually in a matter of weeks. It can be described to be very time efficient. It should be started right at the onset of any sickness.

Acupuncture is equally effective at all ages: in the infants, children young adults and the elderly. In fact, the old people are amazed at its efficacy, as they don't have to live any longer with ailments related to their age.

Acupuncture and Acupressure

Acupressure is an art based on the science of acupuncture where a simple knowledge of the meridians and reflex points imparted to a paramedical worker, a masseur or even a lay person is used by applying pressure on them for energizing the chi for first aid or relief of minor ailments.

Current status of acupuncture in the world

In People's Republic of china (P.R.C) the country's primary health care is based upon the T.C.M. It also supplements all the centers of modern medicine providing secondary and tertiary care. This model has proved its tremendous success as within its limited resources the P.R.C has achieved a health status comparable with the best in the world.

After exhaustive scientific evaluation over 25 years, the world health organization (W.H.O.) has given recognition to acupuncture. The Food & Drug Agency (F.D.A.) and the National Institute of Health (N.I.H.) in U.S.A. having endorsed its scientific basis the various states in U.S.A. offer licenses to its practitioners. In U.K. the National Health Services (N.H.S.) recognizes and pays for acupuncture.

The Process

Traditionally it involves insertion of special hair fine sterile needles at prescribed acupuncture points to regulate the flow of chi in the body and bring cure. There is also a method called non-invasive or needle- free Acupuncture. It's the form of acupuncture where penetrating needles are not used. This modality may be preferred in young children, frail and the elderly, for cosmetic use or when the recipient is afraid of needles. Some of the non-invasive modalities are, however, always used as supplements to the main therapy.

Limitations

Like all other systems, acupuncture would have its inherent limitations in not being able to cure all the patients. A patient in medical emergency needing life saving resuscitations, urgent surgery, serious infection, any life-threatening condition or a mechanical problem must be first directed to a medical facility.

Acupuncture in such conditions would normally be a useful supplement in speeding up the recovery, final outcome of the sickness, and curing the residual\ chronic component of the sickness.

The most important of all is that the practitioner must be competent and know his limitations as not to waste precious time vital for patient's recovery.

Disorders Treated by Acupuncture

- **Orthopedics:** Myalgia fasciitis, periathritis spondylitis, spinal & disc lesions, radiculopathy, osteon & Rhtd. Arthritis etc.
- **Angiology:** Hypertension, CAD, Arrhythmias, Gangrene, Post CABG/PTCA, rehanilitations /neuralgia etc.
- **Pulmonology:** Allergy, Br. Asthma, Ch. Bronchitis, Emphysema etc.
- **Gastroenterology:** Dyspepsia's Ulcers, Hiatus Hemi ach Colitis, I.B.S. Gall stones, Ch. Hepatitis pain abdomen (NYD).
- **Neurology:** Migraine headache, neuralgia paralysis insomnia, autonomic/functional Disorders, etc.
- **Endocrinology:** Diabetes, dyslipidemia, gout, obesity, menstrual disorders, PR. Sterility menopausal syn., oligospermia.
- **Dermatology:** acne, alopecia, allergy, eczema, psoriasis, leucoderma, keloids tec.
- **E.N.T. & Eye:** ac/ch rhinitis, sinusitis, laryngitis, tonsillitis, epistaxis, mennier's syndrome, vertigo, myopia squints, etc.
- **Psychiatry:** addictions, smoking, alcoholism, drugs; anxiety, neurosis, psychosis, psychosomatic etc.
- **General Medicine:** Autoimmune disorders, allergies, viral infections, general debility, shock P.U.O. Etc.

The Tip

Acupuncture being a natural therapy saves one from the side effects and toxicity of drugs. It complements all other systems of therapy. The greatest advantage is that acupuncture cures most of the diseases permanently and activates positive wellbeing of the body mind and spirit.

Acupuncture is a highly efficient cost effective & truly holistic (body-mind-spirit) natural modality for the cure of acute & chronic ailments, especially effective in most of the conventionally incurable disorders. It is highly useful for all specialties.

Its efficacy becomes much higher in combinations with other life-force management therapies like yoga, pranayama, meditation, reiki, pranic- healing etc.

Dr. Ravi. K. Tuli, MBBS MD PhD is a Chief Consultant Holistic Medicine Fmr. Indraprastha Apollo Hospitals & Indian Air Force. From aviation medicine to holistic healing, Dr Tuli's journey has been tremendous. Dr. Tuli is also the founder of "SOHAM" Clinic for Holistic Medicare & Cure. He is totally dedicated to delivering positive health and total wellness: Body-Mind-Spirit, by optimum synergy of drug-free harmless means of the recognized systems of health for CURE of conventionally incurable pain & diseases.

www.holisticmedicare.org

CHAPTER 30

Sujok & Acupressure

Amarjit Singh Narula

The Essence

My journey to adopting and promoting holistic well-being began 3 decades back when I was fresh out of Engineering College. I was working in Gulf from where I returned to India, not able to fully cope up with the challenges of my work, my health started failing. I became seriously sick and every day I struggled with loose motions and bleeding. I actually lost count of my visits to the toilet, and this continued for 6 months until I was diagnosed with Ulcerative Colitis by a Gastroenterologist. I was put on steroids and other medications, instructed not to stop them until advised (Steroids were to be tapered off gradually). A slight recovery and I would opt to stop my medication and my Colitis would relapse, in & out of many hospitals under different specialists, I struggled endlessly with same medication and no lasting relief or effect.

I tried different methods for healing as well, however my suffering was not to end so easily and thus I suffered for 13 long years during which I gave up my job and started working as a civil contractor, which allowed me to remain home on days when I would be unwell. In the year 1999 I read a newspaper article about a combination of certain alternative therapies, with a faint hope I tried it and this time it worked. My health improved substantially in just 6 months. This incident changed my life path altogether and I discovered a new passion, that of helping people end their physical suffering through these therapies. Today I am living an inspired and contended life. I am healthy and thriving in my work and I am glad to share with you more insights about two such therapies.

SUJOK Therapy was first developed by Prof. Park Jae Woo from South Korea in later part of 20th century. It works on the principle that the human body is a form of well-harmonized universe. The body innately has everything needed to maintain itself to its optimum. And indeed this has been proved true as we witness healing miracles every day.

Sujok in Korean language means 'Hand & Foot'. "SU" means a hand & "JOK" means a foot. It is expressed in ancient healing systems that our hands and feet resemble our body structure and certain points on hands and feet when stimulated have a direct effect on the related organ. Stimulation of these points produces an evident treatment and prophylactic effect. These points are arranged on the hands & feet in an anatomic structure of the organism. The body and its corresponding areas interact continuously and when this knowledge is applied in the form of a technique like Sujok or Acupressure the energy meridians of the body are cleared which then helps in resuming the flow of vital energy. As the malfunctioning organ starts receiving the vital energy once again, we see a shift in the functioning of the organ and a consequent relief from disease.

When we are not sick we might not need intensive therapy however good physical activity like walking, running, household work, dance etc. are the best ways to keep these vital points stimulated which can help us maintain good health naturally. However when our health is compromised we can always consider Sujok as accessible and effective method of improving our health, getting fast & markedly curative results. In Sujok it is important that the corresponding points are correctly and regularly stimulated using various appropriate methods, this ensures that we get the desired effect. In some cases we have seen results within a few minutes of proper treatment.

When the natural stimulation of the correspondence system/points and areas becomes inadequate, a person falls ill. In such cases, accurately applied stimulation of points usually proves quite effective. Methods of effective stimulation include Micro needles, Pressure, Electro Stimulation, colors, different edible seeds, Star magnets, and natural minerals, to mention a few. At our holistic healing centre in Mumbai, we offer Sujok therapy not in isolation rather we give it in combination with certain therapies that further enhance the effectiveness of the therapy and the patients get faster and lasting results. Sujok has been found to be effective in diseases like Kidney/Liver failure, High or Low Blood Pressure, Coma, Diabetes, Spinal Disorders, Scaloderma, ENT problems, Nervous

Disorders, Stress & Depression, Hormonal Imbalance, Vertigo, Heart Problems, Skin Problems etc.

Other than Sujok Acupressure is also very effective and simple to administer. Acupressure has been in India and China for thousands of years. The principles applied in acupressure are same as that of acupuncture but no needles are used and stimulation is achieved by applying pressure through fingers. Other bodywork therapies of Asian origin are medical Qigong, Tuina, Shiatsu (Japanese form of acupressure), and hand and foot therapies from Korea, Body and Foot manipulation (both dry and wet) from Thailand etc.

The Process

These healing methods are based on the knowledge of special acu-points/locations or acupressure points that lie along meridians/channels/pathways in our body, which are also present in all higher animals as well. It is said that, through these invisible channels flows vital energy or life force at a fixed timing for a specific period before shifting to another energy channel at a 2-hour interval. These 12 major meridians connect specific organs or network of organs, thus organizing a system of transfer of energy throughout our body. The channels begin at various locations and follow various paths to connect to an organ associated with a certain meridian. Illness happens whenever any of these meridians are blocked or are out of balance. Acupressure and Acupuncture are among many type of TCM (Traditional Chinese Medicine) that helps to restore balance of this energy network in our body, which leads to healing and recovery.

Acupressure practitioners use fingers, palms, elbows/feet, or special devices to apply pressure at acupoints/areas and reflection points on palm and feet. Sometimes, acupressure also involves stretching or acupressure massage, as well as other methods for stimulating the points and releasing the blockages. During the session that lasts between 30 min to 1 hour, the therapist gently presses the points/locations specific to the organs/parts of the body that are affected.

Ancient Indian texts also mention application of a method called 'Shingi' which includes treatment on specific body locations. In this method, the traditional healers create vacuum using hollow horn shells and draw out blood. In modern method this is known as bloodletting, instead of horn shells nowadays plastic vacuum disposable cups are available. Bloodletting has therapeutic benefits and when this technique is well applied gives good relief and result in a wide range of ailments.

The main goal of Sujok, acupressure or other types of body work therapies is to help restore health and balance to the channels of vital force and to help regulate the opposing forces of yin and yang. Apart from physical well being many times these therapies also help restore peace of mind and brings harmony to the spirit. I would like to share few unique cases where our integrated therapy brought miraculous results for the patients.

A 52-year-old man was suffering for 22 years with epileptic fits, which occurred on the 26th of every month and he had to take 3 tablets a day. His seizure would last for 6 to 8 hours and he would lose consciousness. After we administered our alternative therapy including Sujok, his medication was reduced to 2 tablets a day and his fits entirely stopped. At present if he feels a seizure happening it only lasts for 10 -15 minutes after which he is able to resume his work.

A 45-year-old man from Mumbai had ulcerative colitis and he was on medication for past 5 years, which included taking 6 tablets a day along with steroids. Despite the medication he suffered from loose stools with blood and mucus sometimes 10 times a day. After he consulted us, we offered him integrated alternate therapy, now after two years he is off medications and he is able to take normal diet and his condition is very stable.

Another inspiring story is that of a 65-year-old lady from Mumbai who was suffering from knee joint arthritis. She had difficulty in sitting on the floor or folding her legs and she could not even walk without a stick. She was advised to go for a knee replacement surgery however her family was reluctant due to possibility of complications. They approached us and within one year's time there was no pain in her knees. Her surgery was cancelled and she can now walk pain free.

We also witnessed another case of healing where a 40-year-old woman from Ahmedabad who had severe pain and numbness in arms for more than 8 years was completely healed within 1 month of treatment. Her MRI report had shown multiple problems like Cervical Spondylitis, Osteophytes from full cervical and full lumbar to base of spine, however a simple approach of alternative therapy worked wonders for her and she was cured within 30 days.

Another case is that of a 42-year-old man from New Delhi who fell down from stairs and had tailbone injury. He opted for many treatments like allopathic medications, physiotherapy and chiropractic treatment for almost 4 months. However he had no relief and ultimately he came to our centre and we started his treatment. Within 2 months his pain was 50% reduced and within few months he recovered 90%. He is very happy and as his treatment continues he is on his way to full recovery.

One more inspiring case is that of an autistic child who came to us when he was just 7 years old. He could hardly speak and had no response to commands. Within four months of treatment he started forming sentences and he was responding to his parents. His hyperactivity was also reduced.

Every day we are thrilled to witness new stories of healing and recovery happening at our centre. The contentment and joy it brings is priceless. Besides the cases we shared here, we had patients with severe diabetes, spinal problems, rheumatoid arthritis, PCOD etc. and all of them recovered very well from their painful conditions.

The Tip

From my experience I have concluded that in any case a combination of alternative therapies always works better rather than the patient trying various therapies in isolation one after another. Sustained effort and positive attitude from patient's side are also important factors that influence the effectiveness of the treatment. In many cases the Dimension of Space (Vaastu) is also included to help faster recovery.

Life is a journey and like any journey it also has its risks and many times we fall prey to the pitfalls of ignorance. In that, we damage our mind stream, our consciousness which leads to the imbalance of energy in the physical body as well. Any injury or diseases is only a reflection of our imbalance within. The therapies whether focusing on mind or body help us restore our lost balance and when that is achieved healing is the spontaneous consequence.

The realization of this simple process can end our futile search for complex remedies. Nature is simple and so is our body, and it knows how to keep itself healthy and efficient. Only a faulty intervention is what causes suffering which can happen through bad diet and lifestyle, wrong and negative thinking, disempowering beliefs and lack of self-love and self-esteem.

If we learn to cultivate a healthy lifestyle, we will not require any intensive health care throughout our life. Even in severe cases natural therapies have proved their effectiveness beyond any doubt. It is only our own willingness to adopt them that is needed.

My vision is to spread the message about this integrated approach of alternative therapy. Millions of people are dying every year due to physical suffering, which can be easily eliminated. Today more than high end drugs and complex treatments we need a holistic approach and an army of healers that do the work required.

"Without health life is not life; it is only a state of langour and suffering - an image of death." - Buddha

Let us nurture a healthy state of body and mind and be ALIVE.

Amarjit Singh Narula is a civil enginner turned holistic healer having more than a decade of experience in alternative therapies, he regularly offers seminars and workshops on Sujok and Acupressure, Bach Flower Therapy and other methods as well. He has been appointed as a lecturer in Sujok Therapy, Twist Therapy & Smile meditation. He travels extensively to teach and spread awareness about the need and scope of Alternative Healing. He also hosts a daily holistic show on Aastha Channel at 00.40 hrs. He has worked extensively with Shilpa Khedekar (Senior Sujok Therapist) on this article and the process.

www.sujokacupressure.net
www.thehealinghub.in

CHAPTER 31

External Counter Pulsation (ECP) - Creating bypass naturally

Dr. S.S. Sibia

Invasive and surgical treatments should be preserved for patients with crippling disease where other 'peaceful' non-invasive treatments have failed.

The Essence

Maintaining health is more effective and less expensive than trying to regain it. However when disease does occur, mankind has always searched for easy home remedies and when they fail patients submit themselves to the physician for medication. Invasive and surgical means are the last choice of the patient's even if the patient is a doctor himself. External Counter Pulsation (ECP) is one such truly non-pharmaceutical program designed to help cardiac patient recover, heal and enjoy an enhanced quality of life besides offering many other benefits safely and effectively. ECP can be life saving for patients who generally have little that medical science could offer till now.

Procedure

External Counter Pulsation therapy or ECP, also known as EECP is a procedure performed on patients with angina or heart failure in order to diminish their symptoms ischemia, improve functional capacity and quality of life. In various studies, ECP has been shown to relieve angina, and decrease the degree of ischemia in a cardiac stress test. The procedure of the treatment is quite simple. ECP is an outpatient treatment and the patient lies on a comfortable bed. While undergoing ECP, large blood pressure-like pneumatic cuffs are wrapped around the legs and arms are connected to an air compressor preferably having provision for both positive and negative pressure. At the same time electrodes and sensors are attached to continuously monitor heart rate and rhythm and a special sensor applied to the finger or ear lobe checks the oxygen level in the blood and monitors the pressure waves created by the cuff inflations and deflations.

The cuffs are timed to inflate and deflate based on the individual's electrocardiogram at specific times between two heartbeats i.e. mid-diastolic phase when the heart is at rest and getting its own blood and oxygen supply. The cuffs should ideally inflate at the beginning of diastole and deflate just before the next heart beat. During the inflation portion of the cycle, the calf and arm cuffs inflate first, then the lower thigh cuffs and finally the upper thigh cuffs. Inflation is controlled by a pressure monitor, and the cuffs are inflated to about 200 mmHg.

The treatment is usually one hour at a time, once or twice a day, 5 to 7 days a week for 35 or more treatment sessions.

Mechanism

When timed correctly, this will decrease the after-load that the heart has to pump against, and increase the preload that fills the heart thus increasing the cardiac output. By increasing the pressure in the aorta while the heart is relaxing (during diastole) ECP increases blood flow into the heart's arteries. Various mechanisms of action find mention in the research papers.

Repeated dilatation of the arteries has the effect of stretching a rubber band repeatedly till it looses some of its elasticity and remains permanently dilated. The ECP relaxed arteries improve circulation.

The repeated increase in pressure stress in the coronary circulation results in the release of Nitric Oxide and various growth factors.

Nitric oxide is a vasodilator that opens and relaxes arteries, contributes to less arterial stiffness, improved function of endothelial cells and thus help improve circulation. oxide

The Vascular endothelial growth factor (VEGF) is a hormone that helps stimulate angiogenesis, the growth of new collaterals for blood flow around blockages, like a naturally created bypass thus ECP helps grow new arteries naturally and improves arterial function.

Recent research has demonstrated that ECP is also a regenerative therapy. It enhances release released into circulation Stem cells (Progenitor and hematopoietic cells) found in bone marrow, the endothelium (lining of the arteries) and organ tissue to help regeneration of damaged tissues.

The increased oxygenated and nutrient rich blood flow revives tissue in heart and body that have restricted or blocked blood flow and the mechanical external cardiac assistance provided by ECP results in improvement in energy and exercise tolerance.

ECP also improves blood flow to the brain, lymphatic circulation and enhances quality of life (less fatigue, better sleep, more stamina, longer exercise duration, reduced stress, passive exercise benefit as from one hour of aerobics). It is expected to improve longevity with anti-aging effects, decreases anxiety and depression besides antioxidant and detoxification effects

Thirty five ECP treatment sessions increases blood flow to the heart myocardium (muscle) by 20-42% and the effect lasts for three to nine years. However this safe and comfortable treatment can be repeated earlier for enhancement in results.

Indications

The no medication, safe, FDA cleared ECP is approved by many insurance companies and has a significant role and can be life saving in heart patients who have no other treatment options. Some patients who can be benefitted are:

- Patients with severe, diffuse coronary atherosclerosis and persistent angina, shortness of breath or significant silent ischemia burden, such as elderly patients and those with diabetes, challenging coronary anatomies, or debilitating heart failure, renal failure, or pulmonary disease.
- ECP Therapy has also been shown to be effective in relieving angina symptoms in patients with Cardiac Syndrome X.
- Benefits of ECP have been determined in the management of angina in the elderly and in patients with mild refractory angina.
- ECP Therapy is equally effective in reducing angina symptoms in patients with or without diabetes, and in patients with all ranges of body mass index / obesity.

- Who have already had angioplasty, stents, or bypass surgery, but their heart disease symptoms have returned or persisted.
- Are not candidates for surgery due to other medical conditions
- Do not want to undergo surgery
- Are diabetic, asthmatics, have kidney or other problems making them unfit or high risk for other treatment.
- Have small vessels – more common in diabetics and in women.
- Rely on medications or curtail their activities to avoid angina
- Peripheral artery disease and Leg pain
- Erectile Dysfunction
- Stroke
- Sports Enhancement to enhance exercise duration and increased stamina
- Renal Failure
- Fatigue

Patients who may be benefitted are those diagnosed to have coronary heart disease. Patients who have Chest Pain, Shortness of Breath, Pain in the Jaw/ Shoulder/ Arm/ Back or above the Stomach, Palpitation, Heavy Sweating, Fainting Spells on walking or climbing stairs at a normal pace, while performing daily activities such as household chores/ shopping or leisure, after eating or just watching television should have themselves evaluated by a doctor as these may signify underlying heart disease. Some patients may get these features even at rest or are awaken at night with these symptoms.

Contraindications

ECP therapy systems should not be used for treating patients with significant leaking aortic valve, irregular heart beat, bleeding disorders, aortic aneurysm, uncontrolled blood pressure and Pregnancy. Patients with blood pressure higher than 180/110 mmHg or heart rate greater than 120 beats per minute should be controlled prior to treatment. Age, pacemaker, obesity, diabetes, thyroid or other problems is no bar for ECP treatment.

Improvement

Improvement can be seen and tested. The patients feels the improvement and tests can document the changes,

Approximately 80% of patients who complete the 35-hour course of ECP Therapy experience significant symptom relief that may last up to three to nine years. Patients have decreased symptoms of chest pain, shortness of breath, chronic fatigue, tiredness as well as a significant improvement in exercise tolerance and energy. They can walk longer distance and faster more comfortably. Medication is reduced in almost all patients.

Stress Thallium shows increased myocardial blood flow. The new non-invasive Cardiovascular Cartography hemodynamic study maps takes less than 30 minutes to graph improved blood flow to different regions, Oxygen demand reserve ratio and arterial compliance and decreased myocardial burden.

ECP Therapy continues to demonstrate a reduction in hospital admission and re-admission rates in patients with chronic Coronary Artery Disease (CAD) and patients with Congestive Heart Failure.

References

ECP now finds reference in leading medical text books and journals. Numerous presentations have been made in major scientific conferences, reporting results of clinical studies. Harrison's principles of Interna.Medicine mentions "ECP utilizes pneumatic cuffs on the lower extremities to provide diastolic augmentation and systolic unloading of blood pressure in order to decrease cardiac work and oxygen consumption while enhancing coronary blood flow. Recent trials have shown that regular application improves angina, exercise capacity, and regional myocardial perfusion." Where as Braunwald's text book of Cardiovascular Medicine writes "External counter pulsation is another promising alternative treatment of refractory angina. Data suggest that ECP reduces the frequency of angina and the use of nitroglycerin and improves exercise tolerance and quality of life. In a randomized, double-blind, sham – controlled study of ECP for patients with chronic stable angina, counter pulsation was associated with an increase in time to ST segment depression during exercise testing and a reduction in angina. It also reduced the extent of ischemia detected with myocardial perfusion imaging."

Future of ECP

ECP is now available worldwide, There are more than 900 academic institutions and physicians who provide ECP therapy in the U.S. alone, including many renowned centres such as Mayo Clinic, Beth Israel Medical Center, University of New York at Stony Brook, Cleveland Clinic, University of California, University of Pittsburgh Medical Center, etc

Still, ECP Therapy is still underutilized worldwide. More than 75% of all angina patients remain unaware of External Counter pulsation Therapy with less than 5% of cardiology clinics offering treatment for their patients. ECP has great growth potential due to its safe, effective, non-surgical option with a substantially lower cost.

As current healthcare trends are aggressively evolving towards low cost, non-invasive solutions hence ECP therapy is a hot topic in Cardiology.

Dr. S.S. Sibia MBBS, MD (Internal Medicine), Director and Consultant, Sibia Medical Centre, Ludhiana. Sibia Medical Centre is dedicated to care, prevention and treatment by latest patient tested methods. Sibia Medical Centre is primarily a No-Surgery Clinic dedicated to treating various diseases without surgery. What started as a small service to mankind has now turned into a wave and the clinic has treated patients from not only various parts of India but many different countries also. The 'small' setup is now known world-wide for 'big' results.

Schooling: Sherwood College, Nainital; M.B.B.S. - Government Medical College, Ranchi; M.D. (Medicine) - Government Medical College, Patiala; Diploma Lithotripsy (for stones treatment) - Direx Ltd., Israel; Trained Chelation Therapy - Arterial Disease Clinic, England; Trained Bio-oxidative medicine - Arterial Disease Clinic, England; Training Non-invasive testing Cardiovascular Cartography - Centre for Artificial Intelligence and non Linear Studies, Bangalore; Training in External Counter Pulsation – Canton (China); Training in Tissue Engineering with Cytotron to Regenerate and repair joint cartilage.

www.sssibia.com

CHAPTER 32

The Magic of Crystal Healing

Bindu Maira

The Essence

What is a crystal, you might ask. The answer to that question depends very much on whom you ask it to. To a Geologist, crystals of all shapes and sizes reveal astounding Atomic symmetry. A Jeweler will tell you the most desirable crystals are gemstones used to make expensive jewelry. To a Historian crystals are a means to interpreting our cultural heritage finds from the graves of royalty as well as artifacts unearthed from ancient dwellings reveal the changing desirability of gemstones since antiquity.

Priests, shamans and holy men have used them down the ages to help heal body mind and soul. They have been used as weapons, tools, objects of divination in jewelry, as talismans and amulets. They have been worn by emperors, rulers and popes to symbolize authority, spirituality or union. Crowns were set with precious stones, both for their beauty and for the crystal energies to enhance and prove their importance. Pope Clement the 7th in the late 16th century is reputed to have ingested a gem concoction worth 40000 ducats equivalent to more than 3 million $ today in order to heal, harmonize and empower himself. Down the ages rubies were worn in the navel by belly dancers to excite passion. Egyptians used malachite for healing and protection. The Incas used emerald; The Azteks used obsidian; the Chinese used jade; Tibetans and native-Americans used both turquoise and smoky quartz; the Celts used Shale Amber.

Ayurvedic and tantric scholars from India knew the amazing potential of precious stones and used them with vedic astrology; they used emeralds, diamonds, rubies, sapphires for their physiochemical and electromagnetic properties. In Atlantis they were used to power entire cities. The mighty pyramids that still stand in all their glory are said to have been built with the help of huge crystals. Today, Crystals play a vital role in technology, from laser tipped drills, silicon chips in computer chips, credit cards, smart cards, lasers and the programs of domestic appliances and quartz watches.

The Process

Crystals are natural rocks and minerals born deep within the womb of mother earth. They are mineral and solid substances created during the formative cooling stages of earth's development some 5 billion years ago and they have continued to metamorphose as the planet itself changed. They are miniature storehouses containing the records of the earth over millions of years and bearing the indelible memory of the powerful forces that shaped it. Some have been subjected to enormous pressure, others grew in chambers deep underground in layer and others dripped into being, all of which affects the properties of the crystal and the way that they function. These crystals all have some amazing healing properties and are increasingly being used across the globe to heal, balance and harmonize our energies.

How Crystals Work

To understand Crystals we first need to understand who we are. Human beings are basically a mass of pulsating energy. We are actually beings of Light. We have 7 different energy bodies. We have a mental energy body, an emotional energy body, an etheric energy body, an astral body and a physical body. The physical body is the one we can see because it is the densest form of energy, but that too is an energy body. All these energy bodies are constantly interfacing with each other and impacting each other in a negative or positive way. All the energy bodies flow through each other through our chakras, which are vortexes of energy spinning at different centers. We are nothing but energy vibrating at different frequencies, and all energy has a physical as well as a metaphysical aspect to it.

Each Chakra is a certain color, is positioned in front of an endocrine gland and has to do with a certain psychological aspect of our lives. Each color infuses the appropriate soul center with power and vitality. So we are also nothing but different colors vibrating at different frequencies. When this energy is in a state of free flow we will be in a state of Health and when there are blocks, these could be in your mental or emotional energy bodies; we end up in a state of depletion or excess of a particular energy in a certain chakra. This creates an imbalance of energy and eventually it leads to a physical disease. Disease is simply a lack of ease in your auric and energy body which when it gets out of hand manifests as a disease in your physical body. To heal a disease you have to heal the aura and crystals act at the etheric level.

Properties of Crystals

Crystals are manifested forms of light and color. They vibrate at a certain frequency, each resonating with certain chakra and emitting a sonic frequency. This is the music of the crystals, which can be heard by clairvoyants.

Crystals are PIESO-ELECTRIC, which means when you apply mechanical pressure to a crystal it produces electricity, notably the quartz family and if you apply an electric current to a crystal it will move mechanically, i.e. it oscillates.

Crystals also have Morphic resonance. Medicines that we ingest are made based on Bio Chemistry and Biochemistry is underpinned by electromagnetism. We are electromagnetic beings. As we are beings of energy in a constant state of vibration, we absorb the vibrations emitted by different crystals easily at an auric level and the aura will absorb just as much as it needs to. So the energy field of the crystals is actually the energy field of the soul. Working with the energy field of the soul is the highest form of intervention that you can receive, because it is the most efficient way to identify and eliminate the root causes of both the psychological and physical illness.

Crystals can increase the vibrational frequency of a room, and change the frequency of your body and environment. In fact they can reach as far down as your cellular DNA because everything and all matter is vibrating energy.

The ability of crystals to focus energy means they can be used for specific tasks such as directing energy to a specific point on the body or to an emotional blockage .The disease is then gently dissolved and any imbalance corrected. From hurt, grief, trauma, anxiety, to migraines, thyroid problems, kidney stones, back pain to name just a few I have been the happy witness to many magical moments with crystals. Each time a healing happens it feels like magic, and magical it is in the gentle ease and joy with which crystals help us heal. In fact mostly the shifts are so subtle with the healing that half the time one may not even be aware but then one day one realizes that one has actually become much better and one's condition is greatly improved.

Crystals can enhance meditation, deepening attunement with universal energies. They aid manifestation and offer protection. Crystals are all basically Alchemists, in that they catch negative energy, transform and transmute it into positive, and in so doing they bring you into a state of wellness and wellbeing with peace of mind, happiness and good health.

The Technique

Carrying crystals as protective amulets or wearing them as jewelry are the simplest ways to utilize their natural potential. They can also be placed in your rooms, with specific grids to enhance the vastu and fengshui of a space. Gem elixirs are another easy way of utilizing their healing potential.

No matter what healing modality one is involved with, using Crystals alongside can enhance and empower the whole experience. Throughout the world, now crystals are being used to heal. Medical and scientific reports confirm that crystals have healing properties.

Different crystals resonate with different chakras and specific crystals will work for specific problems. There is a method of correct usage, which involves not just the correct diagnosis and recommendation, but a process of cleansing, programming, attunement and connection all of which contribute to maximum efficacy and healing.

Some Successful Stories

- A young man of 27 comes to me saying he has a really bad back problem and the doctors have said he will never be able to gym again. Three healing sessions with regular use of the crystals each day and at the end of the month, he is feeling much better and by six weeks is back in the gym. That was 2 years ago and he tells me he is still doing fine.
- Another young boy was in hospital in the ICU with a bad case of jaundice. His parameters were sinking and the doctors were skeptical of his chances of recovery. I got a frantic call from his mother and sent across some large

crystals to be placed next to him .The doctors couldn't understand what turned but 36 hours later he was better, out of the ICU and within a week out of hospital. Today he is a healthy strapping young man leading a full life. What is interesting to note is that his mother told me one of the crystals I had sent across turned completely yellow in the ICU as the boy simultaneously got better. Coincidence? I very much doubt it.

- The mother of a school boy came to me saying her son was in a lot of pain due to Kidney stones but being in boarding school and in class 10th nearing exams she couldn't bring him home. I gave her 2 crystals and told her how he must use them saying, "lets see where it goes". Three and a half weeks later, the boy is back home, goes in for an MRI and the doctor says, "What stones? It's like sand out there". What happened? I don't try to decipher it. I am just happy he is better.

- A young girl who happens to be my son's friend was upset because her old dog has lost the use of his hind legs, could not move much, was in pain and the vet had advised it may be a good idea to let him go and put him to sleep. My son calls me as I am out of town. I direct him as to which crystal to give to Figo, the dog. We tape the crystal on the inside of his collar and exactly 3 days later I get an ecstatic phone-call from the excited girl saying, "Aunty what magic did you do? The vets called a mini conference. They say they have never seen anything like this." Figo has not only got up, he is walking, running and back to being his old self. It is the magic of the crystals.

- I have subsequently had a number of aging pet dogs who were flagging in their energies, finding it hard to walk actually begin jumping around all over again with enthusiasm. Simply taping a bloodstone on the inside of their collar was what did it.

- I had one of my favorite plants in my backyard beginning to show signs of dying. I dug in a crystal in to the soil right next to it and lo and behold, my plant righted itself and was in a healthy state within a couple of weeks. When I place indoor plants next to some large crystals I have at home, I have noticed it takes a much longer time before they need to be put out again, not only that I have noticed they actually grow more upright and seem to lean towards the crystal as if they want to receive and soak up all the good energy from them.

- They say a crystal ends up where it is meant to be, to the person it is meant to reach and I interestingly experienced this in a most amazing way. I was on a road trip in the interiors of Australia with my family and we ended up in a place called Coonacarabran where it turned out there was this amazing store for crystals, which had been set up initially as a museum by this Australian geologist who had a fantastic collection of zeolite crystals. I was excited to see so many new crystals which at that point I had not had occasion to do back home in India so I ended up buying quite a few. Because of my big purchase the lady at the counter who was the wife of the geologist presented me with a few magnetites, saying "if your husband keeps these in his pockets while flying, he will never get deep vein thrombosis" I remember finding it strange she said that because as a matter of fact my husband did have a problem on his last flight overseas. On our return flight, we made sure to carry the crystals in our pockets, got seats near the bulkhead of the plane where there is extra leg room; he was fast asleep when I woke up to find a woman had collapsed at my feet. She was surrounded by the airhostess and pilot and her partner who was trying to revive her. It took a moment to figure out she had had a stroke. I instinctively reached out for the crystals we had and asked that they be placed one each in both of her hands. I said to her partner that I am a crystal healer and this is all I have with me at the moment and maybe we can try using it.

The next thing I knew there was a big tear rolling down the old mans cheek; shaking his head smiling through his tears he said, "She is a crystal healer too." Well, the flight was diverted to Darwin, my husband and I were sent to other seats and 4 hours later just before we landed at Darwin the airhostess woke me, returned my crystals to me and said " I don't know what these are my dear, but they seem to work." What's the chance that I end up at the crystal store without previously knowing of its existence, am gifted those crystals ensuring I carry them, the lady collapses at my feet, is a crystal healer too and gets to use them at a time when she needed them most. Chance? Possibly. Coincidence? Maybe. Was it meant to be? Most likely, I would like to believe so. One way or other I am convinced to date that the crystals managed to do some damage control that day on the flight all those years ago.

So friends, cherish these crystals, nurture them and connect, for you never know, maybe we hear a similar successful story from you next!

Bindu Maira has been a professional TAROT card reader and CRYSTAL HEALER for the last fifteen years. An English honors graduate from LSR Delhi coupled with a degree in German from the Max Muller Bhawan in Pune; she is a versatile woman who has met with success in various fields. Being an articulate communicator as well as a people's person, she has been a teacher, a trainer and worked as a marketing consultant as well as a voice-over artist for many years. Radio shows, tarot shows on television, interviews on Pragya channel for crystal healing, giving talks to corporates, rotary clubs and international groups as well as being quoted in leading newspapers and magazines like HT and ELLE, are all part of her 15 year repertoire.

www.bindumaira.com

CHAPTER 33

Breath-Work, The Re-Birthing Process

Smita Wankhade

"Without full awareness of breathing, there can be no development of meditative stability and understanding." - Thich Nhat hanh

The Essence

Five years back during Navratras, I began my deeper connection with the supreme Goddess. I was awakened every morning at about 5am with someone calling my name aloud. I would get up and see who had come over so early in the morning. Surprised, seeing no one around I would go back to sleep. It went on all the nine days. The voice would change. At times it would be a recognized voice. I would ponder and then I got the answer! It was Her awakening me, I had to meditate. Oh! I missed the chance I thought. Just before Navratra this year, I thought, I am now ready to heed to Her calling. This has to be a divine Navratra for me. I want to connect. The next thought that came to my mind was that I wanted to attend a good workshop, I want it in Pune and I want to connect to Babaji.

Two days later, a Facebook post flashed an advertisement about a two-hour talk on Breath work by Leonard Orr, the father of Breath-Work. I had taken training in Breath-Work from Life Research Academy and have been practicing Breath-Work since last 8 years, but yes, to get trained by Leonard Orr himself would be great and moreover, I would get to work on myself! I requested the organizer to let me know if they could organize a minimum two days workshop. And to my surprise, a seven days workshop was planned, and with total co-operation from my husband and son to take responsibility of my ailing mother-in-law, I was on my way to the training!

The entire workshop was not only a hands-on training but also a connection to Babaji, as Leonard has been gifted of the Breath-Work by Babaji himself. And he happens to be a believer of the Supreme Goddess and Shiva. The concluding sentence of every topic in the workshop was - '*Jagdamba Mata Ki Jai. Bhole Baba Ki Jai!*'

I learnt and re-learnt that, and what my practice of the last 8 years taught me about Breath-Work or the Re-Birthing Process is that Breath is a miracle. And that, Breath can cause miracles!

BREATH- A word we know, or rather, we think we know.

BREATH-That's what we start the journey in this body with.

BREATH -That which we take before we make our transition to the life-between-lives state.

BREATH-That changes with any and every emotion we experience.

BREATH-That's true *sathi**!

We start breathing when we are born. But does anyone teach us how to breathe? Infact, at birth, aren't we slapped if we don't breathe? NO one corrects our breath. Breath-Work is here now. Just to correct our breath!

Our breath changes to become slow or fast, shallow or fuller, varying as our emotions change. Without realizing, we take the 'Breath' for granted. Many of us are not even aware that we are breathing! We forget to breathe to the best of our capacity. In fact the tragedy is that we breathe just to keep us going.

It is commonly believed that infancy and old age are similar, and that when we grow old, we get slow, inactive and dependent. Senile. Just like a child. And then we stop living. As if old age is a 'waiting for death' period! Dear friends IT NEED NOT BE SO…We are unaware of how much can change with the breath that is taken to its full extent and utilized properly.

We are not just the physical body we identify with. We are multi-sensory beings. We are physical extensions of the Divine Source. We are immortal. The body has the mechanism to heal without medicines and can be cured using the breath and the gifts we are bestowed with by the Divine. We, too, can live like the yogis if we just use our breath to the fullest. Do you know that 98% of our body's cells are replaced once per year? Our stomach lining is new every 5 days. Our skeleton changes every 3 months. We make a new liver every 6 weeks. In fact our body is designed for continual renewal and rejuvenation when it receives proper attention and support. We can also live for millions of years if we follow the simple rules that the God, the Creator has laid down. The Divine Energy is the source of our salvation.

We receive salvation through the **Seven Vehicles of Grace**. They help us to rejuvenate, balance and maintain our chakras. These 7 rules to self-mastery are:

Meditation- Thinking and study

Water- drinking and bathing

Earth- nutrition, fasting, exercises massage and work

Air- conscious energy breathing

Fire- purification

Love- having harmonious relationships, gurus, spiritual community

Rest- pure relaxation, solitude and peace

Our breath is our connection to the Divine Life-Force. It is the primary source of nourishment and helps in eliminating all the unwanted thought, toxins and undesired emotions. Intuitive breathing is a skill that we can learn easily. Intuitive breathing is the ability to breathe energy as well as air. It involves breathing in a gentle relaxed rhythm.

All the traumatic memories from our past are stored deep in the subconscious mind and are reflected in the way we breathe. By changing the way we breathe we can change the way we live.

We have in us worries, tensions, fears, which is known as 'a death urge'. Death urge is a psychic entity that destroys the body by splitting it from the Eternal Life Force. Without the Eternal Life Force, body of beings become stiffer and more solid till the spirit drops the body to become dust. This death urge can be conquered by out-living it by developing habits of aliveness, mantra, yoga, earth, air, water, fire and spiritual community. **Breath-Work releases us from the death urge and increases in us the life urge.**

Leena, a college student, was ragged in the hostel. She tore up all her certificates and stood in a frozen state for three days. When she came to me she would shout at me when I started the process on her. After three days she started becoming calmer. The next week she borrowed from me some self-help books. Ten sessions were enough to heal her and making her the old, rather, a more mature person!

Breath is a vital link between the body, mind, emotions and the soul. Our breath varies according to changes in emotions and the state of the body and soul. And what are emotions? Emotion=Energy in motion. Whenever there is a stimulus, there are thoughts. And they create emotions. Quantum physicists say that our emotions are made of energy particles and if they are not expressed they remain trapped as energy in between the atoms and molecules of the cells of our body.

Moreover, while taking birth the baby is exposed to harsh lights, harsh sounds; it is squeezed through the birthing canal and is manhandled. The birthing process is many times unnatural, i.e. a caesarean birth, a forceps delivery etc. This creates a birth trauma, which creates the first energy blockages in this body. These can be released by way of Breath-Work, and hence, it is also known as The Re-Birthing Process.

Shailesh came to me with issues regarding his career. He was unable to move ahead in life. We started his BW sessions and he responded very well to the process. In the second session itself he could hear someone telling him to die. 'Don't take birth,' the voice said over and over again…And he could see a room with green curtains and doctors in a general conversation. He spoke to his mother and asked her what happened during his birth…Yes! It was the mother herself not wanting to give him birth. It so happened that his father did not want the child and so his mother had come away to her mother's place during that time. In this condition, separated from her husband, she gave birth to the child and the child sensed her dilemma. She was thinking, but for the child she would be with her partner now!

We also have memories of our past-life traumas, which create energy blockages, and these can be understood, processed and released by BW. When we go through traumatic experiences in this life or the previous life, the emotions are stored and these are the energy blockages that hamper our growth on a spiritual and a mental level. Memories as these traumatic moments are not only stored in the brain but it is now widely accepted that they stored in every cell of the body!! These are effective if released by way of the BREATH-WORK or INTUTIVE BREATHING or CONSCIOUS ENERGY BREATHING or RE-BIRTHING.

Rajesh had numbness in his legs and palms since about ten years. He had intense fear of going out alone and felt a gripping fear of death. The BW sessions brought out intense pain in the numb parts of this body and slowly the numbness disappeared and his fears receded. He became independent and very confident.

The Process

Breath-Work or Re-Birthing process is a process of continuous connected breathing... It is the process where there is no gap between the inhalation and the exhalation. The inhalation is merged into the exhalation. It is breathing easily, gently, in a relaxed manner, to take in with air the Prana, the Tao, the Chi, the Divine Energy. It is simply breathing. **Breathing to the fullest.**

Actually, we do not make use of our entire lung capacity. And we feel we have to die to be with God! We don't have to die to feel Him. Conscious Energy Breathing or Breath-work gives us, and is called, *a biological experience of God*. Breath connects us to the Divine Source, the God. It helps us to release all the energy blockages and our energy body is cleansed, and then begins transformation. It produces ecstasy. Conscious Connected Breathing has a healing ability that makes us spiritually self-sufficient. It energizes the body and the mind. The bonus effect of the process is the realizations that we get. Breath-work gives us fresh and pure energy that makes us feel good, creative, productive and peaceful. It cleans the blood and the nervous system. Negative emotions, feelings like anger, hatred, jealousy and sadness can be released just by way of Breath-Work. It releases us from depression and mood swings. Tensions and the emotional energy pollution that we have collected are released. If practiced on a regular basis, ailments like asthma, epilepsy, migraine headaches, cold, AIDS and cancer can be cured by BW. It helps us to release blockages that have kept us away from success.

The Tip

Success in every area of life!! You can do Breath-Work forever once you have learnt it. It can be learnt from any trained Breath-worker/ Re-birther. Ten, one to two-hour sessions are required to be done with a good Re-birther.

It is such a simple technique that it cannot be believed until it is experienced!

So breathe.... Just breathe....

Smita Wankhade is a Breath Worker, a Past life Regressionist, and a Reiki master. She has been studying the benefits of meditation, creative visualization and energy work and past-life regression. After having gone through different experiences in childhood like tuning to different realms, seeing a 'soul', out-of- the- body experiences, her curiosity about the mystics increased and she understood these experiences when she began learning more about this subject. With her questions answered when she was introduced to the world of spirituality, she realized that spirituality is a wisdom that brings joy which has to be experienced, and that, this joy has to be shared with all mankind!

Having benefited from the breath work and past life regression sessions and with a natural flare for teaching, she realized that giving healing to others and spreading the knowledge of spiritual science is her purpose in life! Through her healing sessions, people have found relief from issues, which were preventing them from living a fuller life. Each of them found the purpose of their life and been able to balance their material and spiritual life.

www.pastliferegressionindia.com

CHAPTER 34

Food as Medicine

Dr. Ashish Paul

"Let food be thy medicine and medicine be thy food" - Hippocrates

The Essence

Any nutritious substance that people or animals eat or drink or plants absorb in order to maintain life and growth is called food. Like all living beings we humans had an evolutionary survival relationship with food for centuries. Human beings eat a mixture of plant origin and animal origin foods and these foods sustain us throughout our lives. All indigenous systems of healthcare or medicine around the globe believe in therapeutic value of foods.

Ayurveda is the oldest system of healthcare on the planet and it talks extensively about prevention, rejuvenation and longevity. It is the only indigenous healthcare system that has a whole branch dedicated for this called *Rasayana* and *Vajikarna*. Simple foods of our daily life become therapeutic or medicinal when taken judiciously. For example: Amla Rasayana where Amla churna (powder) is given everyday for a set period of time in a subsequently increasing and then decreasing dosage. This is used as an intensive rejuvenate therapy in many chronic conditions such as diabetes, autoimmune conditions or cancer for its powerful antioxidant effects.

Ayurveda also talks about three pillars to sustain life; food, sleep and biological wastes of the body.

So food is part of the fundamental concepts of Ayurveda. Ayurveda is unique to talk about foods according to our mind-body types or personality types. In Ayurveda, food is eaten according to our body types. We are all unique with our own individual set of chemicals, neurochemicals, hormones, different absorption and adsorption rates, digestion and our unique psychological and emotional patterns. So two people might eat the same food but the effect those foods will have on their systems is completely different. We all know that even biological identical twins can have completely different personality type let alone two different individuals.

The Process

In Ayurveda we have three main dosha types; *vatta, pitta* and *kapha* and three dual types; *vatta-pitta, vatta-kapha, pitta-kapha* and one tridoshic; *vatu-pitta-kapha*. Ayurveda explains each food according to these mind body constitutional types. For example; in a *pitta* personality type hot and spicy foods must always be avoided because these can lead to hot diseases such as ulcers. In *kapha* types there is a tendency for accumulation of weight or water and are thus advised to not eat heavy foods such as bread or cheese.

All the foods in Ayurveda are divided according to *vatta-pitta-kapha*. For example most of the dairy products such as milk, cheese, yogurt are *kapha* producing. Most of the spices such as cumin seeds, paprika, green chillies, cinnamon, black pepper are heating and thus pitta increasing. *Vatta* aggravating food would be beans, peas, cold foods, cold drinks.

Also foods are divided according to their special effects and called *Sattvic, Rajsic* or *Tamasic* foods due to the effects that they have on us psychologically and emotionally.

Ayurveda also talks about '*ama*'. 'Ama' is the non-digested or partially metabolized food in the digestive tract that plays an important role in the pathogenesis of every disease. In Ayurvedic management of diseases '*ama*' is almost always treated along with the presenting symptoms. This concept has been picked up in the Greek-Roman medicine that filtered down to Western Herbal Medicine. Western Herbal Medicine believes that gut or digestive system must be treated in every disease. Even allopathic medicine knows now that most of our immune complexes are made in the digestive tract or gut so it must be the healthiest to keep our immune system optimal. And we all know how bad digestive health is across the globe and we also know that autoimmune conditions are on the rise.

With the compromised digestive health we do not digest the foods that we eat and do not comprehend the vitamins and minerals from the foods in our bodies. This has led us into eating concentrated forms of foods also called super foods to compensate for the lack of nutrition.

There is so much talk about the functional foods or nutraceuticals in modern nutrition now that everyone is taking some form of natural supplement to augment their health. I strongly believe that when we are eating the right kind of food at the right time according to our *dosha* type, the need to eat these nutritional supplements will be minimal.

Today we have a more gluttonous complex sensual relationship with our foods but have forgotten the real purpose of eating it. We are eating more for pleasure or for emotional support and are paying less attention on the qualities of the food. We as a society are eating out more and more for various reasons and take-away foods are made to please the tongue and not necessarily for health benefits of any foods. We have all the scientific tools to substantiate all the medicinal properties of our foods and then use them in our diet. So we are not just eating foods as a cultural or traditional recipe but clearly understand their benefits too.

On a regular basis I have seen this in my clinical practice how quickly and effectively dietary changes bring improvements in patient's symptoms.

Case study:

Women 50 years, has chronic stomach ache after eating food, indigestion and bloating, chronic constipation. Many of these symptoms are typically present in people with Irritable bowel syndrome. According to Ayurveda it is a typical vatta profile. Patient was advised to follow vatta-reducing diet according to Ayurveda. No beans, peas, potatoes at nighttime meal. Warming spices such as ginger, pepper, coriander, cumin seeds to be added to the meals. Good breakfast, good lunch and light cooked dinners. Food must be always cooked and warm and no cold foods. Digestive herbal tea after each meal was given and it generally contains fennel, chamomile, ajwain, and a pinch of hing. Aloe Vera gel was advised to be taken internally regularly. Patient's symptoms improved considerably within first 4 weeks.

The Tip

My recommendation for anyone trying to lose weight or maintain a healthy weight is to have no dinners or very light dinners. People can still have good breakfast and good lunch but as long as they eat light cooked dinner such as soups will maintain a healthy weight. In other words, they also need to avoid kapha-aggravating foods at nighttime. Eating right food is as important as eating it at the right time. This should be part of the lifestyle advice for everyone especially young kids.

Dr. Ashish Paul is a fully qualified Ayurvedic Practitioner (BAMS- Bachelor of Ayurvedic Medicine and Surgery) and a Medical Herbalist (BSc Hons Herbal Medicine). She recently qualified in MSc Herbal Medicine (Scottish School of Herbal Medicine) and training to be a Dynamic Yoga teacher.

Ashish has just launched her new business Ayuva and the aim is to bring awareness to the holistic benefits that people could enjoy by using the ancient Indian treatments and the western herbal medicine. These therapies work with the natural rhythm of the body, treat the cause of a problem and have less adverse effects.

www.ashishveda.uk

CHAPTER 35

Bach Flower Remedies

Aryanish Patel

Bach Flower Remedies are 100% safe and natural. They establish equilibrium between mind and body, the application of specifically related flowers helps in correcting emotional distress that hampers well-being. Dr Edward Bach created Bach Flower Remedies for all ages of individuals and even plants and animals.

The client meets the practitioner at a one-to-one session. Through the course of the conversation, the practitioner determines the client's remedy requirement, and by a process of elimination, narrows down the choice of remedies. The method is known for its simplicity. Certain flowers have a natural healing quality and there are no adverse reactions or side effects. This is the safest and fastest way to find emotional balance.

> *"Disease of the body itself is nothing but the result of the disharmony between soul and mind. Remove the disharmony, and we regain harmony between soul and mind, and the body is once more perfect in all its parts."* —Dr. Edward Bach.

Dr. Edward Bach and the Bach Flower Remedy System: Background

The Bach flower system was the first of its kind and remains the most thorough set of Natural remedies for emotional distress. Failing within the umbrella of complementary medicine, Bach flower remedies can and often should be a part of professional healer's arsenal of interventions. The remedies have been derived from the specific flowers and are used in a number of different health care settings, from various mediums of health care and wellness. The remedies have proven to work in most unusual ways and The Bach system is one of the most recognized natural remedy systems by far. It works on People and animals both. It is 100% safe and non addictive, which are its strongest qualities.

Parents continue to find Bach flower remedies attractive and effective because they are safe, and do not interfere with any other medication. It is said that it "works in conjunction with herbs, homeopathy and medications and are safe for everyone, including children, pregnant women, pets, the elderly and even plants."

I appreciate the way the Bach flower remedies honor the power of nature as healer. Flowers are most commonly appreciated only for their visual and aromatic beauty. However, there is more to the floral kingdom than decoration. Like many other plants, the 38 flowers used in the Bach system also offer the means by which to achieve wholeness and healing. The remedies have led me to think about plants and flowers differently, and with more respect. I do not look at my garden in the same way; and I have a greater appreciation for the mystery of nature's beauty.

The remedies have become for me a system whereby individuals can achieve harmony with themselves and the world around them. I have used the flowers in this way, with positive results. Those I have worked with have similar reactions to the flower remedies. Peace of mind and well being are the most common reactions to regularly interacting with the flower remedies. They are not drugs; they are the means by which to avoid needing drugs.

As a special needs counsellor and educator, I have worked with a lot clients and the use of the Bach Flower System has definitely made my life easier. I have experienced better results in a shorter duration of time and it has helped me overcome my stress cycle as well. I have to constantly deliver results and I get very drained out when I need longer time to work on one case. Now, after using the Bach System on myself as well, I have felt more ease at work and I am able to enjoy my work process without getting impatient. I have had clients who would not have stayed the course of treatment with any other module other than the Bach System. They themselves admit it. It is, by far the most easiest and safest, with the convenience of anytime anywhere and any amount taken. As special needs educator, my challenges with the temperament of children are a common factor along with being bullied. The Bach system addresses them so easily that one does not even realize how the change manifested in the course of ne treatment bottle. My clients have even called 'Miracle in a bottle'.

Using Bach remedies along with other therapies

I had already begun work as a counsellor. The Bach flower essences fit in well with other types of healing I was drawn to, and became a part of a holistic approach that I continue to cultivate today. The Bach flower system is a holistic type of complementary medicine because it "treats the person and not the disease, considering each client as a unique individual rather than prescribing a standard treatment for certain symptoms or diagnoses."

As I started to incorporate Bach flower remedies into the broader rubric of my own healing practice, I became confident of it being used to support in mainstream medicine. It is not important that doctors dismiss many types of complementary care; so long as those methods of complementary care do not harm, they do not violate the Hippocratic Oath. Moreover, the Bach flower remedies are safe. They are effective.

Dr. Bach, whose work converged with early research in psychology, believed also in personality types. According to Dr. Bach, personality types were related to disease manifestation. When using the flower remedies, the practitioner must discern between the issues that are chronic, or part of the person's personality, and the issues that are acute or temporary.

After taking this course, I see the importance of receiving a more comprehensive accreditation in administering the Bach flower essences. While it is not essential that a healer receive accreditation, it is important to maintain an aura of creditability, and ensure patient safety by having a set of standards that Bach flower practitioners ascribe to in their practices. The course will enhance my confidence as a practitioner and also offer me networking opportunities that can be monetized in the future.

The practitioner- licensing course for Bach slower essences has tremendously enhanced my skills as a practitioner, as well as boosted my confidence in administering the right flower remedies every time. Whereas I used to consult my books when meeting with clients, I now know by heart the uses of each flower remedy and can quickly prescribe formulas that are individualized and personalized. Because "individuals with serious medical or emotional conditions should not rely on Bach flower remedies alone for treatment," I am cautious when prescribing the remedies. The course has taught me the ethical parameters of working as a healer, and how to recognize in others symptoms of resistance to healing. I have worked with several individuals who are averse to seeing doctors, and have coached them to overcome their fears and accept what modern medicine has to offer while also relying on the remedies for their mental and emotional well being. I would never discourage someone from taking medication prescribed by a doctor, but I also encourage my clients to rely on their own mental, emotional, and spiritual reserves rather than on drugs. The purpose of Bach flower remedies is to enhance overall healing.

We have a range of Flower essence ingestible remedies for all spectrums of:

1. Dyslexia
2. ADHD
3. ADD
4. Post Trauma
5. Lack of Focus
6. Easily drained of Energy
7. Requiring motivation all the time
8. Nervousness and being easily bullied.
9. Unable to say No to anyone
10. Not able to make friends
11. Self pity
12. Nonstop self talk.
13. Temper Fitz & The Tantrums
14. Perpetual anxiety on anything
15. Lack of interest in present circumstances
16. Lost and running around aimlessly
17. Unable to break habits.
18. Fear of known things and fear of Unknown

19. Babies who are unable to sleep
20. Parents who require energy balance after draining days
21. Teenagers feeling unloved and unwanted
22. Feeling of not looking pretty
23. Self Doubt
24. Monday morning feeling
25. Gloominess posts a trauma of separation and loss of loved one's accidents, financial losses.

- **Remedies also help for Pregnancy stages like before birth, during birth and post pregnancy.**

    Rescue Remedy is a mix of remedies specially chosen to help at times of everyday crisis. It contains five *Bach Original Flower Remedies* for shock, terror, agitation, loss of control, and feelings of faintness, so it's an ideal one-stop solution to take with you into the labour room.

    Rescue Remedy Spray is a convenient way to take measured doses of *Rescue Remedy*.

- **Remedies for sleeping disorders**

    We have a problem getting restful sleep. According to the National Sleep Foundation, about 70 million people experience sleep-associated problems. Almost 40 million suffer from chronic sleep disorders, and an additional 20 to 30 million are affected by intermittent sleep-related problems. Even worse, most people ignore the problem; few think they actually have one. Only half of those polled by the foundation earlier this year were able to say they slept well on most nights; and one-fourth of adults say sleep problems have some impact on their daily lives Richard Gelula, the foundation's CEO, said there's a link between sleep and quality of life.

"People who sleep well, in general, are happier and healthier," he said. "But when sleep is poor or inadequate, people feel tired or fatigued, their social and intimate relationships suffer, work productivity is negatively affected, and they make our roads more dangerous by driving while sleepy and fewer alerts."

Sleeping medications, including sedative/hypnotic medications, like Ambien, are recommended for short-term use, but lots of people take them frequently and become dependent upon them to fall asleep. Sleep-inducing medications, especially when taken over long periods of time, stay in the bloodstream, giving a hangover the next day and beyond, impairing memory and performance on the job and at home. All medications interact with other medications to one degree or another, sometimes with harmful effects. Finding a natural product or modifying our patterns of behaviour to get a good night sleep is a good first approach with little or no harmful consequences.

There are questions about the effectiveness of sleeping pills. A study by researchers at Beth Israel Deaconess Medical Center and Harvard Medical School found that a change in sleep habits and attitudes was more effective in treating chronic insomnia, over the short- and long-term, than sleeping pills (specifically Ambien). Ambien is the most prescribed pharmaceutical product to induce sleep, chemically. Earlier this month, it was reported that some Ambien users are susceptible to amnesia and walking in their sleep. Some even ate in the middle of the night without realizing it. In contrast, Bach well-known "Rescue Remedy", its 38 specific natural remedies and the just released natural sleep remedy, "Rescue Sleep", acts organically upon our feelings and emotions to bring us emotional balance and a sense of well-being.

The original Bach natural remedies have been used confidently in Europe for over 100 years. Among Bach Remedies most visible advocates in America are Jennifer Anniston who says it keeps her cool under pressure. Kate Blanchett and Salma Hayek have been fans for years. Roberta Flack uses "Rescue Remedy" soothing effect for menopausal hot flashes.

The new release, "Rescue Sleep" contains the 5 effective ingredients of "Rescue Remedy" plus White Chestnut. White Chestnut is effective against restless mind.

Case Studies

Description of client – age, sex, marital status, number of children, etc.

A middle-aged lady in her late 50's. Married with one son. Having a pale complexion and thin-built with an aura of stress visible on her shoulders.

Outline of the problem for which the client came for treatment.

A middle-aged lady with an autistic son was worried about their future. She had been wondering if she dies earlier than her son, who will look after him. How will he go on with his life? Her age was catching up and she was not able to do as much as earlier.

Client's knowledge of the remedies.

The client's had observed my earlier client's son having been able to transform his temper and improve overall focus. She asked the parent how the change happened and learnt about Bach Flower Remedies. Her idea of the remedies was that they are safe and can do what allopathy cannot. She had a detailed conversation with the parent who also told her about Dr. Bach's system being about treating the person and not the disease.

First impressions. How the client appeared, behaved, etc.

The client had a nervous disposition and also guilt and embarrassment about having a son with autism. Her in-laws had been hard n her about it. She had lost her spark and was only a shadow of what she once was. Yet, she was open-minded about trying the remedies and comfortable in talking about her situation with me.

My introduction to and explain of the Bach system; the main body of the interview; My interactions with the client and his/hers with me; how I obtained information to enable me to choose appropriate remedies.

I started with introducing my client t to the system –

The Bach flower remedies are natural remedies derived from 38 specific flowers. Dr. Edward Bach, a medical doctor during his early ages has discovered this system and remedies. All of us go through stressful situations in our life. These can be overwhelming emotionally. The Bach system of remedies helps us restore balance.

Interactions

She began to trust me once I showed her how she can find a balance in the situation through the Bach Flower remedies. She spoke about how her married life and overall life had been affected by her having a son with such a disability. With each interaction, she was becoming a more confident and someone who started to look forward to having fun in life rather than just brooding over her problems and more so the perceived problems of the future. She always gave out clear hints of what remedies to go with. Every time I asked her how she was feeling the day she visited for a consultation, her answers were "I am feeling like how will I go on with the day?" or "Today I am more worried than most days, as today my father-in-law asked me what arrangement have I made for my son if something were to happen to me?" or "I am too tired to go on with life and I do not see clear skies in the future."

All of these sentences coming from her were indications so close to the remedies to be used for her. It seemed like at some level she had connected so well with the remedies that Dr. Bach was himself guiding to see which one to give her.

Remedies considered.

The first time I thought of using Pine, Elm, Clematis, and Chestnut bud, White Chestnut, Hornbeam and Mimulus.

The remedies above were the most appropriate choices for my client. When our initials consultations about her feeling what she at that time was clear, I looked at what best to give her immediate relief.

This combination was most appropriate for her situation and she took to it really well. The client was very vocal and clear of what she has come to me for, and right from the start it was clear about how to take course, so there were no changes in the mid way.

Remedies chosen and reasons for my selection. Reasons for not giving other remedies that could have applied.

I chose remedies on the basis of how to relieve her from the stress and magnitude of the burdened life that she was living. I had brought the chart of the Bach Flower remedies and framed and kept in the consultation. I asked her to look at the chart and see what she can relate to with the remedies. I chose for her. She looked at the chart and felt she wanted to go with what I had chosen. She was comfortable with the remedies I had selected for her. Since it was her first time, she also wanted to go with the flow and see how it works out for her. I felt the smoothness of her acceptance to the remedies helped her heal sooner than had expected.

Follow up and progress made. Development of the treatment programme, and changes in mixture with reasons for any changes.

My client came for a follow up after 3 weeks. There was a remarkable difference in her. She had returned from a holiday and had a makeover in her appearance, which was refreshing. I almost did not recognize her. She said the remedy helped her get good sleep and she found herself smiling a lot more and wanting to give herself time as well. She had not complained about her appearance once she started the remedies.

This time, she wanted herself gain more ability to handle situations with ease rather than wanting them to go away. She has also realized how she had inspired other mom's to connect and share their lives and worries forming a group. She obviously headed it and made a page on Face book where there can all be there for each other when needed. The mother who came to me so worried is now helping others overcome their problems.

I had good reason to make changes in the remedy. I changes Chestnut bud, White Chestnut, Hornbeam, Mimulus and pine. They had done their job. She was now steady on Clematis, Elm and Oak. Along with which I felt the need to add Centaury. Though she was refreshed in her life, she also needed to give herself the luxury of being there for herself and not always doing it for other. I really liked the outcome and so did she. She did tell all mothers about the Bach Flower Remedies. Rather, she started the trend.

Overall Progress made during the whole course of treatment or treatment period thus far if still going on.

She made dramatic progress in the first treatment itself, Post the treatment, she did two follow ups and then on it was not necessary as she found a good emotional balance and stayed the course, She also gained her long lost self. I have mentioned the entire progress in the above section.

Present state. His/Her client's expectations, hopes and plans for the future in respect of continued treatment, other avenues to explore, and general development of well being.

My Client and I saw the remarkable difference of the natural remedies by Dr. Bach. She felt alive again after decades. The remedies more than met with her expectations. She joined a yoga and singing class. She was now self motivated and driven to live life and enjoy it. I feel this case was a huge motivation for me too.

Aryanish was born dyslexic, but overcame the challenge at an early age. Showered with love and understanding, she grew up in an environment where individual conditions were seen as mere variations in the human diversity that enriches the planet. As she grew into a talented and accomplished youngster, Aryanish felt obliged to empower others in similar situations.

She went on to pursue a training course in Dyslexia Correction in London. She also embarked on year-long research in the fields of classical Indian music and belief restructuring through neural pathways. To keep herself abreast with international developments in the field, she underwent training in 'Bach Flower Remedies' from the Bach Centre, London. She is the founder of 7Pathways Global, a social enterprise through which she combines her training, her own personal experience and her zeal to make a positive contribution to the world. All her therapies are backed by intensive study. Today, Aryanish has four method patents pending on corrective learning with dyslexia, ADHD, ADD and post-traumatic disorders. She has been featured in numerous journals and magazines such as DNA and Times Wellness. Her products have been well received in Indian and international markets. Her focus is now to reach out to a wider audience and provide innovation solutions on a global scale.

www.7pathwaysglobal.com

CHAPTER 36

Sports and Spirit

Theresia Eggers

A few years ago I decided that I needed to do things I loved to do! Whenever I don't follow this rule, I get stuck, things don't work, or I get sick. Pondering over what I really love doing I came up with: exercise, being creative, believing in a positive energy field, and sharing this with others. The idea of "Sport & Spirit" was born. Being aware of the connection between body, mind, emotions, and spirit, one realizes that we create a positive energy field when we do something we love to do. Exercise is also one of the most powerful tools to feel good. I observed this not just with myself, but also with many people I met and interacted with in my 10 years of professional work as a fitness trainer and spiritual coach. People who do exercise seem to be more balanced, happier within themselves, and also look healthier. Around 10 years back I got really curious about this topic. Why did exercise make such a big difference in people's lives? The explanation of medical research, that our glands release hormones (viz. endorphins) in our body when we exercise, which in turn makes us happy, seemed to be an effect of something bigger – but not the cause. I started to research this topic on a spiritual basis and found that we are dealing with the universal energy itself. When we make the conscious effort of training, we are pulling the pure positive energy through our energy centers into our aura and our body. This has such a powerful effect, that it can clear blockages, negative thoughts, tension, and emotional imbalance.

One of my clients, a woman, started to exercise with me. She was in great turmoil because she'd gone through a divorce a couple of years earlier. She felt unattractive, weak, and was overweight. She'd just fallen in love with another man and doubting whether this man liked her too. It was a long journey of physical and spiritual training to convince this woman that she was lovable.

The physical exercise motivated her so much that she could transform her belief system and get the power to lose weight and believe that she was lovable. Finally, they got together and, are still a couple. There are many stories like this, where people transformed their beliefs about themselves, using exercise to connect to their own power. There is an old saying: "You are what you think." Sometimes we are not even aware of what is going on in our minds since we get so used to our thinking habits. Our emotional state shows us whether we are really happy (i.e. healthy) with our belief system about ourselves or our lives. After a longer period of feeling down, often because of having negative thoughts, the physical body begins to shut down too and you become sick, sometimes very sick. But you have the power to create balance: you are the creator of your well-being. The most effective way to clear your aura, retune your chakras and transform your belief system, is through physical and spiritual practice.

Imagine your aura and body as a house getting stuffy and dirty from too much sitting around, poor diet, emotional overreactions and stress. You start to clean up, open the windows and let fresh air in, take the garbage and broom and polish out. What a feeling! That is what physical exercise does for you. Through exercise, the chakras become activated and draw pure unprocessed energy into the many layers of your energy system and physical body. Congested energy is pushed out, negative blocks disappear, and depleted energy is renewed.

It's not only mental or emotional beliefs that block the flow of energy: poor diet and too much sitting around also weaken you and your self-esteem. One of my clients worked in an office and ate fast food when he found time to eat. His face was gray, his skin showed low blood circulation and, he had no energy left. He could hardly concentrate on his work – so the outcome was accordingly poor. His self-esteem had gone downhill and he knew he had to get help. After one month's physical training, a new diet and spiritual motivation, he transformed himself into a new man. Physical and spiritual work go hand in hand.

After intense research, observations and evaluations, I found the best outcome in training when I worked with the energy of the four elements. They flow through us and can be activated through the four training types, which are directly linked to the four elements. Different intentions create different outcomes.

1. For energy and to feel vital and active: Cardio training; Element: Fire.

2. For strength, muscle tone, posture and self-esteem: Resistance training; Element: Earth.
3. For flexibility, subtleness and self-awareness: Flexibility training; Element: Air.
4. For balance, calmness and inner peace: Relaxation training; Element: Water.

The four elements are the major vibrational building blocks of our Earth. They balance, complement, and also oppose each other. It's the same with the four training types: if you want to create an optimal energy flow, you should combine different training types; or if you really like to work on a specific issue, choose a training type which can help you to best manifest the outcome you are looking for. Effort creates reward and balance. With exercise you are activating your natural potential to look good, feel good, and think positively. But you need persistence and discipline and, if this doesn't come naturally to you, try to become this person. There is nothing more rewarding then turning a belief around. I am talking about my own experience. I have turned many beliefs around – and am still doing it. One of my misleading beliefs was that I had no discipline. But as I look at myself now, I see a very disciplined person. Every belief is changeable. Take your time, start slowly, start steadily, but do it!

Theresia Eggers is the founder for "Intune" Program. Intune- The program is Theresia's vision and interpretation of a holistic exercise program. It works with the energy of Four elements- Fire, Earth, Air and Water, which are a part of everyone of us, and the activation of seven chakras. The goal of this program is to make you feel whole by connecting to all the different aspects of yourself through a training that includes body, mind, emotion and spirit.

www.sportandspirit.co

CHAPTER 37

Say Yes to Money
Create a Happy Relationship with Money

Suresh Padmanabhan

The best month to have Money is December, some of the other months are October, April, August, March, May, January, July, September, November, June, and February - **Suresh Padmanabhan**

Close your eyes and review your money life now. What is it at present? Do you think you have actually had great money potential but somehow money flow is not right. I have been conducting Money Workshops across many parts of the World since 15 years and having spoken to more than a million people, I realize that "Money is an issue deep down with many".

The only difference is some have guts to confront it, whilst others push it under the carpets. Some just do not want to look into the money aspect, some are playing escaping games, and some are praying that money takes care of itself.

You would have observed that people less talented are making more money than you. I have seen highly talented nice people who are skilled in their profession but lost when it comes to money. It gives a lot of pain to watch this. Talent has gone waste. There is a fight between what you love and money flow. What you love might not give money, so you get trapped in a job, profession or business, which is paying but not nourishing. Some day you say, you will do that Job which you love. And sadly that day never comes.

My Own Personal Life Story

I hail from a typical middle class tamil family. My dad was working in a clerical cadre with the Government of India. I was told a family secret in my childhood.

Study Hard, Live Simple, Earn Less but have Good Values and Work Hard. Nowhere in my family dictionary was *Earn Big, Work Easy, and Do Business.*

When I asked that taboo question, my father said a simple answer- "you are a south indian and not a guajarati, punjabi or a marwari."

My life was exactly as per my family standards. Having passed from a management school I joined the world of advertising. I ended up working hard. My whole family was happy but not very Happy because I did not fulfill their dream of working for a government organisation. Everyone was happy except me.

I was seeing the sparkle in my sindhi, marwari, guajarati friends who were making so much money by running their family business. Their life was big, grand and limitless. My life was small, mediocre and full of scarcity.

I wanted all this to change and change Fast. I dared to be different. To start with, I started investing all that I earned into the stock markets. Suddenly I hit a jackpot. Goddess Lakshmi started showering her blessings and my money started to grow. While my dad was happy with his 8 % to 10 % in the FD of a bank or the post office, Here I was making 40% , 60 % and even 200% in the stock market. The going was super good. My family got tempted and they also gave their hard earned money to me to invest into the stock market. My dad's friends, My own friends all gave me money to invest. I was suddenly the blue eyed investment banker to one and all. Everyone was enjoying the ride and I was flying high. I wanted more. Dil Mange More. Greed possessed me. I then discovered the world of speculation. So called F & O (futures and options). I lost caution to the wind. I became possessed, reckless and unguarded.

And one day everything changed. The stock markets crashed, along it my money, my family money and money of my friends. Huge losses. It would have took me years to even come back to zero. My dreams crashed. I kept slipping, making one mistake after the other. And I ended in the darkest phase of my life.

Then I realized the harsh realities of money. I lost my name, face, friends and myself. I was down and out. I started the blame game. Why me? I am honest, sincere, did not do anything bad for anyone and I assumed for sure God punishes only good people and life is unfair. The more pessimistic I became worsen my situation turned out to be. I forgot to read, meditate and be happy with my friends. I had few support and more so from my family. I was in a dark cave waiting for light. Time just went by.

One day it just hit me. I had to take responsibility for my money actions. I have to move on. I gathered courage, became positive in my thoughts and started taking small micro steps towards brightness. I read, re- read, meditated, prayed and learnt more about the stock market. If I had gained once there, I could gain once again. I now had the conviction. I borrowed money from my parents with an assurance that I would get out of all my money Issues. Over a period of time, I emerged stronger. I started clearing all my debts. And soon I was again in a positive cash flow. But it took years, lot of struggle, lot of hard- work. But the experience was huge. I became the hero of my own story. And one day money workshop just flashed into my life. It was a divine blessing by God who possibly tested my patience. It was a prasad he gave me. I got my life back; I got a mission to teach about money to one and all. It is 15 years since and because it is a God's blessing and a moving experience of my own, Money Workshop turned out to be a greatest original authentic workshop on money. Today so many workshops are modeled on money workshop. It makes me immensely proud to have created money magic in so many lives.

Isn't it the Time to Wake Up and Smell the Money?

Money, Money, Money- It is everywhere. If it is not in your pocket, it is in your head. It is part of everybody's life and it is a part of you. It has such great power that it can command attention from everyone.

Understanding Money is Understanding Life

The biggest lie you have ever heard is, "Money is not important in my life." There is enough proof that whatever you are today and whatever you will ever be is shaped by money. It is a bunch of hypocrites who keep saying, "Money is not important in my life."

Everything you are today is an outcome of the money flow in your life — your status, net worth, and self-image...

Money is needed to get you started and keep you going through life. It is very much like the fuel and oil that is needed to keep your vehicle running. Run out of fuel and your vehicle stops. Run out of money and your life could stop. It is as essential as the air you breathe, as vital as mother's milk to a new born baby or the blood circulating in your body. Whether you love it or hate it, you simply cannot live without money.

Forget friends; look at your own shadow. When the sun is shining brightly, your shadow also follows you so faithfully. When it is dark, your shadow too disappears. Without Money you realize "you are a nobody from nowhere."

You may have felt life was just like Maths. *Disappearance of friends is directly proportional to disappearance of money.*

Take Some Money Actions Now!

Develop a Happy Relationship with Money

Drop your seriousness around Money and make it playful and joyful. In a lighter vein we learn the importance of being playful and relaxed. *Be aware* should be the motto for a joyful life and that includes money.

Money too is a natural phenomenon. Being playful with money means that you can see its natural beauty, know the laws it follows, know the rules of games you can devise and enjoy with it. As in any game, the vital elements in the money game are knowledge of the rules and skill of the players. With increasing practice your skills increase by leaps and bounds.

Learn About Money- But Only Once and For a Lifetime

"The illiterate of the 21st century will not be those who cannot read and write, but those who cannot learn, unlearn, and relearn." -Alvin Toffler

Money is like learning to play music. First you play with all rules then you forget the rules and play by the heart. As children we all avoided the subjects in which we were weak and this habit still continues. Plunge into the world of money. Read, watch motivational videos on money and attend workshops. Master this subject once and for all.

Take 100 % Responsibility for Your Money Life

We need to summon the courage to take ownership of all our thoughts, deeds, knowledge, actions, choices, experience, most importantly, our success and failures. Becoming honest and transparent with our issues of money will help us overcome it forever. Encounter and demolish the fears of money. Fear is not just forgetting everything and run. But face everything And rise. As you take responsibility the whole universe sends you resources and power to become successful.

Review all your Belief Systems

Belief is what is true For you. If you believe money is scarce, struggle, tough, it will turn out to be that. People who are healers, tarot card readers, energy workers, light workers, and new age therapist sometimes get this wrong belief that one should not charge money for their work. They create a split personality and conflict with money from inside. Some of them do free work. Deep down they are highly disappointed but just fool themselves that "All is well". Don't fake your life, it is hard work. They get disturbed with smart new age therapists who make good money and also have a lot of clients.

All free or low paid services are not appreciated. Once you set a low standard for yourself, it becomes so difficult to change it later.

Have respect for your profession by giving your very best and also charging appropriately. Remember money is also energy. Become comfortable with it. Then magic happens. You feel good with yourself. You attract the best clients who respect your energy work and most important even your energy flows well.

Brand Yourself Well

When you brand yourself well, the competition becomes irrelevant. It just does not exist. What people think about you, your brand and your service really matters. Your brand is a story that should do the talking. Learn all about technology. Get a good website. Create a powerful presence in Facebook, Twitter or LinkedIn. Write a super blog. Make classy presentations. All your visiting cards, brochures and your promotional material should be done professionally and spell class. Times are changing super fast so adapt or be left behind.

Some Quick Techniques that you can Act Upon Now

Buy a good quality wallet. Buy a cash box for your business or home. Money comes to those who are ready. You send a powerful message to the universe that now you are ready for big money flow.

Organise money neatly wherever it is placed. When Money is scattered life is scattered. Organising Money is organising thoughts about money thereby leading to a healthy money flow.

Do Daily Accounting

Another invaluable practice is that of maintaining daily accounts. Daily accounting is simple. You need to account for each rupee coming and going out of your life. Account as it happens. Each one of us has just about ten to twelve transactions each day. Keeping the bills organised and in one place will enhance the process.

Beware that your mind right now must be telling you, "Hey, what big difference is it going to make?" or "nobody ever became rich because of writing their accounts," or anything else that will prevent you from writing the accounts. Daily accounting is painful, but so was brushing our teeth or taking a bath in childhood. It may seem boring or lot of work, but it's essential for holistic money growth and for a factual picture of your strengths and weaknesses. Through precise accounting, troublesome money patterns like excessive spending or poor savings can be curbed. Even if you now hate figures it's not so hard to grow to love them.

Remember "Daily Accounts" is writing accounts daily and not all the account of the week on a Sunday. And that Sunday never comes!

When the account is in the mind, it does not give a clear picture. As you put it into writing, clarity starts coming in. Now you can see every account as it is. This is called "chunking" (sorting into smaller bits). Now you can see various headings of accounts very clearly — for e.g. Food expenses, travel expenses, communication costs, rent etc. You can exercise control over money only when you have the details. If you realise that the food bills are high then the next month you can cut it down. Most of the times a mere realisation that "Food bills are high" will ensure that the expenses are cut down naturally. I have great respect for my father, who all through his life time maintained perfect "Daily Accounts." He never forgot to write the daily accounts even for a single day. This ensured that he never had to face a big money problem in life.

You may have 100's of reasons for not writing the "Daily Accounts" but once you get into a habit you will be more disturbed if you forget or don't write the "Daily Account." Well you can ask anyone who is maintaining "Daily Accounts."

Personal Money Rituals

Each day carry a min of Rupees 11,000.00 in person. Remember money attracts money. If your mind resists this idea for whatever reason think If you cannot handle a mere 11000 Rupees how will you handle a million.

Always count money towards yourself and not away from you.

The color that attracts money is red and green. Hence our own Goddess Maha Lakshmi is always dressed in fine, rich green or red Saree. For starters you could have a green or a red Wallet.

Remember money day is friday. Shukrawar. The energy that influences money is the planet Venus. You many take powerful money actions on friday which is the money day world-wide. The other auspicious days are full moons where maximum manifestation happens and also money being a feminine energy, the influence of moon is highest.

Free Money Resources

We have created the most powerful mantras in the world on Money and Abundance. They are the largest hits on YouTube. You may access some of them here at http://www.youtube.com/themoneyworkshop

Also we have created the Worlds First 3 D Money Mantra one of its only kind in the whole world. You may search 3 D Money Mantra in youtube.

http://www.youtube.com/watch?v=HhTlpfUhZv4

You may like our facebook page for lifelong connectivity. We have the largest number of fans for any motivational programs which exceeds 11000. You may like this page https://www.facebook.com/moneyworkshop

We have a great website which you may go through www.TheMoneyWorkshop.com

Suresh Padmanabhan is the Creator of the Money Workshop. An Original Authentic Workshop on Money running successfully since 15 years across many parts of the World. He has authored an International Bestseller "I Love Money". Running into a million copy it is now translated into 14 Indian and International Languages. His other books are "Ancient Secrets of Money" and "On Cloud 9" a motivational parable. You may read his blog at http://www.themoneyworkshop.com/blog/

www.themoneyworkshop.com

The Being Approach

CHAPTER 38

Healing Through Hypnotherapy

Suzy Singh

*Hypnosis is not some mystical procedure,
but rather a systematic utilization of experiential learning. - Milton Erickson*

As he emerged from trance, Anand felt all of the doubts and conflicts within him dissolve. The turmoil about the crossroads he stood upon seemed to vanish, and it was replaced by a sense of deep inner calm. He no longer worried about the right thing to do, because the wisdom of his subconscious mind had shown him exactly why this experience was important for his evolution and what he ought to do. He smiled at me and uttered a word of thanks for having helped him discover the power of his own mind.

All of us know that we have a mind but not everyone is aware that we actually have two minds. The western world and psychologists refer to these as the conscious and subconscious mind while the eastern complimentary sciences such as Ayurveda, speak of the inner or deeper consciousness, and the outer or sensory mind.

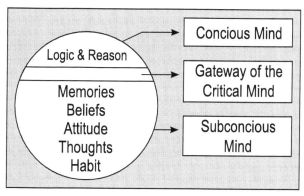

The conscious outer mind that most people are familiar with constitutes only the tip of the proverbial mind-sphere iceberg and is responsible for cognition, reasoning, analysis, evaluation, calculation, judgement and decision-making. It feeds off the five senses to perceive its reality and helps you arrive at suitable conclusions. So when your eyes see an overcast sky, your conscious mind concludes that when you step out of your house that morning, you should carry an umbrella.

The subconscious or inner mind constitutes almost 88% of the whole mind and is the storehouse or repository of all your long term memories and impressions both from this life as well as past lives.

All positive and negative experiences that you have ever had, are stored here and the resulting impressions are embedded as beliefs, attitudes, tendencies and habits which determine the hardwiring of your brain. This is akin to a library where your soul's personal records are stored and maintained.

Now if it so happened that at age two you had met with a car accident on a cloudy day, chances are that even 32 years later, when you see the sky overcast, you may feel anxious and restless. For no apparent reason you may decide that you don't feel like driving to work and prefer instead to take the train. Your conscious mind will rationalise that decision because it must analyse your feelings and may conclude that taking the train on that day makes much better sense because the traffic is always terrible on Thursday's. You end up believing that choosing the train ride to work is an active choice; but is it really?

The reason you are not aware that choosing the train was motivated by the subconscious mind is because these two minds are separated by the critical mind which acts as a doorkeeper of your inner consciousness. It operates as a guard that does not permit entry into the subconscious mind in beta brain wave frequency, which simply stated, is your active everyday ordinary awareness, and hence you cannot recall the memory of that accident at age two.

Bridging The Two Minds

Both these minds interact and engage with each other guiding, directing and affecting how we think, perceive information, behave, act and relate to life's challenges. While the conscious mind is what you are normally aware of, it's the subconscious mind that is really pulling the strings like a puppeteer who controls the puppet, but is never seen. How many times have you decided to go on a diet only to find yourself gorging on that irresistible chocolate cake? Or made a New Year resolution to quit smoking and broken it on the second of January?

The reason is that while your logical mind tells you not to eat the chocolate cake because it is unhealthy for you, the data stored in the subconscious mind sends out powerful signals instructing you to eat it, since all past associations with eating chocolate cake embedded in the subconscious mind are positive. So while 12% of your mind says no, 88% of your mind says a resounding yes. Is it any surprise that you end up breaking your resolve?

The conscious mind makes the intent, but it's the subconscious mind that steers and drives your behaviour. In order to understand why you act and behave in the ways that you do, it is important to uncover the associations and motivations that lie hidden in your subconscious mind. It is these associations that determine your choices and each time that you act them out, they are further reinforced making those preferences habitual or hardwired in you.

So think about this, every time X ignores you it only strengthens your belief that perhaps X does not like you. What you are unaware of, is that you perceive this event through the filter of a past memory which is triggered in your subconscious mind when you felt similarly ignored, albeit a long time ago which you may not remember. You begin to feel uncomfortable around X and start avoiding him. As this continues to recur, there comes a time when even the sight of him stresses you out triggering your defences and releasing a surge of adrenaline and cortisol into your blood stream making you want to run.

Since you don't ordinarily have access to the subconscious mind, you are not aware of the deeper reasons for feeling and behaving as you do. You wonder why you dislike X even though you have no obvious reasons to do so, and you remain stuck in the vicious circle of disliking and avoiding him, feeling unworthy in his presence and by association disliking him even more because you associate X with feeling rejected and unworthy.

If however you could go into your subconscious mind and change the belief that X dislikes you, it could transform your relationship with him. So let's say if you found out that X had not meant to ignore you that very first time you felt this way, but had just received news that his mother was hospitalised and was overcome by grief, you would perceive that situation very differently and perhaps even feel kindly towards him.

Or if you discovered that X actually reminded you of Uncle Tom who never liked you as a child, you could heal that original experience with Uncle Tom and it would change how you felt about X. However the important question is, how can you get past the doorkeeper of the critical mind to reach the subconscious, from where you can dig these memories out and access this hidden knowledge?

Using Hypnosis as the Bridge

Hypnosis can allow you to bypass the critical factor and focus on selective thinking, allowing effective and speedy access into your subconscious mind. It can bridge your past with your present and unravel memories and experiences that compel you to feel, think and behave in ways that easily override your conscious decisions. It leads you into a trance- like, deeply relaxed alpha state into which the subject is guided by the hypnotist, by getting his attention to slip past the doorkeeper of the subconscious or the critical mind.

In this dreamlike state, the subject can now recall information from other times or states of consciousness. He still has a fuzzy awareness of his present and immediate surroundings which creates a kind of elliptical awareness whereby he can be in both states simultaneously, focussed more there and less here and hence, not only recall but also digest information that is retrieved from the past giving rise to insight and integration of the data recovered.

Researcher, teacher and author Dr Joe Dispenza[1] describes this state perfectly when he says that the brain literally becomes unaware of time (because we lose track of time), we lose awareness of the environment (we don't see anything because our visual cortex shuts off), and we don't have any concept of our body. In fact, we don't feel like we are in our body anymore – all we see is that important thought in our mind. This process is called dissociation. It happens when we naturally dissociate from the constant sensations of the body in the external world in linear time. We are no longer associating with our sense of self with our environment.

What is so amazing is that we dissociate all the time in our normal lives like when reading an interesting book, driving on the highway, watching an engrossing film or playing video games. Trance is about learning, and as Elmar Woelm[2] says, it involves learning to go into trance, learning to get into contact with ones subconscious resources and learning to widen ones range of beliefs.

When you are driving on the highway, it's easy to zone out and lose track of time because your mind gets focussed inwards becoming absorbed in either the music that's playing on the radio, or immersed in the scenery or even thinking about that fabulous holiday that you enjoyed last summer. You could become so absorbed in these thoughts that you might even forget that its way past lunch hour and your stomach is growling for food, or wonder how you reached your destination so fast.

This then is the experience of the hypnotic state during which you gain entry into your subconscious mind. During this trance- like state, the external reality is temporarily suspended as the mind turns inwards and focuses sharply on the subject of enquiry. This is a highly creative state and most artistes produce some of their greatest works from this state of consciousness.

Hypnosis which comes from the Greek word *Hypnos* means to sleep. This does not imply that you lose control over yourself while in hypnosis, but that your mind turns inwards and does not engage with the external environment just as in sleep. A skilled hypnotherapist can easily induce such a state of trance in a subject and then proceed to look for the source of his suffering, be it mental, physical or emotional by using effective therapeutic techniques that allow for the healing to happen.

In this highly imaginative and creative state, it is the subject's mind itself that provides the solutions to his problems, as Anand discovered, while the therapist merely facilitates and allows for insights to surface and the healing to occur.

Using Hypnosis for Healing

I remember an amusing incident that occurred on a flight back from one of my healing intensives in the country. There was a dapper gentleman sitting next to me and he spent a long time chatting up and telling me about his ceramic business. When we reached our destination and boarded the bus to the airport building, he casually enquired about my profession. The minute he learned I was a hypnotherapist, he jerked his body away from mine, aghast with fear and almost begged me not to hypnotize him.

Most people have the mistaken impression that a hypnotist will put you under his command, depriving you of free- will and leaving you with no control over the situation. Nothing can be further from the truth. This impression has been erroneously created by the entertainment industry, particularly movies and stage hypnotists whose primary purpose is to entertain, amuse and shock the audiences.

Clinical hypnotherapy uses hypnosis with the sole intention of healing and therapy work. However, there are few aspects that are critical for the success of this approach.

- First and foremost it requires that the subject or client be willing to enter into hypnosis without which it is virtually impossible to create a successful trance. Many a time clients bring their grown up children or spouses to my clinic wanting to help them de-addict or change some unhealthy pattern. However, unless the subject himself requests for therapy, I do not take on these cases because no matter how skilled a therapist you are, you cannot assist in healing someone who does not want to heal himself. Furthermore, such people are unlikely to enter into a hypnotic trance because their subconscious mind will resist it.

- Secondly, the quality of trance is important and this must be ascertained before proceeding with therapy work because different issues need different levels of trance depth. Some therapies are better performed under light trance while others require medium or deep trance.

- Thirdly, creating a good trance only opens the door to the subconscious mind but you now need to determine how to get to the source event or what caused the problem in the first place. The therapist must be well versed to guide and direct the search to the source of the problem.

- Fourthly, the therapist must have enough training and tools at his disposal to successfully conduct the therapy work which is always unique to each

- case and cannot be standardised. Knowledge about mental health and psychotherapy can be greatly beneficial in doing this work.
- Fifthly, you must be equipped to think on your feet and change tracks or techniques as required. For as someone once said, it's like searching for the treasure and if the key you are using to unlock the treasures of the mind does not work, make sure you have others handy.
- And last though not the least, appropriate use of post hypnotic suggestions, and where required, future progressions must be employed to integrate and complete the therapy work. This is why it is commonly said that putting somebody into trance is the easy bit, but knowing what to do after they have been hypnotized is where the real challenge lies.

Clinical uses of Hypnosis

a. Suggestion therapy

There are broadly two major approaches used in clinical work, namely suggestive and analytic. Suggestion therapy employs the use of direct or indirect suggestions under hypnosis to create desired outcomes and to modify behaviour. This method has several applications and is widely used to enhance sports performance, help people to quit smoking, in alcohol de-addiction, reversing the habit of nail biting and enuresis (bedwetting in children), building self esteem, stress release, pain management and dental hypnosis, to name just a few.

I have also used hypnosis quite effectively to improve academic performance in children who either have trouble concentrating or tend to procrastinate and put off studying for their exams. These children have shown note worthy improvement and gone on to score good grades, greatly improving their self confidence.

In one of my cases, I used dental hypnosis to assist a 10 year old boy to remain perfectly calm and relaxed during a series of dental extractions. The blood and saliva flow post the extractions was considerably reduced and he was able to undergo all the extractions painlessly.

Hypnotic suggestions are also useful in overcoming nausea in pregnant women, fear of public speaking in those whose expression is blocked and in speedy post operative recovery.

Several Olympic athletes routinely use hypnosis to enhance their performance. In the year 1956 the Russian Olympic team, took with them a team of 11 hypnotists to the Melbourne Olympics and went on to win the highest number of medals as compared to any other country.3

b. **Analytical therapy**

Analytical hypnosis involves the search for the origin or source of the problem which could lie in either the subject's present life, in-womb state or a past life, and enable its effective resolution through therapy. It involves filtering down from the presenting problem that the client comes in with, to arrive at the real issues which can often be very different from what they thought their problem was.

Once the original source of the issue is found, the emotional charges associated with that problem can be released and any physical body armours related with that initial event dissolved under hypnosis. Relationship issues, fears and phobias, relief from irritable bowel syndrome (IBS) overcoming hyperhidriosis (excessive sweating) and personality based issues such as procrastination, stammering and obsessive compulsive disorders (OCD's) are some examples that fall into this category.

A middle-aged client of mine came in for therapy wanting to heal his IBS. He had been taking medicines to treat the same but relief had been temporary and the symptoms recurred frequently whenever he was under stress. During therapy he discovered a childhood memory under hypnotic age regression in which he was mortified of failing at a sport that his parents really wanted him to pursue. This created a double bind in him because a part of him felt fearful of failing and didn't want to go for the practice sessions, while the other part wanted to please the parent and hence did not express his fear. As a result he continuously repressed his inner feelings and self expression. With each successive practice session as his fear surfaced, he repeatedly repressed it, causing his stomach to churn and knot up.

Through the pre-talk and hypnotic interventions he realised that many years later, as a successful corporate executive in a leadership role, he felt a similar abdominal churning whenever things at work got too challenging, triggering his IBS.

Under hypnotic trance he recognised how he was still operating from his childhood fears and experiencing the double bind situation at his work place. If he expressed his point of view at the management meetings he was worried about sticking his neck out and then failing. If he didn't voice his opinions he was anxious about being perceived as lacking vision or not taking a stand, which as a leader he was expected to do.

Through therapy his fears were resolved by healing his inner child and reframing the source event. Within a month his IBS vanished and he discovered a new found freedom at work where he could openly express his opinions, confront situations which he was earlier averse to, and also became more expressive with his colleagues. It has been two years since, and the client reports that he is free of the IBS and has not required medication during this period.

Hypnosis is very effective in re-engineering negative beliefs. Often negative experiences create limiting beliefs and opinions in the subjects mind about their own selves and others, causing them to think and behave in ways that create disharmony in their lives and prevent them from harnessing their full potential. In such cases the old limiting beliefs must be released or rewritten, substituting them instead with empowering and positive beliefs.

The meanings and interpretations that people attach to their experiences make their lives either happy or unhappy. This means that how people think, affects the quality of their lives. The power lies within them to change their thinking and hypnosis can help in doing just that. For as Mahatma Gandhi so aptly said, keep your thoughts positive because they become your words, keep your words positive they become your behaviour, keep your behaviour positive it becomes your habit, keep your habits positive they become your values, keep your values positive, they become your destiny. So if you want to change your destiny, you can start by changing your mind through hypnosis.

Personally I also find hypnosis to be extremely useful as an adjunct therapy in conditions such as epilepsy, dyslexia, bi polar disorders and depression.

Using Hypnosis For Spiritual Direction

Hypnosis can also be very useful in accessing spiritual guidance from the higher planes of wisdom and knowledge. I have had the opportunity of witnessing some remarkable experiences where clients have received guidance from other dimensions, masters and spirit guides. This proves once again that all answers lie within us and if we search deeply enough we can go beyond the limits of our own mind to connect with our higher wisdom.

The following case demonstrates how hypnosis was employed for spiritual purposes. Here the subject's presenting issue was non-specific and it did not relate to any discomfort or conflict but rather sought guidance for her spiritual growth.

The subject, who I shall call Deepa, was a devoted spiritual seeker training to be a hypnotherapist herself at the time when this session was conducted. She wanted to explore how she could accelerate her progress on the spiritual path.

After inducing a medium hypnotic trance, during the body scan Deepa found an obstruction at the site of her *swadhisthana (sacral) chakra*. At that point I instructed her to look inside the chakra to see what was causing the obstruction.

S: Miniaturise yourself and enter into the obstruction to examine what lies at that spot.

D: I see a small piece of burnt wood. It's black in colour and about 2x2 centimetres in size. It appears empty but is porous and there are interconnecting tunnels inside.

S: When did this energy take shape or come to you?

D: I can see a black shower. It's like dry black rain. I have no shape. I'm just in an energy form. I carry something around me, for protection. It reflects the black rain back, but a small drop enters me.

S: How did the black drop affect you?

D: My defence mechanisms have surrounded it so it couldn't be fully absorbed nor was it completely eliminated.

S: Why did it come to you?

D: The attack was so powerful that my protection couldn't push it back. My shield got pierced and it immediately closed. It regenerates on its own.

S: Who was the attack by?

D: I was not alone. There were many more. I decided to take it all on me. It was meant to be received by more of us.

S: What were you fighting for?

D: It was an energy battle of some kind. I have asked for this black drop to be eliminated so many times in earlier lives also but it remains in me as a reminder that *I don't stand alone. It's not for me to always step forward and take on the attack....* I now see a small child doing summersaults. It wears a cap and clothes. It has no face.

S: Has it ever had a body of its own?

D: I don't think so…it says it is Illusion.

S: Yes I know it's all illusion but how may I address you?

I: *(A change in the tonal quality of the voice is detected here)* I am Illusion.

S: Do you help or disturb Deepa with these illusions?

I: I keep her entertained. I keep her moving, seeking, thinking and creating the WHY'S in her mind.

S: Can you explain to me how exactly you do this?

I: It's not about explanation but experience.

S: What is your purpose?

I: To entertain and keep people busy.

S: You keep people busy so they don't focus their attention on what?

I: On their boring existence.

S: Do you wish to make life more meaningful?

I: I don't wish it, I do it. People would be too lazy otherwise. Inertia would have prevailed if I was not there. So I give them a kick and keep them moving on...and searching. Would Deepa have come this far if she didn't seek answers to her whys?

S: So what lies beyond the illusion?

I: TRUTH. But in your world it is fluid. There's always solid and then there is fluid. I prefer dynamism and I make you flow.

S: So what is the point of being fluid?

I: The point of being fluid is going with the flow. Just go with the flow. Doesn't flow take you to the truth? (*Gestures with the hand to suggest a meandering flow*)

S: How can we help Deepa into the flow?

I: All her problems are helping her to be in the flow. Her problems keep her moving. How did she end up doing hypnotherapy? How did she discover the things that she recently did? All because of the illusion called PROBLEM.

S: Doesn't she have the inner drive to remain in the flow?

I: That is always there. There are forces that are perceived as good and attractive, but actually; they are not as perceived. Then there are those that are painful, and are perceived as bad, but actually they provide the guidance and the push. You must have the drive to keep flowing and aspire for that final target.

S: What is the final target?

I: What you all aim for. What the river yearns for, to reach the ocean and to merge with it. Till that happens you must keep flowing.

S: What does she need to do to progress?

I: She likes to stand in the front and take the fire. She has to learn that it's not just an individual journey, its team work too. You have to work as a team.

S: So what is her lesson more clearly?

I: The same lesson that she had to learn when that energy battle took place. She stood forward to get the black storm. She was hurt in it and she carries that reminder, that no matter how much protection she may have had, she shouldn't have fought alone. In a family, all responsibilities must be divided. *So also in light work it's very important* to identify who is part of your team. You must stand in for each other. Help each other because everyone can't have the same skills. But then identifying your team is itself a great play as well. You can easily be fooled. All of it is merely entertainment, an illusion ... but it is for your own growth.

S: What measures can we employ to identify our team?

I: Your heart will always know it. Expand it and you will connect to the right ones. Otherwise you will just learn lessons.

S: How can we expand our heart?

I: When your heart is pure and clear, the golden light will find its reflection in the other heart.

S: Why is she so vulnerable to foreign energies?

I: The distinction between helping others, and helping others without hurting yourself, is very thin. When your heart is wide open, you have to be discerning and careful.

S: So it is right to be so open?

I: It's very difficult to say what is right and wrong or positive or negative when you work with such energies. The line is so thin.

S: How can we make sure that our protection is strong enough?

I: So the shield being of white light should not be crystallised it should be *Masterized*. So that when Masters give you the shield they know what is right or wrong, positive or negative.

S: How can we *Masterize* the shield?

I: Just request the Masters to create the shield around you. Imagine you are in a ball of white light and then ask for the shield to be *Masterized*. If any negatives are inside the shield they should be helped to go out.

S: So is M*asterization* a technique of visualisation where the Masters put the appropriate armour on each person? Will the Masters tune the intensity of each person's shield according to his or her vibrations?

I: Yes. Some may require more and some less. The more progress a person makes, the stronger is the attack on them. It's not about quantity but the quality.

S: Does not one reach a time, when one is powerful enough not to require a shield?

I: Yes, but working with protection during growth is important.

S: Does everyone, all healers specially, need a daily shield?

I: It's good to do it not only for yourself, but also for the people around you as well. Family shield must be done daily. They definitely need it. All light workers must do this. You've got your sensors a little more sensitive so you will be able to detect these energies. But focus on your work and don't waste time focussing on these energies. Wear your shield and let the Masters protect you.

S: Does calling out to the Masters' amount to wearing a shield?

I: Those connected to the Masters are already protected but it is good to be safe.

S: What are the instructions for Deepa now?

I: She needs to be her true self first, for which she must be free of these energies that are blocking her inner vision. Also, practising regular inner work will help her in establishing a much stronger connection with the divine and working with other people will strengthen that connection.

S: What is her special talent?

I: Giving

S: But didn't she give too much of herself at the black shower fight. Isn't that her lesson? When does a talent become a detriment then?

I: There is a very thin line

S: How can she find that balance?

I: Her connection to the Source needs to be stronger, her shield *Masterized* and her actions divinely guided. Only then will she find the balance. But if she is guided by her emotions, then she will not get there.

Deepa emerged from the session with a feeling of great joy and peace at having gained a deeper insight into her issues and felt a renewed sense of purpose. During the three hour session she received a lot more information about her spiritual journey through several lives and planes of existence, but I share here only the more immediate guidance that she received.

- She understood that her so called problems were merely an illusion that kept her searching for better and more powerful methods of healing and they actually kept her on her chosen path of being a healer.

- She also grasped that she must keep flowing and not let challenges stop her from moving on.

- She realised that she had to work as a team player and not stand apart as an individual or a leader, like she had done in several earlier lives.

- She recognised the importance of daily personal and family protection, which was of particular importance given the nature of her work. The concept of *Masterising* the protection shield was a revelation to her.

- Deepa understood that her empathetic behaviour sometimes worked against her and she decided to be more discerning in the future. She became aware that choosing who she works with, was very important, and if she did not choose wisely, she would continue to suffer and learn lessons until she wisened up.

- Most importantly, she received a powerful reminder to do her daily spiritual practice, balance her giving and not become overwhelmed or driven by her emotions.

When we gain extraordinary insights into our everyday ordinary problems and limitations by delving into the submerged depths of our minds we can truly harness the power of our subconscious. Hypnosis empowers you to deep dive into those limitless boundaries of your all-knowing inner space, to access the wisdom of pure consciousness.

For me, this is perhaps the most exciting application of hypnotherapy, for it awakens multidimensional perception that can help you discover new realms of consciousness, learn about your soul lessons and why you have incarnated, help your discover skills and talents you may already have mastered in previous lives, visit the life-between-life stages to comprehend your soul's journey and use these insights to heal yourself at the deepest core.

Why Hypnosis is the Preferred Modality

- Although there are several other trance inducing modalities such as breathwork, magnetic passes, storytelling and regression bridges; the reason I prefer to use hypnosis is because it can create a really good trance faster than any other method. A skilled hypnotist can easily create a somnambulistic trance in a subject within 3-5 minutes allowing for more time to do the real therapy work.

- I also find it easier to induce trance in children who lack patience and whose attention span is short. Most children respond very well to hypnosis. If a trusting and playful rapport has been established with them during the pre-talk, they can achieve very good trance levels within a matter of minutes.

- When the memories are particularly painful or if the client is uncomfortable about revisiting them consciously, yet eager to address the deeper issues, hypnosis can be an easier and gentler route to bridge them to the original memory. I find this method useful in working with addicts where there is a strong tendency to hide or report occasions of substance abuse.

- In cases where there is little or no verbal communication during trance because of some internal barriers to the subconscious exploration, use of ideomotor responses taught in hypnotherapy can be very helpful in letting the therapist establish direct communication with the subject's subconscious mind.

Ideomotor activity occurs despite your will, involuntarily, just like kinesiology and it allows the therapist to speak directly with the subconscious mind once the appropriate ideomotor signals are installed.

In an interesting case of a lady, who had still not recovered from the post traumatic shock of a car accident, it was ideomotor signals that facilitated entry into a past life through which she understood how that accident was part of a soul contract that she had with the others involved in that accident.

Her fears and stress related to the event was so severe, that without the help of ideomotor signalling we may have had to abort the session until she was more ready to deal with this issue. It was ideo- signalling that helped in by- passing her critical factor and enabled her to find the answers that she was seeking.

- In cases where the client has a fear of the dark or is uncomfortable about keeping his eyes closed, inducing a hypnotic trance through eye gaze fixation or other suitable methods allows the therapist to do the therapy work even while the subject keeps his eyes wide open, and yet maintains good trance level. This is even more relevant in cases where the emotional charge is missing and hence cannot be used to bridge the subject back to the source event through other methods.
- Sometimes while scanning the energy bodies if aggressive ego states are encountered it's easier to work with such personas under hypnotic trance because it permits catalepsy in the subject in which the limbs are relaxed into a state of immobility like in deeper meditative states.

In Conclusion

The possibilities for healing with hypnosis are as vast as the therapist's imagination, commitment and creativity. This modality gives you the power to investigate and explore endless possibilities existing in the subconscious mind to heal either your own self through the use of self- hypnosis or assist others in their healing.

From the esoteric and fascinating, like speaking to body parts and organs, looking inside chakras to identify and heal blockages, removing and freeing entities and foreign energies, reconstructing a fragmented psyche and retrieving soul parts, to the ordinary and routine such as resolving everyday conflicts, reducing stress, overcoming insomnia and experiencing deep relaxation, everything becomes possible with hypnosis in a safe and non intrusive way.

No matter what you might be seeking or hoping to resolve, hypnosis can help you find answers, just as one of my clients Nandini did. In her words, *I had been suffering from acute knee pain before I came in for therapy. It was so bad that I would wake up in the mornings with terrible pain and my knees would creak. But now,* that pain has miraculously vanished. I am now cured of this pain that had plagued me for so long.

Also the sudden and acute shoulder pain that I episodically experienced has decreased substantially after a hypnotherapy session during which an incident from one of my past lives was recovered and healed, in which I was severely beaten up and dragged by my shoulder.

In the multiple sessions with my therapist, I have undergone several hypnotic regressions into past lives, experienced spiritual hypnotherapy and energy releasements. During these experiences, I discovered information about some of the relationships that were troubling me and learnt how to take care of them. I was also able to understand and dissociate from the various unreasonable fears and anxieties that I earlier suffered from.

I have undergone a major shift in attitude towards a major lesson that my soul must learn. I now recognize my life patterns and these have helped me understand, what I should do, in order to dissolve my karmic baggage.

I have also discovered what some of my key soul lessons are in this lifetime. And thankfully, I have glimpsed my soul state and probably met my soul guide too. I have been able to enrich most of my important relationships as a result of this therapy work.

The efficacy of this healing modality is enhanced by the fact that it is non intrusive and yet has powerful healing effects. As noted parapsychologist Dr. Hans Holzer[4] says, it is quite superior to conventional chemical agents because it leaves no residue, has no side effects, and reaches the very centre, where all activities originate.

Hypnotherapy gives you the power to change your limiting beliefs and re-engineer your life to fulfil your dreams. It helps you discover your potentials so you can experience limitless success. It opens your mind to create harmony and intimacy in your relationships. It enhances your performance and productivity. It allows you to heal your body without medication or invasive procedures. And it can also help you discover, what your soul purpose might be in this lifetime.

To my mind, this is undoubtedly a master healing modality which can put each one in touch with the powerful field of divine consciousness in them. Just as twentieth Century psychic and medical clairvoyant, Edgar Cayce[5] did, by putting himself into a sleep-like state by lying down on a couch, closing his eyes, and folding his hands over his stomach. In this state of relaxation and meditation, he was able to place his mind in contact with all time and space — the universal consciousness, also known as the super-conscious mind. From there, he could respond to questions as broad as, "What are the secrets of the universe?" and "What is my purpose in life?" to as specific as, "What can I do to help my arthritis?" and "How were the pyramids of Egypt built? It is through these readings that he was able to help and heal thousands of people across the world. With Hypnosis, you too can aspire to do the same.

If you are enamoured by the mind body connections and wish to explore the unexplored realms of the subconscious mind as Cayce did, or if you yearn to understand this phenomena called life and why humans act and behave as they do, hypnotherapy is an essential tool that you must have in your healing toolbox.

Suzy is a Certified Clinical Hypnotherapist, Wellness Mentor, Spiritual Teacher, Channel and Author. She has spent 32 years researching and experimenting with consciousness. She works with a range of alternative and complimentary healing modalities employing a holographic approach in her work. She combines her rich experience in Corporate India with the insight and creativity of a psychic medium. She has authored the ascension e-book, Awaken, which can be read free of cost on her website.

www.suzyheals.com

References

1. Evolve your Brain by Joe Dispenza D.C.
2. Hypnotherapy and the Inner Judge – Relevance, Methods & Spiritual Aspects by Elmar Woelm
3. http://www.examiner.com/article/sports-hypnosis-1
4. Hypnosis By Dr. Hans Holzer
5. http://www.edgarcayce.org/are/edgarcayce.aspx

Chapter 39

Integrated Healing Through Hypnotherapy

Anjali Chawla

The Essence

Life is a beautiful journey. We learn everyday new experiences from our lives. It teaches us the art of becoming a better human every day. We have our own set of patterns, which we acquire from our parents, from our environment since we are born. These patterns are also the conditioning we make in our minds about life through the experiences of others in our lives. As we grow, we start having our own experiences in life and with the awareness these patterns and conditionings start breaking and new, better thoughts start making our new realities. This new reality which we make ourselves becoming more aware and conscious about our life purpose and the spiritual being within us gives a new perspective towards others and ourselves.

In my journey of Life, it has been very experiential. Initially I used to feel that why I have been chosen to live a harsh circumstantial life. But gradually with time and awareness I came to know that this is the way I am choosing it. The day I decided for myself that enough of drama, now I want to live a happy and prosperous life, things changed. The more we think of lack in our life, the more we manifest the same. Always count on your blessings and see how beautifully Universe unfolds the mystery to support you in different ways. The only thing you have to do is make right decision at right time. Rest all is taken care of always.

My journey with Hypnotherapy started way back in 2009. Before that I already knew that there is something more to what I was doing. Something I really wanted to do for the humanity and myself. Hypnotherapy changed my life in a way that while I was learning, I started realizing how much I have stored in myself

Holistic Wellness in the New Age

as the emotions like anger, guilt, fear etc. Guilt and fear, according to me are the two major emotions that can create lot of unhealed emotions and blockages in our system. The more I started to learn that life is a flow, at certain point how we react to a certain situation is all based on our awareness and consciousness at that point. How we behave at the age of 15, we don't behave same way at the age of 25. Why ? Because, we have mature thoughts at the elder age and more understanding for the situation. So, it is useless to keep regretting on the past events and experiences. Rather, learn the lessons from past events and move on for a better life with new and better experiences. All the events happening in our lives are created by our own thoughts. We are the creator of our reality. If you don't like your reality then understand how can you change your reality? Answer is very simple, by monitoring your thoughts and by thinking only about what you want in your life, rather than wasting your precious time in thinking about what you don't want. How can we monitor our thoughts? The answer is again very simple, here comes in picture the tools like SELF HYPNOSIS, through which you can give positive affirmations to yourself and become self-dependent to change your reality.

The Process

Hypnosis is a state of altered awareness in which access is available to the sub-conscious mind. The process is initiated by an overload of message units, leading to break down of the inhibitory processes of the critical mind. This in turn triggers the flight-fight mechanism and ultimately results in hyper-suggestible state, providing access to the sub-conscious mind.

Body-Mind Correlation

In a crisis, the mind perceives the danger and the body responds by letting the autonomous nervous system takes over. Originally, the thought comes and then it gets converted into an emotion, then the emotion (energy in motion) gets converted into action in the physical body. This is simple explanation how our body takes action at every thought. The mind again is divided into two parts, Conscious mind and the sub-conscious mind. It has been found that the conscious mind is 10-12% and the sub-conscious mind is 88-90% of the total mind. Originally, the primitive man functioned completely by instincts. He did not have inhibitions. With the passage of time, man started developing the ability to think. Amongst the first things, the man thought about was survival. Man came to the realization that he did not have to act on every impulse that confronted him. He then started to develop CONSCIOUS CONTROL. At this point, the fight mechanism started to become anxiety. He started to feel in his body. The modern way to look at this is action vs. reaction. The flight mechanism also developed a modern way of coping. This can be seen as repression vs. depression. The modern flight mechanism is depression.

Model Of The Mind

When an infant is first brought into the World, he/she does not have the logic, reason or inhibitions. To make their needs known, the child uses the more primitive mechanisms. The child has a more of primitive mind, with flight-fight mechanism. The baby is born with only two fears, fear of falling and fear of loud noises. Everything else is learned by the associations and identifications. From the age, zero to eight years, the child develops a library or a store house of these associations and identifications, he learns that some of these are good as in positive associations and some are bad as in negative associations. These associations form the pillars of our conditioning which in turn govern our responses to life's situations. Between the ages of eight and twelve, the child starts developing the logic and reason. The child is capable of taking decisions and developing will power. This becomes the CONSCIOUS MIND, which represents 10-12% of the total mind power. The SUB-CONSCIOUS MIND is made up of remaining 88-90% of the total mind power. It includes the modern memory (where the library of associations is stored) and the primitive mind.

Age Regression In Hypnotherapy

Age regression is basically based on the model that everything that has ever happened to us in our lives is recorded in our minds like a recorder. Age regression therapy operates from the assumptions that many of our problems as an adult stem from traumatic experiences that happened to us early in life and that were responded from conscious memory by the sub-conscious defence mechanism of repression. Such a model is commonly held among traditionally trained psychologists schooled in the Freudian tradition.

For example, in my practice, there was a client, whom I should name Pragati, came for the reason that she was very scared of going to hospitals. Even though she was at the best of her health, she had the feeling that she will not live for long and will not survive. For no reasons this girl would not go to hospital even to visit a close relative. She came for the session for her problem that when she is so healthy and fit, why does she feel that she will not survive and what was the reason for so much of hatred and fear to go to the hospital. Under Hypnosis, she regressed to the age when she was newly born and due to some allergy during the birth, she was kept in incubater for one week. Then she saw that her parents were being told by the doctor that this girl will not survive. But due to good medical help and the will of the parents and the child, the girl survived. But the sharp comment of the doctor became a memory for the girl that there are less chances of survival for her. So throughout her life till the latest age of 28, she has been thinking the same way without any ill health. And in the next session, she discovered that she was by mistake locked in a washroom of a hospital at the age of three years. Already having the belief system that she will not survive(from previous experience) and spent few hours locked in hospital washroom, with all pungent smells of medicines, got these two traumas affecting her so much. After the successful session of Age Regression, she became absolutely fine and few affirmations were given to her to have Faith in the process of life.

Another very profound example of healing through Age regression in my clinical practice is of a girl, age 37, whom I should name Parul. She had a very indifferent relationship with her mother. She never used to be comfortable talking to her mother and they never shared any much of physical touch. She used to feel that her mother doesn't love her and she doesn't love her mother either. The hatred was becoming strong day by day which of course neither Parul, nor her mother were liking. They were suggested to visit me by a common friend. When I spoke to the mother, she had her own part of the story to tell and when I spoke to Parul, she had her own story. Even though I counseled them separately but common issue came up between both of them was that what may they were trying to patch up with each other, nothing was working. I suggested Parul to go first for the session because she was more receptive to my suggestions. Under Hypnosis, Parul regressed to her age of four, probably her fourth Birthday party, where she saw her mother being ready for the party and suddenly she saw her uncle entering the room and they both became intimate. Parul, in deep hypnotic state could feel the pain and she hated her mother for doing this. Then she being a small child at that point of time, did not understand and went to her father and told him what she saw. Her father asked his wife what child is telling so mother manipulated things and went off. But the next day her mother brought all her anger up and beaten Parul with broom. This was very traumatic for Parul to experience in Hypnotic state again as if it was happening again. But that is how the therapy works. With age she have had forgotten the incident but the hatred for her mother was becoming stronger day by day. After the session and therapy, Parul got the wisdom and she accepted the situation with a mature understanding. She didn't become loving towards her mother but yes, she was at peace with herself.

The memories which we register in our minds in early childhood, they become very prominent beliefs in later age. Once the right approach has been taken up by the therapist to reach to the conclusion what age of the client is the trauma coming from. Once that trauma is re experienced by the client and the therapy has been done, it can lead to a better life.

Past Life Regression

Past life regression is a technique, a therapeutic process that uses Hypnosis to recover the memories of past lives stored in the sub-conscious mind. Past life regression therapy is typically undertaken either in pursuit of a spiritual experience or in a psychotherapeutic setting. Past life sessions can proved to be excellent if the subject (client) is receptive and the therapist's intentions are very clear to guide the client through the therapeutic process. There are many blocks that can be cleared from the mind of the client with these sessions by making them understand the reason of what is happening in current life with a different perspective.

A client came to my clinic for a session of healing and therapy with the complaint of having severe pain in shoulders for no reasons. I should name her, Srishti. She had been taking medication for cervical thinking that this pain was due to that. But she was not getting relieved at all. A friend of hers suggested her to go for an alternate healing modality and referred me to Srishti. She was a young girl of 22years. When asked that since when does she had this pain. She could only recall the age of 10, when the pain started and it had been aggravating by every year. While counseling and talking to her, I discovered that there was no physical injury or damage in the shoulders. I took her for the session and under deep Hypnosis, she regressed to a past life where she saw herself as a middle aged woman working as a laborer in a building under construction. She kept on seeing few details and then I guided her to witness that major event which will give her the wisdom about this pain. She saw that one day she was working on the site and suddenly, a huge wall fell on her back and her last thoughts were that " this pain is terrible, it is killing me". Then she was taken to the Higher Self to get the wisdom and therapy was done completely on her. For another one week she had to continue medication for mild pain but after that she got absolutely cured from the pain. There was no further pain. The beauty of the session was that sub-conscious mind exactly opened the file or folder of that past life which had got the wisdom for her to get relieved from the pain.

Another case I would like to share is in 2011. There was a couple being married for good fourteen years but shared a very cold relationship. The wife came to me for the therapy as she was at the verge of getting collapsed with the situations in her life. I should name her Divya. When she came for the therapy she had tried all her best ways to maintain the marriage. She had been staying in a joint family and had one daughter. When I asked her that could she recall good memories with her husband, she was so frustrated coping up with the situations that she had no answer but cried a lot. Release of emotional charge is very good before or in between the therapy. Divya had a major complaint that her husband behaved very different with other people and different with her. She herself said that her husband is a very good human being with no bad habits according to her, he was a good son and a very good brother. But when it used to come down to the relationship with her, he was very indifferent. She also explained that she always see hatred in her husband's eyes for her, which was a very strong statement. I never wanted to manipulate her mind and reactions so I was simply listening to her complaints without making any judgments. Divya was then regressed and in very deep Hypnosis, she saw herself in England, in very old times. She could not make out the year though but the dresses she was mentioning and the chariots etc. she was visualizing were all pointing towards the fact that she was visualizing the very old era. She saw herself in a very beautiful English attire and like a rich lady. Then she visualized herself falling in love with some average status guy. In next few minutes, she could recognize the guy, it was her current life husband. They were madly in love with each other. Then she progressed in that lifetime and saw that there was disharmony between both of them because of money. Divya, in that lifetime was a rich woman but this man was not that wealthy. But the man loved her madly; he was ready to do anything for her. I guided Divya to progress to the major event of that past life which had a major impact on her current life. She saw that she had started liking another man in that lifetime, who was very rich. She was in a way cheating on her boy friend. The last event that she witnessed was that she sat in a chariot of the new guy and eloped with him. While she was leaving the city, her current life husband encountered her and was very angry with her. He confronted her and she very rudely told him the truth that she would prefer money over love. The guy shattered and in his eyes Divya could witness the same hatred that she used to feel in her current life's Husband. Then Divya saw her death scene and her last thoughts were of guilt and regret for what she did with her current life husband. Then she was guided to her Higher Self to get the wisdom why she saw that particular past life. The therapy was done and she got the wisdom and improved the relationship with few affirmations given to her for acceptance of the situation and moving ahead in life with a new perspective of life. The beauty of the process was that the wife got the wisdom from the session but the husband's awareness also shifted after the healing.

Another case I would like to share is of Anita, age 28 (name changed for privacy) She came to me for a healing session for relationship issue. She was in relationship with a guy since five years. The guy was three years younger to her. She was madly in love with him and he was also equally in love with her. The problem arose when she started earning better than him and the guy couldn't take it. The male ego of the guy was making the relationship go haywire. She was very upset but wanted to save the relationship. While counseling her, I noticed that the girl was very insecure about taking decision about this relationship. She already had a heartbreak few months back and now she was trying to hold on to the guy. Under deep Hypnosis, she regressed first to her early childhood days, where her whole life as child was spent in lack of love and compassion. She witnessed two incidents in early childhood, which were very evident to make out that she was a child without being loved by anyone the way she wanted. Even though her parents would have loved her to their capacity and understanding of the emotion but she felt the lack of love and created a void for herself. At that point of therapy, I guided her to heal the INNER CHILD personalities of hers that surfaced and integrated those inner children with the current aged, mature Anita. Then my concern was to guide her about the current relationship issue. The main concern was that her previous relationship also broke because of money. In that relationship, her boyfriend was financially much better than her so used to put her down always and in current relationship, the guy was feeling insecure that she earned almost double the money he earned. So in the further session, she regressed to a past life where she saw herself as a queen of some kingdom and due to some circumstances had to get married to a not so rich guy. She saw herself suffering because of lack of money and lack of love in that past life. When she was guided to see her last day of that life, she saw herself dying in misery and the last thoughts were that she had a miserable life because she married in love with a not so rich guy. So two prominent thoughts that money is very important and love and money are related. Then she was guided to her Higher self to get the wisdom from that lifetime. After the session, few days later, she got married to the same person without any insecurity about love and money.

The more I have taken up these sessions the more I have realized that Life is a beautiful journey and every person, every situation that comes in our lives is an opportunity to learn and grow. Even though when we are in any circumstance and we see no hope at that point of time, there is already a bigger and a better plan been made by the Universal force of energy. We just need to trust in the process of life.

The Tip

I am giving a few affirmations for healing below. I have believed in affirmations and experienced a major shift in mine and other's lives. I am sharing a few here for the purpose of self healing.

"All is always well in my life."

"I trust the process of Life."

"Abundance flows to me in all areas of my Life."

"I am a Divine Being. I am limitless. I have the power within."

"I forgive myself and I forgive others. I am thankful to all the people in my life."

"I love, accept and approve of myself."

"I release all the past guilt, all the fears and insecurities. I am always safe."

"I know all my needs are always taken care of by the Universe."

"I am at peace and in harmony with my own thoughts and actions."

Anjali Chawla has been connecting intuitively with the Divine Beings (Angels) since childhood. Professionally, she facilitates Hypnotherapy workshops and healing sessions. She also does Angel Healing, Reiki and many other alternative healing modalities. She has done her training in Hypnotherapy with CHII. She is a certified trainer in training for integrated hypnotherapy foundation course by Ekaa.

www.kalpavrikshakriya.com

CHAPTER 40

Transformation Through Past-Life Regression

Smita Wankhade

'As you live deeper in the heart, the mirror gets clearer and clearer.' -Rumi

The Essence

"It's burning." "Something is burning." Dr. Rakesh kept saying. I looked around in the surroundings for any smoke coming up but there wasn't any. He had come to our center in Nasik from Mumbai for a 2 days workshop on Past-Life Regression Therapy. And he was getting the clear smell of smoke for about seven hours. That was the day when the Mantralay i.e. the government secretariat building had caught fire in Mumbai!

Sumeet, in one of the sessions, saw his boss asking him to attend an interview from their head-office in the U.S. And he was asked to report immediately to head a project undertaken by the company. And it happened in reality exactly after ten days.

Yes this is one of the bonus effects of PLRT sessions! Time and space travel. It just happens if we are ready for it...

We heard loud shrieks on the staircase! It was time for my next appointment at the NewAge World Wellness center in Delhi. The door was flung open and a boy about five feet tall dashed in, walked past us and started exploring, scrutinizing everything that came his way. Following him the parents came, to stop him, but in vain! As he moved further I simply slid a sketchbook in front of him and some color pastels. And that did the trick. He sat glued to it for about twenty minutes, which gave us enough time to speak to his parents. Sujeet, a fifteen-year-old boy suffers from Autism, a neuro-developmental disorder that creates an imbalance in the mental growth. In school Sujeet frequently sketched a car and violently scribbled red and orange strokes on it. On asking what it was he would say, "The car is on fire. Dehradun. Traffic jam." In school he would be assigned to write a story and he would again sketch the same picture and that's when the school consulting psychologist recommended him to consult me.

I guided him into prolonged sessions of breath work and color therapy, which is used to release, pent up emotions and to balance chakras, as PLRT was difficult due to his inconsistency. But he repeatedly sketched the same pictures and also a bus with the same strokes of red and orange which validated the fact that it was his pattern. He might have died in this manner repeatedly.

After the sessions there was a remarkable change in his behavioral pattern, the most important change being that he became sure of what he wanted, which was one of the intentions with which his parents had come to me.

Yes, we live lifetimes of patterns, which need to be broken to bring about transformation. The sessions brought about changes in him but what is the intention of the soul when such a differently abled child chooses a life like this, to learn his own lessons? Teach them? And his parents are they in a karmic cycle completing some incompletions? To gain a deeper understanding of such karmic relationships the parents also need to go through the sessions. It can reveal to them deeper insights about the relationship than they can consciously comprehend. This helps them to open their hearts and be with more compassion with the child and with others!

PLRT has a profound effect not only on differently abled children but also on persons suffering from depression, mood swings and such other psychological disorders. Breath-work or Re-birthing Process and Inner-child-work can be effectively used along with PLRT to release unknown blockages that we carry not only to heal the issues but also to bring about ascension on a soul level, mental level and physical level.

Fifteen year old Nina was guided to her past life where she saw herself as a woman running away from a few men and she was actually eating papers of her house ownership. She then jumped into a well and died. Later on, her parents shared that she had a habit of eating papers and would consume an entire notebook. During that time she would faint for no apparent reason. This too was cured completely after the sessions.

PLRT can be used to get answers to the 'why me.' It gives us an understanding and facilitates healing of issues related to health, relationships, fears and phobias, all that keeps us from leading a fuller life in the present.

We are not our body, our thoughts and our emotions. Our body is in fact our first environment. It is the carrier of our soul. We are the soul, the spark, and the particle of consciousness or the divine source. The soul manifests into the earth plane or many such realities, in order to experience. Through these experiences we learn lessons and ascend till we reach to our Godliness. Before coming down on earth, we pre-plan that life time, choose the parents who will teach us the lessons we have decided to learn in that lifetime. We also come here to teach whatever we have learned and to enjoy what we have created. And we also come here to enjoy creating! The lessons we learn are those of trust, patience, forgiveness, faith, acceptance, unconditional love and many more which eventually lead us to opening of the heart, to be with compassion to one and all. So, we are the sum total of all our experiences from many life times.

At the time of birth, the soul enters the chosen body and that is the time when our entire history or past data is inserted into the body that we have chosen, just like a chip with data is inserted into a gadget. This data exists in every cell of our body, known as "cellular memory". We choose lessons to be learnt in every lifetime. But when we come down here, we forget to learn the lessons and there begins the blame game --- of blaming others, god, destiny or our karmas.

'Karma' is a Sanskrit word, which simply means action. As Jesus Christ says said, 'As ye sow, so shall ye reap' or we know that 'every action has an equal and opposite reaction'. But Karma is not a reward or a punishment system. We sow what we reap because of the guilt that we carry. It is we who punish or reward ourselves for our negative or positive actions. As a result what we did yesterday shapes our today, and what we do today shapes our tomorrow.

The Process

By reincarnating we are completing our karmic cycles with other souls, though we actually ought to learn lessons that the other person was/is trying to teach us. **Every experience is trying to teach us lessons and with every lesson learned, the soul is ascending to a higher plane of consciousness.** Hence we need to take up the responsibility of our life and see what each experience, each event, each person is trying to teach us. PLRT helps us to work on ourselves, to find the lessons, and free our selves.

Relationships

It is relationships that teach us lessons. They help us to evolve.

Simran, a forty year old, had issues with her mother-in-law. Initial trivial arguments between them blew up into a lot of anger and resentment. The mother-in-law controlled the finances of the family and when she gave Simran money even for household expenses, she would literally throw the money in front of her. During PLRT sessions Simran saw herself as a queen in an ancient lifetime, wearing a gown, and tied to a pole in a market place. She could literally see flames coming up toward her. She was being burned to death and she could literally feel the heat of the flames. On being instructed to go to another significant moment of her life, she saw herself walking along with the king, followed by a retinue going through a narrow lane. The path way was made of stones with small houses on either side. An old lady suddenly came out of one of the houses and begged before the queen. The arrogant queen kicked the old lady and moved on. "You will come into my hands and I will show you," said the old lady. When she looked into the eyes of the old lady, Simran could clearly see the face of the mother-in-law. In another incident of that lifetime, she saw herself and the king enjoying themselves in the well-protected fortress and the subjects were left to protect themselves from an attack of the neighbouring country. It was after that incident that the enraged subjects pulled the ruthless queen into the market square and burnt her alive.

She could now understand why her mother-in-law treated her in that manner which helped to forgive her and their relationship started improving. But that was not all. We worked on their relationship from different angles which made her aware of the larger picture and she got her answers to her 'why me'. Her health issues, the root of which were the burning of her body, were released as well. The sessions taught her to take responsibility of all that happened in her life.

These sessions work on a deeper level and help to release blockages. The transformation within facilitates a transformation on the outside, which includes situations, persons, places and everything around the person. What anyone says or does is not important. What is important is what we need to learn from them. By letting go of the blame game, Simran learned the lessons of acceptance, patience and above all compassion.

In relationship issues we find that situations are repeated and we realize that it has actually become a pattern. PLRT helps to bring about a higher understanding as we now see the bigger picture. Every troublesome relationship can be reformed into a love-based relationship. The process helps us to forgive, accept and then love the other person. We realize that most of the people in our life have been with us in other lifetimes too. The previous life explains why we feel instant attraction or resentment towards certain people. The 'why me' dissolves when one sees 'what I did'.

Health

Re-living is relieving.

When Varsha's oncologist broke the news of her tumor being malignant, her family and friends were devastated. In a PLRT session, she saw herself as a butterfly that was caught by a bearded man and shoved into a sack that he carried on his back. "I can actually feel the sack swinging as he is walking and it's painful," she said. He reached a hut and forgot all about the butterfly, only to open the sack two days later. He simply picked the half-dead, de-hydrated butterfly and threw it away. The butterfly just died. When I asked Varsha to find similarities between that life and this, it dawned on her that she felt captivated and stuck in the sack and she had an exactly similar feeling in her current job. She was at that time at the peak of her career and had worked hard to be there. But during the session she realized that her body was signaling her to make changes and PLRT helped her to take the hard decision to resign and to do things that she wanted to do now. Thereafter, her body responded well to the treatment and she was healed!

In another session she experienced astral travel and connected to Lord Krishna. Rays of bright light flooded from his hands to her body and the vibrations of the energy were felt in the entire room. This was an overwhelming experience for both of us. She now works as a freelancer and has authored a few books. She is now her own master. "I feel liberated now that I am living life on my own terms" was her response, months later.

PLRT helps us to get rid of health issues. The memories of traumas are stored in the cells of the body. This 'cellular memory' is the reason why body creates diseases, deformities, birthmarks and scars. They come from our previous lifetimes. Even when the tumors or injuries or diseases are healed, they can recur due to these memories. Also, the body speaks to us. We simply need to communicate and find out what the body is saying. This therapy works very well on cases where diagnosis is not possible. Even cases where there has been recurring sprains, when people are not able to conceive, migraines, arthritis etc. have been cured by PLRT.

By way of this therapy, healing can be instant or due to the blockage released, the process of healing begins and actual healing happens after some time. By re-living the trauma, the symptoms disappear. Even repressed traumas of this lifetime are released through this process.

During a free group session for the NAB students, Rashmi, a 22 year old instantly connected to a past life. In the Indo-Pak partition era, she saw herself as a young female standing on the roof of her house. People were killing each other all around and a mob armed with swords entered her house. She came down and saw bloodshed all over the house and her near and dear ones had been massacred. "I don't want to see anything" she said, and a sword struck her too. After the session, her eyesight did not return but she felt as if a big weight had come off her shoulders.

Every person going through these sessions feels the removal of a burden. Yes, the last thoughts determine the next lifetime. And they profoundly affect the next lifetime.

Abundance

Manish, 35 year-old seemed confused and felt helpless when he came to me. In spite of a lot of hard work, he did not get success in his career. Going to the root cause, he saw himself as a 50 year-old male sitting in a cold cave. Three men with faces hidden by rugs entered the cave and stabbed him on the right side in the chest. He shouted aloud as he actually felt the acute pain in his chest as the blade of the knife pierced through his flesh. Surprisingly he had always complained of a pain in the right side of his chest to the extent that his relatives teased him of having a heart on the wrong side. After this session, his life changed completely and he came out of the stagnation that he was experiencing in all areas of life, especially in his career. In one of the sessions, he connected to his father's soul and received messages from him. This made him feel very light, relieved and empowered.

The sessions helped us to resolve issues related to abundance and remove hurdles in career because they help release the energy blockages that keep us from enjoying abundance.

Concentration and Focus

Amit, a 9 year-old boy was unable to sit still or indulge in any activity even for 5 minutes. There was some kind of an uneasiness and fear in his eyes. In a session, he saw himself as a middle-aged man, clad in white, being trampled by an elephant. Even after he died, the enraged elephant kept kicking his body. After going through the process, the boy was much relieved and became calm and peaceful. He is now able to focus on his activities.

Yes, PLRT has been used successfully for children and elders with an unexplained uneasiness and an inability to focus on matters. Children have a tendency to sleep a lot after the session but a lot of healing takes place on a subconscious level even in sleep.

Fears and Phobias

Many persons have irrational fears and phobias and after reliving the root cause, they can be effectively released.

Surekha, an English teacher had a fear of snakes, so much so that she couldn't even utter the word nor see a picture of it. In a PLRT session she saw herself as a soldier on horseback passing through a jungle. He fell into a pit where there were innumerable snakes. With snakes wriggling all over him, he took his last breath. Towards the end of the session she asked me, "How do I know my fear has gone?" I subsequently guided her to go into the pit again and lo and behold! She said, "I can see snakes all over me but I don't feel the fear now." When I checked with her after a week, she did not feel the fear any longer.

Root cause of a fear of height, water, fire, closed spaces can be traced to past life traumatic experiences and going through the process helps to release them. Generally these fears are traced to traumatic death due to falling from a height, drowning in water, burning in fire, death in an enclosed space etc. During such a traumatic death event when there is an emotional charge and energy block is created and this emotional charge is carried to the next birth, which instigates these fears. These blockages not only create the fears and phobias but also stop us from progressing in many areas of life. They can be effectively released on very deep levels through the process of reliving.

The most important fear that is released during this process is the fear of death, death of loved ones and our own death because when we see ourselves dying and yet existing, we know that we always are.

Talents, Abilities and Purpose of Life

Nikita was a middle-aged woman who did not enjoy her profession any longer and felt extreme uneasiness. In a session she saw herself as a painter and her life changed thereafter. She now pursues her talent not only as a hobby but has made it a full-fledged profession and the uneasiness she felt has gone away completely.

Through the PLRT process, past life talents, abilities, and wisdom can be retrieved. Moreover the purpose of our life can be found which can help us to live a meaningful, joyous and fulfilling life.

Along with PLRT, Breath-work or Re-birthing can be effectively used to release unknown blockages and remove depression, negative thinking and death urge. Inner-child work releases blockages created due to traumatic events in childhood.

Anita, in her late thirties conceived sixteen years after marriage when the root cause was traced to an abuse during childhood. Seema, who was addicted to smoking could stop it completely after the root cause was traced to the time of her birthing when she was not handled carefully and made comfortable after birth as her mother had a schizophrenic attack and the doctors got busy attending to her. During inner-child work, the abundant inner-child during the traumatic events is retrieved and assimilated into the self to get a feeling of completeness and wholeness.

There is no side effect of these sessions but we certainly experience bonus effects. Though starting with the intention of releasing one or two core issues, a lot more issues come up and are released during the sessions, as they are all interlinked to the prominent core issues.

Holistic Wellness in the New Age

On a larger canvas, PLRT is contributing in the promotion of global peace as people see themselves born in different nationalities and religions, which increases their understanding of others and brings about a feeling of oneness. PLRT also makes us open to all possibilities and helps us to be with peace and calmness. Every reincarnation we remember increases our comprehension of ourselves as we are.

The Tip

> *"If you dont believe in karma and reincarnation, don't worry, probably you will in your next life." - Dr. Bruce Goldberg*

All the case studies mentioned in this article are with prior permissions from the respective persons and their names have been changed to safeguard their privacy.

Smita Wankhade is a Breath Worker, a Past life Regressionist, and a Reiki master. She has been studying the benefits of meditation, creative visualization and energy work and past-life regression. After having gone through different experiences in childhood like tuning to different realms, seeing a 'soul', out-of-the-body experiences, her curiosity about the mystics increased and she understood these experiences when she began learning more about this subject. With her questions answered when she was introduced to the world of spirituality, she realized that spirituality is a wisdom that brings joy which has to be experienced, and that, this joy has to be shared with all mankind!

Having benefited from the breath work and past life regression sessions and with a natural flare for teaching, she realized that giving healing to others and spreading the knowledge of spiritual science is her purpose in life! Through her healing sessions, people have found relief from issues, which were preventing them from living a fuller life. Each of them found the purpose of their life and been able to balance their material and spiritual life.

www.pastliferegressionindia.com

CHAPTER 41

Cellular Rhythms in Regression – A new paradigm to healing and integration

Aasha Warriar

The rhythm which is necessary for our cure is brought about by bringing the circulation of the blood into a certain rhythm and speed -Hazrat Inayat Khan

Be it classical, folk, reggae, country, rock, or any other genre and whether it has lyrics or is plain instrumental; I realized that one of the biggest influencers of our belief system is the music we listen to. And if we listen to a particular genre over and over again, neural pathways get generated and the emotional reactions get etched in our sub-conscious. Eventually, these neuro-pathways become the story of our lives, creating and re-creating our realities to match these imbibed beliefs.

Whilst working on cases and understanding the human mind and programming, I started working with the music people listened to and once again the results were astonishing. People who were deeply affected by sad, emotional songs developed depressive reaction patterns and helplessness. Continuous hard rock and songs with loud banging music created a trance-like state and leave people vulnerable to influences of belief systems that may not even be their own.

Basic theory:

There is an innate rhythm within our body, its cells and with the environment around us. Our Thoughts, Emotions, Energy and the Physical Body which are controlled by the mind need to function in alignment for the body to be at ease.

If this alignment is disturbed at any level, there is dis-ease. The endogenously generated rhythm is a 24-hour cycle in our physiological process in the cells although, it can be modulated by the external environment. We already know that there are clear patterns of brain wave activity, hormone production, cell regeneration and other biological activities linked to this daily cycle and is controlled by our states of consciousness. Therefore, cellular memory can be tapped by focusing on the rhythm of this alignment to bring up positive as well as traumatic images leading into regression for healing at all levels.

Since ancient times, music has been used to put people in touch with their emotions which are the cornerstones of our existence. At a broader level it is said that music tones the soul. And at base body level, it has been noticed that the cell frequency changes with change in external rhythm and music. Enlivening music causes the cells to vibrate at a frequency which is very different from that of melancholy or sad melodies and these are all different from peaceful mantras. The mind and body are so deeply connected that our own beliefs affect the way in which these emotions get embedded in the body cells.

Research has shown that all sounds and especially human sound affect the chakras and aura. Since, a thought is eventually stored in the body by virtue of the emotion it generates and the energy carried by that emotion, it is possible to work on any of these three layers to bring about a change in the physical body and bring it back to harmony.

I found that clients were able to auto-regress into events that are relevant to the issue which bothered them the most during that time. Once the imaginative bridge was established, the somatic could be brought up and regression session completed. Since the work began with energy-work and ended with regression, I have learnt to close the session with the opposite frequency of music and emotion - eventually collapsing the anchors.

Excerpts from my book:

Case I: Neena (Inner Child work)

This case has been a wonderful experience for me as a therapist because it was one of the first experiments of how healing with music works.

Neena is a dear friend and on that day was feeling a bit low and felt as if she was missing something in life. There was no particular thought pattern or ailment. So, I asked her to be relaxed and take a few breaths

T: Notice now that a song will begin to play in your mind…simply tell me which song it is…

C: Strange, I would never think of this song…anyway, it is *"zindagi ke safar mein guzar jaate hain jo maquaam, woh phir nahi aate…"*

[This means - so many opportunities / events pass us by in life and once gone, they never come back.]

T: Which are the words that strike you the most?

C: "wohphirnahiaate…" [I.e. they never come back]

T: Just repeat these words till you feel it in the body…

C: "wohphirnahiaate…,wohphirnahiaate…" (I notice tears)

T: What is happening Neena?

C: It's funny; maybe I miss my college days and my friends, I am not sure…

T: It's okay, just be there.

Here, Neena started crying and spoke about her college days when she was spontaneous, carefree and did what her heart desired and now she has changed so much, she is stressed most of the time.

T: Just repeat the words one more time, Neena and let me know if there are any images that come up.

C: I can see myself in the Biology laboratory in my college…(she smiles)

T: How old are you?

C: 18 years.

T: What is happening there?

C: I am with my friends and we are having a lot of fun…it is such a carefree environment…we are laughing, enjoying…hmm…

T: Can you bring 18 year oldNeena with you here?

C: No, she refuses to come with me…she says "this is the best time of life and it may never come back"

Here, I did an intervention and worked with the inner child simply holding her hands until, Neena finally said, "I miss this part of me"

She was crying just recognizing that she was still living in college and hence, resonated with the words of the song.

When I asked her to integrate this part with herself, a strange thing happened.

C: She doesn't fit into me…actually I need to merge with her….she seems bigger than me, more confident and she is inviting me

And before I could say anything, she hugged 18 year oldNeena; "this was missing, this was missing"

T: (pausing, giving enough time) What is happening?

C: Now she is growing up to my age and I feel as if my spontaneity is back, I am myself again - we are walking out of the college together and being the woman I am today…(she hugs herself)

After she had settled, I asked her to listen to the song playing in her head now… it was another song the lyrics of which represented being a spontaneous, lively and happy woman.

Neena opened her eyes with a sparkling smile and zest in life that had been missing.

Case 2: Cynthia (using Past Life)

Cynthia is a young, beautiful woman for whom life has been quite a puzzle. Her reason to meet me was the issue of her marriage. The client had been through a divorce and was about to re-marry when she realized that the man was duping her. He was not only married, but also had a family and had hidden the details from her. Cynthia was planning her wedding and this discovery came as a rude shock to her and the family. The wedding was called off and the bitter experience caused her a lot of grief.

The words kept echoing in her space: Marriage causes grief. With this background, Cynthia lay down on the couch in the therapy room.

T: Hear that a song is playing in your mind and tell me what it is that you hear...

C: Actually, here is an image of me and my sister cycling in the park and its drizzling...and I am listening to music...

T: What are you listening to?

C: *kuchh khaas hai kuchh paas hai, kuchh ajnabee ehsaas hai, kuchh dooriyaan nazdeekiyaan kuchh hass padi tanhaiyaan...*

[Meaning: it is something special and near, a strange feeling, some sort of distant nearness, loneliness has smiled]

T: Hmm...what are the images that come up when you repeat this in your mind?

C: I am in a battlefield...

T: Okay...and what is happening?

C: I am falling off my horse...I am hurt...and it is drizzling...

(I begin to feel goose bumps)

T: Are you badly injured?

C: Yes...I am dying...

T: What are you thinking...are there any last thoughts?

C: Yes... I wish I had told her that I love her..."

T: Told whom?

C: Naazneen...my fiancé...I had told her that we can never get married...

T: And the reason is...?

C: That I am the king...I have battles and battles to fight...if I die, she will be in grief, just like my mother...(sighs)

T: Hmm...what happened to your mother?

C: My father died in a battle...I have seen them crying and then living in grief...

T: Who is 'them'?

C: My mother…my step-mother…my step-sister and all the people in the kingdom…but I did not cry.

T: How old are you at your father's death?

C: 15

T: And you are not crying…?

C: No, I am the crown prince…the next king…I cannot be weak. [Long pause as if observing the scene of his father's death] I have decided that I will not marry…it brings grief to the survivor. (This time the voice is very assertive)

A decision made in an emotionally charged state has the potency to carry across lifetimes and maybe with a vengeance. In this case, "I will not marry…" seemed to be the crux of the issue and almost like a vow.

T: Hmm…what is happening next?

C: Nothing…I am crowned king and I take charge of my people.

T: Okay. Go to the next significant event.

C: I am telling Naazneen that I cannot marry her…(tears roll down the client's cheeks); although I had proposed marriage to her…that is the reason I cannot hurt her…

T: (pausing) whenever you are ready, go to the next important moment.

C: It's a battle…I am hurt

T: How old are you?

C: 16…it's my first battle…we have won but I am hurt

I worked with the battle wounds and then checked the story of grief that bothered my client so much.

T: What is the next significant event?

C: It is the same last scene…I am dying…I wish I had told her I love her…

T: Is it possible, that not marriage but death brings grief…

C: [thinking...as if exploring this possibility] yes...that is true...(sighs) yes... my father died and so my mother was grieving...my family was grieving...I was not allowed to grieve...and I carried it into this life.

We worked to release this vow and then asked the client if the song was playing again. This time too it was the same songs but the words held a different meaning for her now.

It was time to bring her back to the present reality and since, it was drizzling outside; I asked her what was the relevance of this drizzle...it was drizzling in the park and in the battlefield...

The client was quiet for a long time before the king revealed "when I had proposed to the girl I loved in that life...it was drizzling"

Cynthia suddenly opened her eyes and was surprised at what had come up.

Music makes the soul come alive. Our body has an innate rhythm and even heart has a specific beat

Aasha Warriar is the Founder-Director of the Clover-Leaf Learning Academy Pvt. Ltd. Certified Regression Therapist from Tasso Institute (Netherlands), Integrated Clinical Hypnotherapist (California Hypnosis Institute, Irwine, California) and Inner Child Integration Therapist from the Earth Association of Regression Therapies (recognized EARTh, UK). Author – "From Mediocrity to Madness".

www.cloverleaf.co.in/www.aashawarriar.com

CHAPTER 42

The Journey™ To Healing

Dr. Rangana Rupavi Choudhuri

The Essence

I was devastated and shocked in 2001 when I received the news of being diagnosed with abnormal cells and a chronic hormonal condition, requiring immediate surgery and medication. Although I had a PhD in Cancer Research from Oxford University, UK, I never expected a similar fate to have developed in my body. I still remember the phone call from the hospital. I was driving from home to work in the early morning and I had to pull off from the fast lane into a derelict building site, which backed onto the Florida coastline blocking it from my view.

As the news of the diagnosis sunk in, and while my head was still reeling from it, I also had a gut inner knowing that surgery was not for me and there was another way. I just did not know what the other way was. Or yet how I would find it.

It was a year later in December 2003, after my father had passed over, when I discovered "The Journey", a book written by Brandon Bays. As I read the book, I knew what was written in the book was going to be responsible for healing my body, mind and spirit. I started to make the connections between unresolved past events and limiting thoughts that may have led to the abnormal cells and shut down of my reproductive system.

I used the Journey™ described in Brandon's book to heal the abnormal cells and they literally flowed out of my body and my reproductive system reset to its proper functioning self. The doctors and nurses were astounded and I was now living proof of healing with alternative methods, without the need for drugs or surgery.

The Journey™ is about freedom. All of us sense that deep inside us lies huge potential. We long to experience it, yet something holds us back. We long to set ourselves free, but we don't know how. With The Journey™, you finally learn how.

When Brandon Bays was diagnosed with a basketball-sized tumour in her uterus, she was catapulted into an extraordinary, soul-searching journey. Determined to heal naturally, she took no drugs, underwent no surgery; but six-and-a-half weeks later she was declared tumour-free. Going beyond current mind-body wisdom, she discovered a powerful means to get direct access to the soul – the unconditional love, the boundless peace, the living presence within us – and pioneered a revolutionary paradigm for healing.

Tens of thousands worldwide have since used The Journey™ to awaken to their own infinite potential and free themselves from lifelong emotional blocks and physical illnesses.

With practical, easy-to-use techniques, The Journey will enable you to:

- Dive into your own soul and tap into your own inner genius
- Uncover and completely resolve emotional and physical blocks
- Uncover repressed emotions and cell memories that can lead to illness, and clear them
- Heal your being, your emotions, and your body
- Experience the boundless joy, peace, and love within
- Live life as an expression of your highest potential
- Become truly and ultimately free

"An amazing Journey, a gift to us all." – Jane Seymour, O.B.E., actress, artist, and writer

"Brandon's book is inspiring, exciting and a look deep into the heart about how to live abundantly in a world that often gives too little and takes too much, including the health that sustains us. Her work is a gift to us all." – Timothy J. Forbess, president, The National Foundation for Alternative Medicine, Washington, D.C.

"The Journey offers a remarkable and innovative approach to accessing important inner resources that can powerfully support the healing of body and mind." – Walter Jaros, M.D., M.P.H., Chief Medical Officer, Natural Health Link, and Director of Professional Training, Green Medicine Company

The Process

The Journey™ is about freedom – freedom to live your life as you've always dreamed it could be.

Deep inside all of us a huge potential beckons, waiting to open us to the joy, genius, freedom, and love within. This presence is calling you home right now, longing to set you free. Yet all of us have issues we have felt trapped or limited by. We hear the whispering of our own soul calling to us, but feel unable to access that greatness. Instead, we feel covered or blocked in some way, limited by our issues – anger, fear, depression, grief, hurt, anxiety. It may be as simple as feeling there must be something more to life, or as complex as feeling a complete failure. It may be as debilitating as an addiction or as life threatening as a serious illness.

No matter how deep the issue is and no matter how much you have struggled with it, the possibility exists for you to become absolutely free, whole, and healed. You are capable of getting to the root cause of these issues, resolving them, letting them go completely, and setting yourself free to live your life at your highest potential, as a full expression of your true self.

Across the globe, tens of thousands of people from all walks of life use Journeywork to discover true freedom in their lives. They're discovering their own answers and uncovering their own deepest truth. They are cleaning out past emotional blocks and physical challenges that have held them back. And they are finally healing on all levels of their being. Ordinary people are getting extraordinary results. It seems that no matter what your background is, how old you are, what your culture or upbringing has been, everyone knows there is a huge untapped presence inside, and we all secretly long to experience it. This presence is awake while you're asleep at night, making your heart beat, cells replicate, and hair grow. Part of the extraordinary gift of my own healing journey was to discover and pioneer a simple, yet powerful, step-by-step means to get direct access to this infinite wisdom – a wisdom that can reveal to you old emotional patterns and memories stored in your cells, and a healing energy that is capable of resolving and clearing those old issues completely so the body and the being can go about the process of healing naturally.

Today I travel all over the world with Journeywork, giving workshops and advanced programs. I'm always delighted that it attracts people from all the helping professions, both traditional and alternative. I give talks and seminars at hospitals, hospices, abuse centres, homeopathic colleges, healing centres, spiritual organizations, and to cancer support and addiction rehabilitation groups. Everywhere I go, people successfully incorporate Journeywork into their professional programs with ease and grace. I believe we all recognize that there are some issues that simply require more in-depth, roll-up-your-sleeves healing work. We know it's important to address an issue at the deepest level to finally clear it out and resolve it completely. Together we understand that Journeywork is a way of bringing about pro- found healing, wholeness, and a deep sense of wellbeing – no matter what our backgrounds are.

Research by the American Centre for Disease Control states that 85% of all illness is emotionally based. So at times of stress and distress it's no surprise that heart disease, cancer, depression, asthma, burnout and many other illnesses are on the increase. Our emotions, thoughts and words influence our bodies and the effect our cells, DNA and ultimately our health.

Over the years numerous scientists and medical doctors have studied and subsequently verified research in support of The Journey Method. Dr Bruce Lipton, Candace B Pert, PhD and Deepak Chopra MD and others, have shown that at a molecular level, suppressing emotions can lead to individual cell receptors becoming blocked. These blocks then interfere with the normal healthy communications between cells, and this impairs many body functions. Conversely, allowing the feelings and emotions to flow unblocks the receptors and helps maintain health.

Dr Deepak Chopra, in his book Quantum Healing, published the theory that trauma and suppressed negative emotions are often stored as 'phantom memories' in our cells. He argued that these cellular memories act subtly over long periods of time, and can cause disease and illness many years after they have first been put in place. What Brandon discovered was how to access specific cell memories and, more importantly, how to actively resolve and let go of the stored issues.

Your emotions play an important role in your physical health

Renowned cellular biologist Dr Candace Pert has established that when we have repressed emotions, or issues we've buried or swept under the carpet, it creates a body chemistry that can block our cell receptors in certain areas of the body. If those cells remain blocked over a long period of time there is an increased likelihood for illness to be created in the specific areas where the cells are blocked.

The key to cellular healing is to uncover the repressed trauma, or the unaddressed cell memory, resolve it and clear it completely. Then your body and your being can naturally go about the process of healing and you are left soaring in a boundless peace, wholeness and wellbeing that is your own essence.

The illness starts where your cells are blocked

"What science has found is that when you're at the peak of a strong emotion, if you suppress it at this time – for example as people do when they go into shock or have a trauma – a biochemical reaction will go into the bloodstream. If over time cells remain blocked, that's where illness is going to start. The Journey Method helps you go through a process of releasing the trauma." – Brandon Bays

Your thought patterns can strongly suppress your immune system

"Psycho-neuro-immunology research has produced compelling evidence that our thought patterns directly and instantaneously affect our whole body chemistry, and can suppress our immune system. We all 'know' that angry people get more heart attacks, and stressed-out people get ulcers. Only happy is healthy, and some evidence even links grief, fear or resentment to cancer.

The Journey is a method of cellular healing that can be experienced in an initial 3-day seminar. During the 3 days you will learn the exact same skills that Brandon Bays and Dr Rangana Rupavi Choudhuri (PhD) used to heal themselves from abnormal cells without the need for surgery or drugs.

You are ready for the Journey if you are

- Longing for inner calm, health and balance
- Feeling stuck or that there's just got to be more to life
- Wanting a solution to heal fear, stress and anxiety
- Holding onto repressed emotions or just long to find peace and harmony at every level
- Fed up with the war zone of the mind, emotional stress and bodily tension
- Dealing with ill health or ongoing physical issues
- Depressed, flat or even hating life and want a deeper more permanent connection
- Wanting more fulfilment in your relationship, career or health
- Searching for your own authentic greatness, your infinite potential, your deepest truth

Case studies with The Journey

Many of the participants who attended the Journey program have stated that their lives have been positively transformed. Some noteworthy stories include overcoming longstanding anxiety, instilling hope in healing from cancer, and regaining hearing after 20 years!

This is what they have to say...

I feel happy within and no longer need to take daily anxiety medication

"For me, attending the Journey program was nothing short of a miracle. I was going through the toughest phase of my life. Depression, anxiety, stress, abuse, trauma, lack of confidence, an inferiority complex, a suicidal tendency... I had them all. I had a very abusive childhood, both physically and emotionally. I used to feel trapped, as if I was locked up inside a box, unable to breathe. This led to my developing high blood pressure at a very young age, as a side effect of anxiety and excessive stress. I then attended the Journey program and it cleared all my doubts and made me free from the bondage of negativity. The Physical Journey process has helped me in clearing many blockages. After attending the Journey program, life has changed a lot for me

and is still changing everyday. I no longer take medication daily for my anxiety attacks, I feel a sense of completeness, I am happy from within." –Navolina Patnaik, Bangalore, India

Cancer won't win: combating colon cancer by clearing emotional baggage

Having been fighting colon cancer for four years, Ashi Chandra's hopes of recovery were at their lowest and her spirit at its dimmest. It was then that she discovered the Journey.

"I completely buy Brandon's proposition that diseases are the net result of piling up negative emotions within us since childhood, that's when the process of shutting down begins."

Journeywork has helped Ashi to clear the layers of built up hurt and rejection, and to let go of all the excess emotional baggage that hampered her from moving ahead. Today, a deeper understanding of what could have caused her disease and the knowledge that real healing lies in her own hands, has given Ashi a new confidence that she can and will win the battle against her condition.

Excerpt from article published in Mind & Body, Heart and Soul, June 2012

After 20 years, The Journey gave me back my hearing!

"Over 20 years ago, I had an accident where I fell on my ear. I had lost all hearing function from my left ear after it bled profusely. About 3 weeks ago, I attended the Journey Manifest Abundance Seminar. After the retreat, on the flight back to Delhi, I suddenly realised that I was able to hear my iPod through my left ear. I deliberated and tested it for about three to four weeks, before I contacted my lecturer, Rangana, to let her know the good news and express my gratitude to the Journey and the founder, Brandon Bays." –Nita Gupta, Delhi, India

The Journey gifted me an alternative to chemotherapy

"The Journey arrived in my life as an answer to a prayer that I put out to the Universe. I was diagnosed with lung cancer and western medicine had only 'chemotherapy' to offer me. Having undergone five cycles of chemo, I was desperate for an alternative healing method. The universe gifted me with Brandon Bays' Journey Process.

In my first physical journey I visualized my lungs already healing, which gave me the strength and positivity to go on. Though I had not intended to progress further than the Journey Intensive, life and Grace pulled me to attend Manifest Abundance. I began to experience miracles. As each and every Journey process dissolved some part of the disease, 'chemo' left my life. I felt energy shifts in ways that cannot be explained.

I have now signed up for the complete practitioner program. It is as if Grace was calling me, telling me that this is my healing path, and that I will be sharing this healing process with others who need it. Through the cancer I was given the message that I have in me the power to bring about miracles. This cancer is curable and it's already being cured. I will soon be able to update this story to tell you that my body is completely healthy and free of cancer and all illness... Thank you." –Vibhavari Bhosle, Pune, India

The Tip

The Journey is a method of cellular healing that gets to the root cause of an issue enabling physical and emotional challenges to be resolved. The process was developed by mind-body-health expert Brandon Bays to heal her from a football-sized tumour.

The different forms of Journey processes are as follows:

- Physical Journey – for physical issues like illness, pain, tension, anxiety, addictions, depression and health challenges

- Emotional Journey – for emotional issues likes fears, heartache, sadness, grief, hurt, guilt and unhappiness

- Abundance Journey – to clear everything and anything in the way of abundance in life, health, career, relationships, financial and spiritual life

- No Ego Journey – to clear limitations in the way of self-realisation, spiritual development and personal enlightenment.

- Healing Journey – for phobias, fears, limiting beliefs, vows, pain and self-sabotage

- Designer Journey – this is totally customised to individual requirements and can include any and all of the above for getting to the root cause and clearing any issue.

The Journey is being used to enable healing from issues such as:
- Chronic pain
- Anxiety
- Grief and loss
- Anger and frustration
- Fear and stress
- Addictions
- Illness
- Depression
- No life direction
- Lacking spiritual connection

What makes the Journey unique is that it combines emotional healing with connecting with the body's infinite intelligence, known as Source, to heal cell memories, creating a space for forgiveness and healing. When Deepak Chopra analysed data from tens of thousands of case studies from survivors of serious illness he noted those that healed had two things in common:

1. Ability to access their infinite healing potential or 'source'
2. They uncovered and healed past cell memories

These two components are also part of the Journey process, allowing degenerative memories to be no longer passed onto the next generation and for either spontaneous or incremental healing to occur.

To find out more you can download a free booklet on The Journey with a chapter by Brandon Bays - *http://vitalitylivingcollege.info/free-resources/*

"Dr Rangana Rupavi Choudhuri is the perfect presenter for The Journey – a genuine embodiment of the work, having used the method to heal from abnormal cells without drugs or surgery. She teaches with such love and humour and her wisdom and depth are an inspiration to all who sit with her. Radiant and compassionate she creates an environment of acceptance and safety where all participants can easily open

into their own process work in an effortless way. And her expertise and experience in journey work creates a cradle for our minds to relax and allows us to "Dive in" deeply." Brandon Bays, Founder & Creator of The Journey

"Awesome, inner stillness, lots of gratitude, inner cleansing, peace. Meeting Rangana itself is overwhelming. Thank you so much. God bless. Thanks to the team." – Bindiya Shah, teacher

"It has helped me clear a lot of physical and emotional clutter, heal, help, and forgive in the true sense. Forgiveness could be so simple was a true realization today. And yet how deep." – Amishi Kothari, teacher

Rangana Rupavi Choudhuri (PhD) is the Founder & CEO of Vitality Living College ® and delivers trainings and seminars around the world. She is an international author, dynamic speaker and heart centered mind-body expert. She is totally passionate about motivating people – about boosting their confidence and helping them to achieve their true potential.

Dr Choudhuri's clear and proven coaching style has encouraged audiences around the world to move out of their comfort zones – inspiring them to meet and exceed their personal and professional goals, over and over again.

For information about The Journey Seminars and our other training courses please visit http://vitalitylivingcollege.info/bookme/

© *Rangana Rupavi Choudhuri (PhD) & Vitality Living College 2010 - 2015*

CHAPTER 43

Working with Angels

Susan Chopra

"Angels Have Completely Transformed My Life, It Is Your Turn Now"

The Essence

I am deeply delighted to connect with you through this article and it is my genuine intent to introduce you to the Magical World of Angels where Miracles are guaranteed.

Before I talk any further on this subject, one thing is evident that you are- right now -surrounded by your Angels. In fact, I want you to consider this article as a personally drafted message from your Angels meant for you alone. They want you to be aware of their presence so that you can start to work with them consciously to manifest a wonderful life for yourself. They want to gift you a life of your dreams. Angels brings to us extension of God's love and blessing.

Even though I am closely connected to this loving world ever since I was a young child, my most profound OOBE (Out of Body Experiences) many years ago, fully awakened me as a Psychic and Heightened Intuitive.

Since then, I am living a fully inspired life with my Angels and today as an Advanced Angel Practitioner by Profession, I am making a smiling difference in many lives through my renewed teaching /healing abilities. Even today, I feel that no words of mine are enough to describe their MAJESTIC magnificence.

Working with Angels offers you the opportunity to develop wisdom, strengthen self understanding and overcome obstacles by connecting with your inner light, which is a direct pathway to GOD. When we integrate our body, mind and spirit into one cohesive entity we not only raise our vibrational rate, but also the vibrational rate of the whole humanity and of Earth itself. In my experience,

Angels help us evolve spiritually by helping us reunite Heavens and Earth within. These light beings are always with us, watching over us and they want to help us personally so that we can attain our natural state of peace, which can lead us to experience all the other joys of life.

In my therapy sessions, I am awed till date at the WOW ways the Angels are rehabilitating and helping humanity uplift itself from the clutches of Fear. To sum it up, Angel Therapy is the fastest, easiest and most powerful healing remedy amongst so many other Alternate Healing Therapies existing above the EARTH. As a Spiritual Teacher I have virtually tried, studied, tested a large variety of therapies and found Angels as a perfect Gift for Humanity.

Angels remind us that we being the children of GOD are naturally blessed with the ability to easily see, hear, feel our Angels' presence, communicate and interact with them to receive constant guidance and healings for all situations and circumstances.

The Process

- **Ever wondered who and what are 'Angels'?**

    Angels Are Heavens Intermediaries. In a simpler understanding; the word Angels is derived from Greek word 'Angelos' meaning Messenger and their job is to bring to us heavenly guidance/ messages/ solutions from our creator GOD for all the situations at hand that are bothering us. They are light beings – i.e. they are made of Pure Light and Unconditional love and are created by GOD to help you and me and all on the planet live a life of love, peace, joy and so they are delighted to help us achieve all that we feel stuck with on our way to LOVE, JOY, PEACE. They bring us Answered Prayers, Gifts, Blessings from Heavens in the fastest, easiest and most powerful ways.

- **Why must we invite 'Angels' into our lives?**

    We all go through life's crest and trough, and each one of us has encountered many situations sooner or later where we felt literally pushed through the mangle. During such times, we frequently seek a trust worthy authority, figure or power that we could easily connect with and turn to in times of distress and turmoil and so **'Angels' Is The Answer**.

Holistic Wellness in the New Age

- **How do Angels help us?**

    Angels can bring an end to all our struggles almost immediately. They provide us with greater insights and clarity to deal with all life circumstances with much ease. They help us by delivering timely messages, guidance, health remedies and some times life saving measures.

    Angels help you make improved decisions that will take you towards your desired goals rapidly thereby bringing in peace, happiness and success. Life today is too mechanical and fast paced and the demands on us as individuals are many. It is easy to go split and loose connect with our spirit, the essence that is constantly in-touch with Heavenly Angels. With Angels, you can powerfully restore this connect so that you operate through all life stages just easily and happily.

- **Angels can empathize with you** - they understand that if our minds are stuck on worldly material focus then we are automatically disturbed and our peace of mind is compromised. So they help us with money solutions, can offer health remedies, help us with child issues, woman issues, career, business, property and the list goes on for you to add.

- **Angels are super powerful healers** and can help us with almost anything. The best part about them is that even if they cannot alleviate a problem completely due to KARMIC accounts, they can surely lighten suffering in miraculous ways; removing the pain and agony involved and bringing us internal peace. So an individual finds himself much stronger and in control of all that surrounds and with this renewed energy and state of mind will start to attract good into his life again.

- Thus, it is right to conclude that **angels can lighten your karma- cause and effect and many personalized ways they can help each individual on earth.**

    The good news is that as we consciously become aware of Angels, the veil between our world and theirs becomes thinner. Even though not every one can actually see an angel, all of us are naturally able to feel them around us. However, with the personalized psychic exercises I impart in my workshops, you can awaken your Spiritual sight -Clairvoyance, completely so that you have profound Angel visions.

The Technique
Here is What You Can Do Right now to Sense the Presence of Angels

1. Make an intention to connect with Angels. Be open to the process and enjoy.
2. Sit in a comfortable place where you will be completely undisturbed. Light a candle by your side or incense. You can sit in a cross-legged position or on a chair with back erect, supported and head leveled.
3. Now start to breathe deep through the nose and exhaling out of the mouth. Breath out any tension in the body, doubts, worries, anxiety and breath in peace, calm, more peace, more calm.
4. Next, as you breathe in imagine you can breathe energy up and down your spine.
5. On the in-breath taking in the earth energy up from the root chakra to the crown chakra and while exhaling bringing the heavens white light beam down from your crown to your root chakra and pushing it further down and out from the soul chakras. Repeat a few breaths and see all your worries and blocks being removed by the powerful Angelic light.
6. Next, as you see the energy going up –send blessings and love to your Angels and the Angelic Realms and breathe in bringing down their love and blessings and light, see your entire being and cells illuminated in this delicious rainbow color light that renews you completely on all levels. You may now like to extend and expand this wonderful energy out of the soles to Mother Gaia beneath you and see it ooze out of your millions of pores of the skin. See yourself as a light being radiating a rainbow color Aura.
7. Now focus on your heart chakra that is Rose pink in color. This is the place where your Angels connect with you most strongly. Ask your Angel to draw closer to you.
8. You may suddenly see your Angel, or feel the pressure around your head shift /increase, a sweeping feeling will take over you and your body may start tingling. You may also start vibrating at certain areas of your body.

9. Enjoy this overwhelming encounter with your Angel and see your Angel enfolding you in its wings.
10. Receive the unconditional love your Angel directs towards you.
11. You may like to ask a question or Guidance –Now. Breathe and trust what you receive for an answer.
12. Thank your Angel for this encounter and slowly bring yourself back to the waking consciousness.

Remember, you can never go wrong with Angels and you are always SAFE. So GO ON and HAVE FUN with this whole thing.

Because my life is totally Blessed and filled with DIVINE MAGIC, it is my mission to connect you to your Angels so that, you too can reap the infinite rewards of Heavens and manifest Greater Peace, Abundance of Money, Success, Dream Career and all that your heart desires. Angels can help you easily raise your vibrational rate which ultimately helps to reunite us with our own GOD Consciousness, which once we have experienced it, is so transformative that there is no going back.

"May Your Life be Carried upon the Wings of Your Angels."

Channeled Messages from your Guardian Angels...

"Fear not sweet child for you are not walking alone ever, for you are completely protected and embalmed in our love amidst all the seeming cruelties of life. We are here ever since and we are eternal, immortal beings of light who are here under god's authority and we take delight in protecting and empowering further everything that comes from god including you. So hesitate not sweet child in our wonders and claim as yours peace, happiness, joy and all that you seek for we are working unstintingly for you, to protect you and guard you and purify you so that what only remains eternally is god's light and love in you and around you. We love you for who you are. We Are Your Guardian Angels." www.godheals.in

Date – 20 November 2013
Time – 12:38 Hrs
Conduit- Susan

Susan Chopra is a natural clairvoyant and works closely with the Powerful Angelic Realm, Ascended Masters, Guardian Angels, Fairies, Crystal Energy, Reiki, Human as well as Animal Spirit Guides to heal all aspects of human life. Susan's journey into the psychic development started about 9 years ago and she ended up training as a professional intuitive few years ago. The world of Angels was calling out to her at a very young age. Susan's life changed dramatically when one night a 9feet tall angel carried her away to the HEAVENS – a land of Golden light. (Read more.... Susan's Tale of transformation)

Susan is an Advanced Angel Certified Practitioner trained under Charles Virtue and Tina Marie Daly and channels messages/ guidance from the Angels to heal Finances, Relationships, Medical issues, Health, Housing, Child issues, Career, Life purpose guidance etc. She is Certified Reiki Grand Master, Kundalini, Karuna Reiki Teacher and Healer certified by renowned Grand Master Teacher Mrs. Shabnam Juneja, a Certified Crystal Healer from Hypnotherapy School of India. She shares a close bond with animals/pets and receives guidance from the Animal guides for their healing issues.

Susan can help you unlock the gate to the future you desire and loves to lead people down a path of greater Joy, Prosperity and Abundance by healing any blocks in their Aura, Chakras that prevent them from living to their true potential . She is greatly involved in conducting Counselings on all issues of life, Channeling healing messages from the Spirit World to clients on a one-to-one basis, as well as group settings . She conducts experiential workshops on Reiki, Angels Healings, Intuitive Guidance, Crystal Healings, Angel Power Manifestations, Law of Attraction, Angel Professional Card Readings, Angel Chanellings , karuna Reiki, and Kundalini Reiki.

Her Chief Goal in life is to help people awaken and develop their innate powers which will steer them towards fulfilment and improve their life in practical ways. Her experiential trainings cater to people in all walks of life, from business persons to flower essence healers to psychics. Psychologists to UFO investigators ,in short for all those who deliberately decide to learn and grow. You will learn to trust intuition, heightening awareness and honouring the emotions. As an Energy healer, she feels that the only barrier in our way of healing is—our own decision to release these barriers and believes that for any healing to effectively occur the receiver has to be willing to be healed.

www.godheals.in

CHAPTER 44

Akashic Records - An Illuminating Healing Journey

Bhavya Gaur

We are all visitors to this time, this place.
We are just passing through.
Our purpose here is to observe, to learn, to grow, to love
And then we return home — Australian Aboriginal proverb

Till this day I remember the serene humongous place filled with misty white light and pillars so tall that they seemed never ending. I can still feel the awe from the first time I visited this place in my dreams as a child. Despite the powerful authority in its being this hall had a very sacred, soothing, loving, sublime energy. Everything seemed bathed in glowing, misty white light as if it the place was made out of clouds. At the time I did not know what I was tapping into but I do remember I wanted to stay there longer.

As far as I can recall even as a child I was always intrigued by the cycle of life and death. I had a deep awareness of a bigger plan and purpose. Visit to the misty white halls during sleep as a child and waking up with messages of wisdom beyond my earth age was mind boggling for my parents to say the least. I felt an unexplainable connection to these misty white halls and was pleasantly surprised when I consciously accessed the Akashic records for the first time many years after. It was a feeling of Déjà vu, a feeling of coming home. I knew I was aligned to a very sublime sacred energy. As soon as I accessed my Akashic records soothing sound of chimes and harp greeted me. A great feeling of love emanated from the records and I could feel the loving joy in my heart. Surrounded with love I witnessed visuals and words that resonated within me, physically as well as emotionally. It was like watching a 4D PowerPoint presentation.

Who are we?

Most of us are seeking answers regarding our soul journey to explain who we are, what our soul purpose is, why do we suffer, why certain things, issues, patterns are so persistent in our lives? Why no amount of effort is good enough to change them? It's like being caught in a vicious circle where the variables (people, places, and situations) change but the patterns persist. They just change form but don't disappear.

Our essence is divine. We embody the Source, representing the highest vibration of love. We are an integral part of Universal Consciousness and are never isolated. Earth is our school where we take human form and incarnate lifetime after lifetime to learn lessons for soul advancement through life experiences to manifest the spiritual perfection we embody at a physical earthly level. Through these experiences we continue our journey of spiritual growth and evolvement with the latent desire to align ourselves with our ultimate soul purpose - to be one with Source.

I remember during my first conscious journey in the Akashic records I was looking for answers to some relationship issues. I was definitely not expecting the insights that came through from not one but three previous lifetimes. Saying that I was taken by surprise would be an understatement. I had no idea the issues affecting one relationship was a string of patterns that were manifesting in other areas of my life as well and they were definitely not working in my benefit. The origin of these issues was totally unexpected and it took a little while for the awareness to sink in. With awareness came healing followed by a sense of liberation. Ever since I started connecting with the energy of Akashic records, I have been able to see past the illusion and make life choices that have opened (still opening) new doors and opportunities that I couldn't have dreamt of earlier.

What are Akashic Records?

Akasha is a Sanskrit word which means ether, primary or primordial substance out of which everything is formed. It surrounds us in entirety. Akashic records or hall of records as referred to by some is multi-dimensional library of light wherein all the information and wisdom pertaining to each and every soul ever incarnated is encoded in light. The wisdom of the Akashic records is very sublime and for centuries was only available to seers, saints and highly evolved souls. It is a responsibility that was only entrusted to the ones who were capable of respecting its sacredness with integrity. However, in the Age of Aquarius as humanity is evolving we have come from a state of dependency to a state of responsibility, taking conscious ownership for our spiritual growth and evolution.

Akashic records have existed from the beginning of time. Even though the name is derived from Sanskrit these are recognized and interpreted by different names across different cultures and belief systems (in 'Torah' as the book of remembrance; in Bible as the Book of Life). According to Garuda Purana Chitragupta tracks and builds a record of every action of each life form from birth to death. In mystical traditions these documents are referred to as the Akashic records, said to contain every action that has ever taken in the universe. Edgar Cayce (1877-1945) the American mystic also known as the 'sleeping prophet' used the trance channeling method to access the records and relayed information and wisdom pertaining to spirituality and human evolution. Besides Edgar Cayce, theosophist Helena Blavatsky (1831-1891) referred to "indestructible tablets of the astral light" recording both the past and future of human thought and action; anthroposophist Rudolf Steiner (1861-1925) also referred to the Akashic Records in his writings. According to quantum physicist Ervin Laszlo –"it is the electromagnetic imprint of everything that's ever happened in the Universe". In simple language it would be fair to call Akashic records a vibrational filing system where every thought, word, emotion, action generated by soul experience since its beginning is recorded which translates directly to past, present and future possibilities. Whether you come from a scientific or spiritual perspective or both the energy of Akashic records is deeply healing and liberating.

Akashic records are not set in stone. They are ever evolving and this trait can be attributed to Karma. We are all too familiar with 'Karma' - the concept of "action" or "deed", which causes the entire cycle of cause and effect. Commonly used in Hinduism, Jainism, Buddhism, Sikhism, and Taoism; it is synonymous with "what goes around comes around" and "one reaps what one sows" in western culture. It refers to the totality of our actions and their reactions in this and past lifetimes, all of which shapes our future. As we live through life experiences we take advantage of the gift of free will and make choices based on many tangible and intangible components, as a result of which the records are ever evolving.

Where are Akashic Records located and how they can be accessed?

Akashic records exist in the higher realms of Consciousness in Akasha above the astral plane and are guarded by the powerful beings of light. These gatekeepers of the records have never been incarnated. They do not have physical bodies or names and their strong energetic presence can only be felt. Their responsibility is to ensure the sacredness and sanctity of the records is protected and maintained.

While accessing information about past lifetimes we tap into the seventh vibration and above where all the information pertaining to past lifetimes is stored. Here we get a chance to meet with parts of our soul with the option of integrating with them if this is beneficial for the soul on its journey in this lifetime. At this vibratory level we also get the opportunity to meet with parts of our soul that have already mastered lessons we may be struggling with currently.

We can learn to access the Akashic records by learning techniques to open the records. There are various ways of accessing the energy of the Akashic records like trance channelling, meditations, sacred prayers, breathing techniques etc. I use a sacred prayer as received by Source during meditations to align with the energy of the records. This sacred prayer gives us the attunement or the key to fine tune the messages and wisdom being received from this sublime realm. Once the Records are opened the Keepers of the Records direct the course and as guided the information that is most valuable for us or others (when we are working in someone else's records) is retrieved. By opening the Akashic records with a sacred prayer, we get access to the higher realms of the Akasha protected and guided by Source, Keepers of the Records and Ascended Beings of Light.

In the sublime energy of the Akasha all inner sensory receptors are awakened and intuition is heightened. As we open to Divine guidance we allow ourselves to receive the illuminating wisdom that comes from the ascended beings of light and learn to translate it for our greatest and highest good and for others when we are working in their records.

How can accessing Akashic Records heal?

In search of answers we go outside of ourselves to anyone who can give us a ray of hope and explain to us the causes of what we are going through, not to mention a quick fix as remedy. While the energy field and vibration can give us some information, the long lasting healing power lies deep within our soul.

I don't believe in coincidences. I believe that when one is ready to grow and evolve the Universe orchestrates and aligns everything to support it. It has always intrigued and impressed me how upon accessing the records the information pertaining to current life situations is always highlighted and forefront even when one is unaware of it. During an Akashic record session with Augusta I kept receiving guidance in form of pictures. I asked Augusta for confirmation but since it did not resonate (as I was told) with her I started asking for information on a different topic. This was a strong message and even though I was trying to move past the picture I was repeatedly being brought back to it till I started seeing the words all lit up. It was something like trying to skip a slide on PowerPoint without success (phew!). When I shared this information with her she validated it. The session was not only a breakthrough into invisible patterns but was also a big healing experience for her. What I love about accessing the records is that they are like online resource (if you think about it they are literally like a virtual library) and the more questions we ask the more clearer answers we receive.

The past lives specifics like who I was in the past life or what I did in that life is not important. What is important is the wisdom that comes from accessing those lifetimes, the insight into any karmic debts, blockages or patterns that are still manifesting in the current lifetime as a result of those previous lifetimes.

The records point out the origin of such karmic debts, patterns or blockages which in most cases can be traced back to previous lifetimes. Some of these are linked to unfinished business or pending lessons that the soul has yet to learn. In some cases these are the triggers to remind the soul of lessons mastered in previous lifetime that are waiting to be activated through memory in this lifetime.

Akashic Records provide all the information and understanding so one can take appropriate action. They empower us so we can create a change in our life, release self-limiting beliefs, transform relationships in our inner and outer Universe and embrace peace as a way of life. They never tell us what to do. The guidance comes from a non-judgemental place of love and compassion providing opportunities for growth and direction for soul's advancement.

The Akashic Record Connection

Learning to access one's own Akashic records is the most empowering tool as we can align with the energy of our own soul's records to gain insight, guidance and wisdom regarding anything to overcome issues and challenges so we can live our life fully and abundantly. It gives us a sense of accountability for our own self and a deep healing as we peel through the surface layers to discover the root system of self, outside the constraints of time and space. Accessing records of others is a very enriching experience because it's not only an opportunity to assist someone progress on their life path but also many times the messages received contain wisdom applicable to our own life situations. One of the most common feedbacks I receive after Akashic record session is "feeling light as if some weight is lifted off."

The wisdom and knowledge encoded in Akashic records is sacred. To strengthen the relationship with the records it's important to work with integrity in the records. Free will is a gift to mankind and it is absolutely required to respect this gift and not infringe on one's free will by accessing their records without their consent. Last but not the least, when we work from a place of pure, unconditional love without interference from our Ego we are able to receive and translate the messages clearly making amazing progress possible.

Bhavya Gaur, Usui/Tibetan Reiki Master/Teacher, Akashic Record Consultant/Teacher, Master of Crystology, Integrated Energy Therapy Master Instructor, Reconnective Healer and Angel Therapy Practitioner. Bhavya Gaur is a spiritual healer and counselor walking the spiritual path dedicated to healing for over 15 years. Bhavya was born intuitive and having mastered different alternative healing modalities she integrates these as intuitively guided to assist souls blossom into their true magnificence. Having escaped the corporate world after years of enriching experience in India and Canada, Bhavya is devoted to healing and has happy, satisfied global clientele. Besides doing private sessions Bhavya runs spiritual workshops and retreats in Canada, Europe and US. She is traveling to India bringing this opportunity for the first time in summer 2014. www.kindredsoulzs.com

CHAPTER 45

Feng Shui

Meenakkshi Jain

The Essence

Feng Shui is an ancient Chinese Science. It was originally known as 'Kan Yu'. Feng Shui is pronounced as 'fung schway' literally translated it means 'wind and water'. Feng Shui is not a religion, philosophy or superstition.

Feng Shui has gained increasing recognition world over, as the benefit of practicing the metaphysical science and art have been self-revelatory and unchallenged. Here is what you achieve:

- Creating positive career opportunities
- Getting a new job, raise or promotion
- Promoting business success
- Promoting wealth and prosperity
- Bringing respect and fame
- Increasing motivation
- Increasing creativity
- Improving health
- Eliminating depression
- Warding off addiction
- Getting pregnant or preventing miscarriage
- Promoting better sleep

- Promoting peace of mind
- Releasing stress and strain
- Feeling more in control
- Getting married
- Promoting love and romance
- Promoting happy relationship
- Promoting effective networking
- Guarding against separation or divorce
- Creating harmonious relationships
- Stimulating social life
- Developing better study habits
- Inculcate positive attitude and habits in children
- Keep children guided and self-motivated
- Improving a problem child
- Preventing accidents
- Preventing law suits or malicious influence
- Finding a new apartment for home or business

Feng Shui brings much more than all this. It is about achieving life fulfillment and holistic well-being. Thereby, meaning that Feng Shui, when applied correctly and skillfully, can bring fulfillment in our life.

Feng shui has the power to add one-third luck to an individual's luck. This concept has been explained by 'The cosmic trinity of luck'. As per this, there are three types of luck: -

1. **Heaven Luck:**

    Heaven luck is the luck we are born with. It is our fate, our destiny. It is believed that we cannot change our heaven luck.

2. **Man Luck:**

    Man luck is our 'Karma'. It is our handwork, devotion, dedication, education, our virtues and deeds. This luck comprises of the choices we make in our lives and therefore, is within our control.

3. **Earth Luck:**

    The place where we live and work influences our well being. This is called earth luck and can be easily controlled by using Feng Shui.

Therefore, it is quite clear that Feng Shui significantly contributes to our luck factor. Feng Shui adopts the principles of 'Yin and Yang' to create balance. Yin and Yang is the fundamental concept of Feng Shui. It is the concept of equilibrium and harmony. Ideally, for all things to happen smoothly and swiftly, everything should be in a state of balance and equilibrium. Problems start if there is imbalance. Yin and Yang are opposite forces but they complement each other. There is eternal interaction between Yin and Yang. Yin and Yang can never separate. There is a little yang in all yins and vice – versa. There are different degrees of Yin and Yang in everything in the universe. Like life is gray, not pure black or pure white. There is a little seed of yang, a little white, in yin. Similarly, there is black tone, a little yin, in yang. Nothing in the universe is completely yin or completely yang. Everything seeks a state of harmony and balance. On a human level, yin symbolizes feminity and yang symbolizes masculinity.

The Process

In Feng Shui, application of the concept of Yin and Yang brings harmony, balance and good future. If the Yin and Yang are not balanced in your home and workplace, their imbalance can cause physical, mental and emotional problems. Very darks rooms can cause depression and fatigue. On the other hand, extremely bright rooms can cause headache. Feng Shuing your house should be simple. Feng Shui is the art and science of living in harmony with nature. By living in harmony with our environment, we can harness the beneficial energies known as 'Chi' to promote prosperity and vitality. Chi (Pronounced Chi) is described as the air we breathe, earth's magnetic field, cosmic radiation, sunlight, spirit, our luck. Chi means all this and much more. Chi is 'Life's Breath'. To Japanese Chi is 'Ki', to Hindus Chi is 'Prana' and 'Ankh' to Egyptians. The concept of Chi is known to all cultures.

Chi governs our health, wealth and happiness. Feng Shui harnesses the positive aspects of Chi for our holistic well being. Chi rides the wind (Feng) and is retained in water (Shui). Feng Shui enables us to harness the Chi of our living places like home and offices.

The Tip:

To a dark room, add more light. If a room is suffocating, open the windows.

Working places should have more yang energy, so that the staff remains active and works effectively.

Children rooms and living rooms should have more yang energy.

Bedrooms should have more yin energy to induce tranquility and good sleep. However, do not forget the key word is 'balance', so do not overdo!

Yoga, martial arts, Qi Gung cultivates Chi in our body. For refining the Chi of our mind, meditation works the best.

In feng shui, the importance of clutter clearing can't be stressed enough. Welcome every Diwali and New Year by spring clearing your house. Clean each and every drawer with more zest. This will also ensure an organized and efficient functioning for your day-to-day life. You should not just de-clutter your physical surroundings, it is also equally important to do clearing at an emotional level. Shed all emotional baggage so that you can move light into a brighter future.

In your living premises, it is important to remove stagnant chi and bring in fresh chi into your home. A very simple technique to do this is to rearrange furniture, sweep, mop, scrub and dust. Do a thorough and complete spring-cleaning. This removes the old, degenerated stagnant chi with fresh and new chi.

Use space clearing and space purification to remove stale energies. This involves opening the door and windows of the house to refresh the chi. Space purification involves going around the house with bell, incense and chanting mantras pertaining to one's faith. One can also play religious music.

Light up your house. Brighten up your house with lights. Use the fire energy of diyas, candles and lamps. Use red Lanterns. Display a huge bowl full of oranges on the special days like Diwali and New Year. Oranges in feng shui symbolize good money luck. Hang wind chimes in your house. Wind chimes are an excellent enhancing, energizing and positive tool.

Use an auspicious signature to attract prosperity and success. Create a new signature, which begins with a positive upward stroke and ends with an upward stroke. This type of a signature denotes a positive beginning and a positive end to every project undertaken.

Keep a positive attitude and try to keep your thoughts positive at all times. If a negative thought comes, always remember to say 'cancel'. Stay happy and smile a lot. This always attracts positivity and more happiness.

Happy Feng Shuing !

Meenakshi is a qualified Feng shui consultant, besides being an architect. She has completed her master practitioner course in Feng shui under the tutelage of Lillian Too, the internationally renowned Feng shui expert. After which she pursued her higher studies in Feng shui from the great grand master Yap Cheng Hai from the internationally prestigious institute, Yap Cheng Hai, Centre of Excellence, based at Kuala Lumpur, Malaysia. In addition to this, she went through a further and rigorous spate of studies at Mastery Academy of Chinese Metaphysics, Malaysia.

Meenakshi has appeared as a consultant on Zoom TV, Zee TV, Aaj Tak, DD National, Pragya TV etc. She has been a columnist for prominent newspapers like Hindustan Times, Navbharat Times and also for magazines -Designer mode, Destination worldwide, Construction and Material, Indian Empire etc. She has also been a Feng shui consultant on indiatimes.com. She has held corporate talks for HSBC, ICICI, Tata Housing Development Company, Du pont, Deautche bank etc. She has provided Feng shui consultations at Radisson hotel, Shangri la hotel, Jaypee hotel, Uppal's Orchid, Delhi.

meenakshijain@gmail.com

Chapter 46

Colour Therapy

Meenakkshi Jain

The Essence

Color is an experience, that we are uniquely privileged to enjoy. We are bathed in color all our lives, we grow surrounded by color in our environment and home, we dress in colorful clothes, eat colorful foods and make color related choices everyday. We learn to interpret our environment as much by color as by shapes or sounds. Our response to color is so basic that till the age of six or even later children sort colored shapes according to their color rather than shape. Throughout our life we continue to use color as a cue for interpreting what we see: a red apple tells of its ripeness, red traffic lights brings us to a halt, Grey hair tells us of middle age. Color codes guide our travels, administration etc.

The colors we see around can noticeably affect our state of mind and feelings. For example, a red colored room produces very different sensations from a room painted blue. Color is therefore, strongly linked to our emotions. Often we describe people as "purple with rage", "green with envy", and "yellow with cowardice". These are the most common color association we use and they have more truth than we realize. Such associations are only a small part of our lifelong relationship with color, as we live by the rhythm of color changes that denote the passage of time and the cycle of seasons. As the day passes, the hues of the daylight color keep changing. The paler blue light permeates the morning after the deep blue of the sky before dawn. The afternoon is taken our over by a more yellow hue, followed by the red light of the evening. These shifts are so subtle and gradual that they are hardly noticeable, but nonetheless they color our perception of the passing day. The seasons also, highlight very different colors, with the fresh greens of the springs darkening as the summer progresses to provide a beautiful blaze of orange, gold and yellow after a few months. Winter brings along with it a stark note and sometimes a spread of snow, reducing the nature scape to a contrast of light and dark. Today's modern homes offer light all the time, whether day or night and heat or cold throughout the year as desired, because of this we sometimes loose contact with the natural, rhythms of daily and yearly cycles.

Light and its constituent colors have a strong effect on both body and mind whether we realize or not. We always respond to color at all the levels: mental, emotional and physical. The red end of the spectrum tends to make our body tense and an excessive exposure to red increase the blood pressure. On the contrary, blue relaxes our body and lowers the blood pressure. When we see a red room, it appears smaller than a blue one. Emotionally, red excites us whereas blue calms us. Of all the colors, red and blue light have the most significant and marked effect on our body. Red light increases blood pressure, respiration, muscular activity and heart rate. Blue has an exactly opposite effect, relaxes the body, calms and soothes the mind and helps insomnia sufferers. Exposure to blue light over the whole body has long been a cure for children with jaundice.

Our general health and wellbeing is affected by too much and too little light. People who do not get adequate light because they spend too much time indoors in artificial light, which does not provide the full spectrum found in the natural daylight or because they live in latitudes where the sun is absent for long periods during winter, are prone to the 'winter blues'. On the other hand, excessive exposure to light speeds development and can even induce an ageing effect. The best example of this is that the girls residing in cities and towns where nights are artificially lighted begin menstruation earlier then girls from rural areas who experience a normal day night rhythm of light and darkness.

Color is a therapy that can be easily used in conjunction with any medical treatment, be it allopathic, homeopathy, Ayurveda etc. to assist healing. It is simple, user friendly, cost effective, beautiful and safe. Bringing in the magic of color in your living spaces is the great way of making your living environment colorful and the same time therapeutic. Adding color in your living space is simple and fun!

The details given in these guidelines apply to colors seen in rooms in broad daylight. Ordinary bulbs add a reddish-yellow appearance to colors and white fluorescent lighting also distorts colors and makes the color seem more bluish. The effect of pale colors is similar to their respective colorful counterparts. However, adding white always tones down the impact. A room painted strong red is over stimulating and tiring but a pink room increases alertness and is mildly stimulating. Do not forget that it is very difficult to find paints in its pure colors. Colors are mixed together and may not result into the real color and may carry only a subtle tone of the original color. This certainly alters their effects, even if it does not become immediately apparent to the user.

The Process

Red

- **Effect** - Keeps us alert, enhances activity, stimulates inhalation, brings in passion, energy, warmth, optimism, increases pulse rate, enhances activity, facilitates judgment, danger.

- **Pitfalls** - Becomes oppressive, tiring and overpowering when strong and dense. This can lead to headaches. Use it in moderation, in the form of a tint or shade if need to paint a larger area or simply reduce the surface area to be painted. Paint only one wall red or use it in the form of accessories.

- **Usage** - Can be used in activity areas and passages. Use in dinning rooms as it promoters sociable and lively feelings and stimulates the appetite.

- **Avoid in** - Baby room, bedroom, offices, stress area.

Blue

- **Effect** - Releases Stress and calms mind. Combats tension, nervousness, insomnia and asthmatic conditions. Promoters intellectual thought. Induces sleep and associated with loyalty, authority and protection. Prevents nightmares and keeps hunger at bay.

- **Pitfalls** - Can make a room appear cold and unwelcoming. Dash a little warm color to make sure that the room does not induce in a feeling of chill and cold wave.

- **Usage** - Use in bedrooms, bathrooms, studies, offices, treatment rooms and stress area.

- **Avoid in** - Entertainment and sociable areas like dining rooms.

Yellow

- **Effect** - Suitable for mature minds as it stimulates the intellect. It brings in a feel of sunshine and energy and induces a feeling of nervousness and detachment.
- **Pitfalls** - Can induce feelings of emotional distress. It does not make a restful bedroom.
- **Usage** - Kitchens and dining rooms. Best is to use in small quantity in rooms.
- **Avoid in** - Bedroom, offices, study and work area.

Green

- **Effect** - Associated with balance, careful judgment, energy, calming, restful, stability, security and nature.
- **Pitfalls** - Encourages indecision, makes people lazy. Room appears flat, dead and empty. Add a little red or orange color to counteract these feelings.
- **Usage** - Bedrooms, in operation theatres and other places, which require balanced judgment.
- **Avoid in** -Activity areas

Orange

- **Effect** - Encourages warmth, joyfulness, lightness, pleasure, reassurance, stimulates movement.
- It aids digestion.
- **Pitfalls** - Can lead to insomnia in a bedroom. Make a room appear smaller.
- **Usage** - Living rooms, entertainment areas, dining rooms, passages, dancing halls. Bring in lot of light in an orange room.
- **Avoid in** - Bedroom, study or stress area.

Pink

- **Effect** - Associated with feelings of love and romance.
- **Pitfall** - Appears girlie and sweet. Counteract this feeling by using a hint of black.
- **Usage** – It is suitable for bedrooms. It makes the bedroom peaceful and restful.

Turquoise

- **Effect** - Refreshing, soothing, cool and calming, good for nervous system, cures loneliness
- **Pitfall** - Reduces movement
- **Usage** - Kitchen, bedroom, bathroom, treatment rooms and offices.
- **Avoid in** - Play areas, dance halls and activity area.

Violet

- **Effect** - Encourages spirituality, meditation prayer, dignity, purpose, and leadership. Balances and calms mind and body.
- **Pitfall** - Brings in spiritual arrogance and snob value.
- **Usage** - Bedroom, Kitchen, Bathroom, Offices, treatment rooms.
- **Avoid in** - Play and active areas.

Magenta

- **Effect** - Brings in spiritual fulfillment, contentment, self-respect, and completeness.
- **Usage** - Lecture rooms, chapels, Entrance halls.
- **Avoid in** - Entertainment area.

Purple

- **Effect** - Joy, fertility, creativity, magic, sex, evil, and death.
- **Pitfall** - Overpowering.

- **Usage** - Bedrooms

White

- **Effect** - Purity, de cluttering, fresh beginnings
- **Pitfall** - Looks bare and needs to be compensated with plants and accessories.

Black

- **Effect** - Drama, eccentricity, death. It heightens emotional response.
- **Pitfall** - Depressing
- **Usage** - Moderation
- Use to soften girlie colors like pink.
- **Avoid in** - Base colors

The Tip

Color scheme for interiors works well if we limit to a choice of three colors while designing the interiors of a premises. Choose one warm color, one cool color and one neutral color. You can throw in a dash of metallic color like gold and silver in small amount and variations. The warm colors are red, orange, yellow, red-violet, red-orange and yellow-orange. The cool colors of the spectrum are blue, green, violet, blue-violet and blue-green. The neutral colors are white, black, grey and brown.

Bring into your home and office appropriate colored flowers and plants. In your office, choose desktop accessories of your choice. In bedrooms, use bed sheets of different colors to absorb the color vibrations of your choice. Use colored lighting in your premises. Use Potpourri in your bedrooms and other living spaces. Bring in colored candles and aroma candles in your house.

Adding color in your living spaces is a great way to increase certain positive personality traits. Your color preferences are a definitive factor in determining the choice of rooms coloration, with color therapy, the actual function of color takes on greater importance. Therefore, if there is color that you prefer to decorate your space with, make sure it provides the support your life requires!

There are many other ways to absorb color, to promote good health and overall well-being. You can choose whatever suits you and what blends with your personal lifestyle. The different methods that can be employed to bring the magic of colors in your life are: -

- Color in clothes
- Color in Feng Shui
- Color in Food
- Color in Chakras
- Color in Crystal
- Color in Aroma
- Color in Music
- Color in Chanting
- Color in Breathing
- Color in Visualization
- Color using Silk
- Color using Energized Water

As you continue to experiment with different methods employed in color therapy, you will gradually discover your own personalized and unique way to work with color! Color dominates our senses, our wellbeing and our world. May be it is appropriate to say, without life there is little color, without color there is no life.

Meenakshi is a qualified Feng shui consultant, besides being an architect. She has completed her master practitioner course in Feng shui under the tutelage of Lillian Too, the internationally renowned Feng shui expert. After which she pursued her higher studies in Feng shui from the great grand master Yap Cheng Hai from the internationally prestigious institute, Yap Cheng Hai, Centre of Excellence, based at Kuala Lumpur, Malaysia. In addition to this, she went through a further and rigorous spate of studies at Mastery Academy of Chinese Metaphysics, Malaysia.

Meenakshi has appeared as a consultant on Zoom TV, Zee TV, Aaj Tak, DD National, Pragya TV etc. She has been a columnist for prominent newspapers like Hindustan Times, Navbharat Times and also for magazines -Designer mode, Destination worldwide, Construction and Material, Indian Empire etc. She has also been a Feng shui consultant on indiatimes.com. She has held corporate talks for HSBC, ICICI, Tata Housing Development Company, Du pont, Deautche bank etc. She has provided Feng shui consultations at Radisson hotel, Shangri la hotel, Jaypee hotel, Uppal's Orchid, Delhi.

meenakshijain@gmail.com

CHAPTER 47

Astrology - A Tool For Healing Energies

Dipikka Sanghi Gupta

The Essence

Everything in the Universe is Energy. All events are energy driven. This statement comes from the scientific adage that every effect has a cause and that every happening has a force behind it. In other words, it is safe to understand that energy drives the events.

Astrology explains the energy in our life and its potential challenges and possibilities; one can evolve from one's own chart. It is we who choose the way to respond to these energies, based on our thoughts, words and actions. **Astrology is about making a choice between free will and destiny.**

Astrology relates itself to planets and to the two luminaries namely Sun and Moon. In modern science, we know, Sun is a star and is the prime mover and, therefore, secondary sources of energy depend upon its energy. Sun sends in its energy directly to the Earth and, also, as reflected energy from the Moon and other planets. This energy may be light; heat, magnetic, gravitational or any other that may be discovered by Scientists in the coming years. The energy reaching Earth comes from the Sun and other planets both in direct and indirect ways.

Astrology is the mother of all the sciences. Astrology is marvelous science if one has a patience to understand it. Astrology is easy to learn but can take a lifetime to master. It is purely scientific as based on astronomical calculations. It is an ancient practice that assumes that the position of the stars and planets has a direct influence upon people and events on earth.

Throughout history, famous people have studied astrology and used it for varied purposes. The Three Wise Men in the Bible were astrologers and learned that Christ would be born at a conjunction of planets. The Bible is filled with astrological information. Pythagoras and Sir Isaac Newton were astrologers.

In India, Astrology is the part of Vedas. Veda means original knowledge and truth. Vedic means, of the original knowledge and truth. Astrological principles were written 12,00,000 years ago by 12 famous Maharshis like Narada, Bhrigu, Vasista, Parashara, Jaimini, etc. These Maharishis are acknowledged as having been instrumental of preserving the ancient knowledge. Vedic chart is a road map depicting history, genetics and karma, of a person.

Our Vedic astrology has details of the horoscopes of Lord Krishna, Lord Rama and many other ancient Indian kings and queens, recorded thousands of years ago. The Bhishma Parva and Udyoga Parva chapters of Mahabharata mention many astrological descriptions and omens just before the Mahabharata war. It also describes a period of draught with several planetary combinations. There is also a very clear reference about two eclipses, a solar eclipse and a lunar eclipse occurring, creating a rare 13 day lunar fortnight. In Ayodhya Kand of Ramayana, it is mentioned that Lord Rama was born in cancer lagna. Sage Valmiki has given detailed information about the planetary position in the chart of Lord Rama.

For centuries, humans have looked to the heavens for guidance. History proves the truth of astrology. We can find reason for everything in astrology. When all the great sciences in the world failed to explain the reason for a particular thing, Astrology speaks. Astrology as science, used for fortune telling and understanding the personality is only a very limited part of astrology and does not highlight the complete value of astrology. The generalized zodiac sign stuff that is read in the newspaper is also not astrology. There is a need to move beyond our daily horoscope to uncover the complexities and intricacies of astrology.

The Process

Whenever I sit down and talk to someone about a chart, it strikes me afresh just how interesting and unexpected people's stories are. Everyone's life is not just one story but also a whole necklace of tales threaded together by one soul. Those tales, of course, weave in and out of other people's lives, creating a huge tapestry of humanity.

Here are few interesting and amazing stories I have come across during my reading of charts

1. **Astrological Chart can "See" all**

    A well to do businessman once approached me. He had twins, one son and one daughter, the son died; this left the businessman very upset. He was upset because he was a very religious and god fearing person. He also believed a lot in charity, helping the poor and needy, so he was surprised how such a thing would happen to him? After checking his charts, I was surprised to read that the young boy's death occurred at a pilgrimage due to hunger, some accident, due to water drowning and some tree. Moreover, just before his death the young boy must have made huge profit or achievement.

    It looked strange that a child of such rich family would die of hunger? When I told the client, he confirmed that his son got the job he wanted in the US and before going he wanted to visit Kailash Mansarovar along with his friend. On the way they all were hungry but it was cold, so they decided to get some food packed and eat it in the hotel. On the way they took lift from a biker. The bike met with an accident and the boy fell down in the river, later after flowing for some time he got stuck in a tree where he was found. It was surprising how his chart could tell me all this about the boy even before the father could narrate the incident.

2. **Astrology Consoles A Worried Mother**

    Once a woman came to me with a problem, her daughter had got divorced within 3 months of her marriage. Her birth chart showed problems in married life and it was best for her to complete her studies. The mother took my advice and sent her daughter to USA to do her masters degree. She also did the Vedic healing of planets. By god's grace this showed results, the girl completed her masters, started doing a job of her choice, married someone of her choice in the US and is happy now.

3. Astrological Healing Helps Family Get Their Son Back On Track

In India most of business families are joint families, which means parents live with their married children, in short, the whole family lives together in one home. The case that came to me was interesting and different. Here, the father-in-law co-existed with his three daughter-in-laws . The eldest and the youngest sons were financially well to do while the middle son was poor. He used to feel upset about this; his problems grew so much that he soon went and had an extra-marital affair and started drinking heavily. They came to me and got the astrological healings done. Today they are living happily, both husband and wife are earning well.

The logical greatness of astrology can be realized through many other examples. Like, during the full moon children are more hyper, more cars break down and most important, mental patients show change in mood and reactions. This could not be a coincidence. A psychologist may fail to explain this, but astrology can explain this in a simple manner. In Vedic astrology moon is the indicator of mind and heart (Chandrama manaso jathaha). The moon affects the tides of the ocean. The moon rules our emotional nature, and our body is made up of 85% water.

I would also like to draw your attention towards medical field, which is very much scientific. When a person is sick, they go to see a doctor. The doctor inquires a lot to find out about the disease and then prescribe a medicine. If patient is not cured then the doctor changes the medicine. If still there are no signs of relief, patient is advised to take many tests. Again new medicines are prescribed. Sometimes operation is suggested or patient is left on the mercy of God. We, 21st century people are more logic based, accept this by thinking that the doctor has tried a lot. Sometimes the patient goes to another doctor and whole cycle repeats again. But on another hand, while going to an astrologer, we expect that the astrologer should tell everything about family, occupation, children, inheritance, prosperity, diseases, etc. .The knowledge, accuracy & the experience of the astrologer are the factors responsible for the correctness of the prediction. Out of many predictions, if a single prediction is wrong then we blame that astrology, as a science is, fake.

There are several advantages in studying astrology like, learning to understand and know yourself better, understand hidden knowledge, current influences on one's life, learning interpersonal skills, seeking self development, enjoying good health, prosperity & spiritual advancement, developing analytical faculties of children, developing leadership qualities, analyzing and strengthening relationships etc.,

Human beings in their life face a lot of pain, misery and troubles, which affect them both emotionally as well as physically. To avoid pain and to seek pleasure has been one of the major objectives of our lives. The other major objective for a selected few of us is to know our true self and to know the ultimate reality and be one with it. Whether the objective is material or spiritual, as per one's destiny there could be a lot of hurdles.

Jyotish Vidya shows the path and result of karma done in past and freedom to make the future through the position of nine planets. When in exaltation, the impress of the planet can be gentle and often very spiritual and suggests the karma of positive qualities from the past endeavor. In the same way, a planet in a bad position suggests traits that may have been misused, neglected or acted upon in an erroneous manner in previous life creating problems is present life, thus the chance to work on them is accorded in this life. Particular house, compatibility, incompatibility and aspect of planets also play an important role in suggesting that how particular energies have blended and worked together in the past, whether in a harmonious or antagonistic way.

Vedic astrology has not only given us tools to determine what destiny has in store for us but also ways to avoid the hurdles in achieving our material or spiritual goals. Remedial Measures allows one to solve his or her problems by modifying the karma in a systematic way. These measures help in solving karmic problems.

The Tip

- In astrology, wearing a gemstone ring is very common because a ring is a circle, symbol of eternity, unity, reincarnation and the universe. In ancient times, rings were associated with Sun and Moon, hence it was an object of protection, a magical guard that warded off negativity through its continuity.

Rings bind the person with power, energy and keep them in body and so inhibit the release of power.

- Colour therapy is another scientific tool for healing in astrology. Yellow colours rules solar plexus and is useful in study rooms. Blue helps to cure heat, anger, passion as it is the colour of peace. Use of Indigo helps in diabetes, impotency, urinary troubles etc and helps to adapt a practical approach towards life. Violet being a mixture of red and blue helps researchers, aspirants of mystic sciences etc.
- Reciting mantras at a particular day and time has dramatic results in one's life.
- Fasting is another scientific method of healing in astrology.

Dr. Dipikka Sanghi Gupta is very gifted and famous astrologer based in Delhi. She is a pioneer in the field of Astrological consultancy services, Numerology, Tarot Card reading, Palmistry and Vaastu Shastra. She is the author of a book on numerology "Numerology - An Amazing Science", published in June 2011.

www.deepikaastro.com

CHAPTER 48

Mantra Healing

Ashok Angrish

The Essence

What is Sound: We can say that **Sound** is a vibration that propagates as a mechanical wave of pressure and displacement, through some medium (such as air or water). Sometimes *sound* refers to only those vibrations with frequencies that are within the range of hearing. However, we understand sound to be an ordered motion of the molecules of the medium through which the sound propagates.

Can we define Sound as a manifestation of energy spontaneously erupting then dispersing back into the Universe! Our own voice vibrates and creates its own energy. Each thought-wave produced by the mind, therefore, emits a certain sound and that sound is the combined sound of the various acoustic roots associated with the various propensities active in that thought. What the yogis then discovered was that if an acoustic root or combination of acoustic roots was repeated in the mind it would create a sympathetic vibration that would activate the corresponding mental propensity. By repeating the acoustic root for anger, a feeling of anger would arise in the mind. By repeating the acoustic root for compassion, a feeling of compassion would be induced. The closer the sound repeated was to the actual acoustic root, the stronger the wave of that mental propensity that would arise in the mind. It was these discoveries and investigations that led directly to the science of rhythmic chanting.

Our bodies are made up of particles of energy, and there is a vibration that is constantly pulsating through them. Stresses, imbalances, and weakness can cause these energy particles to change the vibration of our body. Sound acts as a solar massage for the entire body and nervous system. This occurs on a cellular level and, as we know, our cells are constantly changing; so, our body is never the same. With the use of rhythmic chanting, we can build a new body that beats to a higher vibrational level by instilling that vibration in the building blocks of our body.

Each and every expression of Universe, each and every wave creates a sound. The sound is called the "acoustic root" of that expression. Can we give a 'meaning' to Sound? Probably not or certainly not! We can give meaning to words and not to sound(s). It is because words are a result of civilization of mankind. Words came later and are products or expressions of collective-mind of mankind; as, words were developed for a convenient and effective means of communication. Sounds came prior to civilization; they came along with the human beings and living beings. Sounds are more primitive than the living beings or human beings. The earlier human beings, when words or the language were not created, used the sounds, essentially, to convey their emotions e.g. the emotion of love, the emotion of fear, the emotion of anger, and likewise. What we need to understand is that such sound or every sound has a specific source (or part) where it is created in the human-body and that specific part of the human-body represents that specific emotion created by the sound.

This linkage of the emotion vis-à-vis the sound was understood and mastered by the Eastern World thousands of years ago. The Eastern World or the Ancient India had a very advanced culture intellectually and spiritually; and a language, 'Sanskrit' was developed which itself means "refined, well done." The alphabets in Sanskrit are perfectly designed for the human vocal apparatus, and are pronounced phonetically. Sanskrit was essentially designed for sound and it is an exquisite language from ancient India. It is considered divine, originating from the meditations of ancient Sages. Sanskrit is pronounced accordingly as it is written, and no sound is dropped while uttering its written word(s). For thousands of years, the profound teachings of India have been chanted over and over, preserving the essence of their meaning. Chanting Sanskrit word(s) forms a direct link or an acoustic root to the vibrations through sound.

The Process

The ancient Indian Seers discovered fifty principle acoustic roots (or matrikas*) which, either alone or in combination, are at the root of all psychic expression.

These fifty roots, on which they based the fifty letters of the Sanskrit alphabet, correspond to the fifty principle natural tendencies of the human mind, such as fear, anger, compassion, etc. These fifty natural tendencies combine together to give rise to the infinitely rich matrix of human thought. One or more of these natural-tendency is always active in the human mind at any given point of time, to one degree or another, and the combination thereof produces the phenomenon that we know of as human thought. When these fifty natural-tendencies become completely quiescent then the pure consciousness shines in its original, unaltered state.

Among the various psychic-tendencies, those acoustic roots which awakened the core tendencies of the individual mind became the subject of intense research and with the passage of time **the processes of rhythmic-chanting or the mantras** were born which tuned not only the mind and the emotions, but the body and its glands as well to the subtle wavelengths of the 'Self'.

The rhythmic chanting forms a complex pattern of vibrations meant to activate certain centers in the human body by repetition of the mantra. Each Mantra holds the ability to open your energy body, emotions, and soul to a higher vibrational level. Silently repeating rhythmic chanting creates a mental vibration that allows the mind to experience deeper levels of awareness and leads into the field of pure consciousness from which the vibration arose.

One thing more worth giving attention seem to be that the world does not exist as we see it; it is merely a huge mass of vibrations. In the system of existence, there are bodies of condensed vibrations having enormous potential(s) which are beyond the understanding of normal human beings. In a higher probability, these bodies-of-condensed vibrations are the deities given names which indicate the nature-of-powers represented by them e.g. Kali, Durga, Lakshmi, Indra, Bhairava, Shiva and likewise. A Mantra is not merely a sound but essentially, a process to put us in the vibrational-layer of the specific deity. Each human being is in essence a mantra, a very unique yet cosmic mantra vibrating at its own level, rhythmic-chanting of Mantras attune us to the layer of vibrations of that specific deity and we acquire the powers of that specific deity as his/her grace.

The exploration of relationship between the sound and the consciousness can lead to a whole different understanding of the world we live in and the world we create. When we have this perception about ourselves, we cannot help but let go of old patterns and obstacles and enjoy the wonder of being part of the cosmic symphony.

This is an example which indicates that India has a lot in its Belly and Brain….. and while saying so, I am not referring to the physical boundaries of India. In fact, I am referring to the unfathomable depth of spiritual history of this Nation. When I say 'India has a lot in its Brain', I refer to the potential of creativity a mind cultivated in above referred Indian-ness can have; and, when I say 'India has a lot in its Belly', I refer to the 'secrets' which the rich spiritual heritage of India is carrying in its ancient scriptures. As stated above, the Ancient Indian Sages have given us potent mantras and seed-mantras which have the potential of working directly on our karmic-impression and giving us the key to re-write our destiny.

The Seed Mantra (or the beej mantra) is a very potent set of sounds which can have a vowel, a consonant and an element of vibrating sound imbibed in it. The vowel is 'the-carrier' which carries the sound energy (created by consonant) in the intended energy-centre in the body; for example the sounds having 'EE' type-pronunciation travel towards 'lower chakras' centered near sexual-organs in the body; and, sounds having 'O' type-pronunciation travel towards 'upper chakras' centered near throat or the 'third eye' (middle of the eyes) in the body. We therefore find that, generally, most of the shakti-mantras have 'EE' type sound in them which strikes the 'energy dynamos' centered near sexual organs. As a result, we create the type of power (or energy) needed by us to meet all the worldly affairs be it sex, money, fame etc. We further find that the mantra having 'O' type sound in them strike the energy-dynamos centered near 'upper chakras' and as a result the journey of soul tends towards purest form of compassion, spirituality and moksha.

Here is an example, which indicates the presence of a Seed (beej) in a Mantra:

There is a Sloka in Shree DevyaAtharvaSheersham which is as under:

"वियदीकारसंयुक्तं वीतिहोत्र समन्वितं
अर्द्धेन्दुलसितं देव्या बीजं सर्वार्थसाधकं"

ViyadiKar Sanyuktam VeetihotraSamanvitam
ArdhEnduLasitam Devya Beejam SarvArthSadhkam.

When we expand the meaning of the above sloka, it becomes:

THAT which includes Viyat = Ether [(h) sound] and 'EE' sound; and also includes Veetihotra=Fire [(r) sound] and is decorated with the ArdhChandra [(mmm) vibrating sound], THIS seed of Devi is capable of fulfilling all desires (sarvaArthSadhkam). Now, what we get in this sloka can be summed as under:

It is sound of H, Combined with R, Combined with Vowel sound of EE and decorated with the MM vibrating sound =

H R EE M = Hreem (the result is beej mantra = Hreem).

This seed-mantra 'Hreem' is a Shakti-Mantra, the rhythmic-chanting of which activates the hidden powers of a Sadhak and places him in a higher level of vibrations. With the patience-practice of this seed-mantra 'Hreem', life of the Sadhak gets totally transformed touching new heights of worldly achievements and spirituality as well.

Another thing which needs to be kept in consideration is that there are a number of seed-mantras which are yet to be deciphered or yet to be given an explanation of their actual genesis or their being the way they are. While the quest to understand the genesis of seed-mantra cannot be denied but at the same time what is more important is getting beneficial impact of the seed-mantras given in ancient texts rather than mere searching for its genesis. Had the Adam thought of first knowing the genesis of the fruit Apple, he would not have been able to eat it, forever.

The last but not the least, mantras are based on sound-vibration-energy and this energy has no religion; hence, mantras are equally effective for every human being following any religion on this Earth. The only requirement is that these are to be done under the guidance of a competent Guru.

The Tip

In Tantra, the fifty or fifty-one letters including vowels as well as consonants from A to Ksha, of the Devanagari alphabet itself, the *Varnamala* of bija, have been described as being the Matrikas themselves. It is believed that they are infused with the power of the Divine Mother herself. The Matrikas are considered to be the subtle form of the letters *(varna)*. These letters combined make up syllables *(pada)* which are combined to make sentences *(vakya)* and it is of these elements that mantra is composed. It is believed that the power of mantra derives from the fact that the letters of the alphabet are in fact forms of the goddess.

The 50 Matrika Kalas are given in the same account as follows: **Nivritti, Pratishtha, Vidya, Shanti, Indhika, Dipika, Mochika, Para, Sukshma, Sukshmamrita, Jnanamrita, Apypayani, Vyapini, Vyomarupa, Ananta, Srishti, Riddhi, Smriti, Medha, Kanti, Lakshmi, Dyuti, Sthira, Sthiti, Siddhi, Jada, Palini, Shanti, Aishvarya, Rati, Kamika, Varada, Ahladini, Pritih, Dirgha, Tikshna, Raudri, Bhaya, Nidra, Tadra, Kshudha, Krodhini, Kriya, Utkari, Mrityurupa, Pita, Shveta, Asita, Ananta.** Sometimes, the Matrikas represent a diagram written in the letter, believed to possess magical powers.

Ashok Angrish is a Vedic Scholar who teaches Healing through mantras. He is a faculty of

Angrish Astro - a team of dedicated astro-experts make use of a fine blend of ancient Vedic astrology and a unique system of Predictive Astrology popularly known as Nadi Astrology. The astro-experts of AngrishAstro *have been using the most advanced and accurate system of astronomical calculations like use of Raphael-Ephemeris, the most accurate calculations of Moon's Ascending Node and Descending Node, the accuracy of Moon's placement meets the most accurate standards at 0.001% error, use of Placidus system (the most accurate system so far) to cast NBC Chart; and so on.*

www.angrishastro.com

49 CHAPTER

The Wellness Concept

Prof. B.M. Hegde

"The establishment defends itself by complicating everything to the point of incomprehensibility." Fred Hoyle

It was in the year 1733 that Charles Scharschmidt, a brilliant young professor of medicine in Vienna, wrote the first textbook of medicine. While writing about diseases with constriction of the vascular bed and agitation of the mind he had the best prescription for those days, which looks contemporary, even to this day. Change of mode of living, tranquility of the mind and drugs rarely, if needed at all, were the three points in his textbook. Listening to the debate on the March 3rd 2010 morning where President Obama gave his last dose of wisdom to the people of America as also to his colleagues in all the political parties about his "so called" *health care reforms,* I was a bit confused as **he was talking only about disease care reforms and NOT about health care reforms**.

In a recent symposium sponsored by Deepak Chopra Foundation at San Diego we were deliberating on the newer, inexpensive and safe vectors of human healing. Scientists and spiritualists from all over the world who are working in this area were invited, as speakers and I happened to be one of them. We are bringing out the abstracts of the talks and papers presented there in this issue of JSHO. The full symposium will eventually be uploaded to the JSHO website in all details.

America is suffering from overmedication and over intervention of all sorts resulting in the abuse of the disease care facilities which cost the nation trillions of dollars; most of which could be well spent if only the powers that be understood the difference between *health care* and *disease care*. The *euboxic* medicine practised in the US, where all the computer boxes in the patient case record will have to be perfect, lest some one should sue the doctor in the unlikely event of patients' death or disability, makes medical care prohibitively expensive. Market forces dictate the management and not science. The whole population of the USA *needs urgent health care* but a microscopic minority really needs disease care. This truth is being kept well wrapped up in pseudo-scientific jargon, myths, half-truths and disease mongering efforts to earn billions from the gullible patients or their caregivers. It is much cheaper to keep the well healthy rather than let them get diseases and then target the disease. This is the rule in the USA as also in other places like India where American medicine is being encouraged.

The above difference is simple enough to be understood by the lay public. However, today the common man on the street thinks that he needs doctors and hospitals to remain healthy and that there is a pill for every ill. **What is to be brought to the knowledge of the population is that if they lived a healthy life style, which will be described below, they could expect to live well and healthy till they die. No one should try to be here forever, as s/he will never succeed.**

It is only in the unlikely event of the body's inbuilt immune guard getting overwhelmed do symptoms of diseases make their appearance. It is only then that the medical profession could help by: "curing rarely, comforting mostly, but consoling always", as was enunciated by the father of western modern medicine, Hippocrates. There are *no silent killers*. All killers announce their intentions loudly in human physiology. Studies have time and again affirmed that treating diseases in their "so called" asymptomatic stage only would harm the patient since nature has built the immune guard with elaborate repair mechanisms to remodel every deviation for the normal, which is the asymptomatic stage of illnesses. Any interference at that stage from outside, that too with chemical drugs, can only harm the former and might result in disaster.

Healthy life style and tips:

No one can help another to adopt a healthy life style. One has to *be the change* and no amount of preaching will help. One has to take charge of one's health and wellness. The methods are simple and could be adopted by anyone in any walk of life howsoever busy one might be! Human body is a nonlinear, dynamic device, continuously run by food and oxygen with the help of the electromagnetic energy from the sun. Some physiologists believe that the body water, which forms around 80-85% of the body, needs to be stimulated (burnt) to release energy.

- Human beings are not just their bodies; they have their all-pervading mind and their spirit. All three of them need to be kept healthy for total health and wellness. Usually it is not what one eats that kills her/him; it is what eats one (one's negative thoughts) that kills. The best bet to keep good health is to have a healthy mind, which, boils down to practicing universal compassion. To get into that state of mind (consciousness) Yoga and the breathing techniques would help a lot. Yoga has very little to do with any religion and could be practiced by all.

- To be healthy one has to change (be the change) but can't expect the world to change overnight. Therefore one could expect others to hurt us sometime or the other. There again the best anti-dote for hurt is to cultivate the greatest asset of forgiveness. "If you can fill the unforgiving minute with sixty seconds worth of distance run, this earth shall belong to you my son, and…more, You shall be a MAN," wrote Rudyard Kipling years ago in his celebrated poem, IF. This is the best health advice that I have been able to find in the western literature.

- Eating in moderation, the foods that please one, without too much change in the food quality from its natural state, would go a long way to help the immune system to keep the repair mechanism in excellent shape. Worrying about the micro-contents of the food is of lesser importance as long as one does not pick and choose foods, thanks to the modern food fads and corporate advertisements.

- Preserved foods are a curse. Let the food be as fresh as is possible. Small frequent feeds keep the metabolism on even keel. Large meals at long intervals are not conducive to body physiology. Each region, ethnic group and race has had its own food habits that kept mankind going in 50,000 generations. The food habits evolved over thousands of years, thanks to our ancestors' observational research. Modern nutrition does not have a strong foundation and the reductionist cohort studies being fed to the gullible masses lack the backing of good science. That is exactly the reason why we get conflicting advices now and then! If Mediterranean diet is good for them in their habitat, it does not mean that it will be good for another race in another continent. Meal times should be happy times and family get-together at mealtime is the best bet to get benefit from foods.

- The two enemies of human health are tobacco and alcohol, both of which must be kept at a distance.

- Regular exercise, moderate in quantity, the best being a daily walk for an hour, would be the ideal tonic for the immune guard. Very heavy exercise might not be good for the system. The key word in every human endeavor should be moderation in everything one does. Extremes are always dangerous. Swimming is another excellent exercise but is not universally applicable and could be expensive to the majority.

- There is no substitute for hard work as another good immune booster. If the hard work involves physical exertion additional regular exercise is not needed. The only qualification is that one should *love* one's work to get the benefit. Hating one's work and working under duress could destroy health.

- Spirituality has very little to do with religion. Spirituality for good health is just *sharing and caring!* Sharing provokes the immune system and hating others depresses the same. A small child smiles 400-500 times in a day. If we take a lesson from that the world would be a better place to live. Natural smile releases so many healthy bio-positive endorphins from the brain.

Conclusions:

If one were to follow the above-mentioned simple daily routine, the wellness concept, the chance of falling ill are negligible like following traffic rules on highways can reduce fatal accidents. That said, I must hasten to add that even those who follow the health rules enumerated above might get illnesses as diseases are only accidents. Medical science or any other science will never be able to answer the million dollar question as to *why* a person gets sick at a given time although we have elaborate details to frighten the gullible people as to *how* they get ill, in our disease mongering, medical (health) *scare* system. A Nobel Laureate physiologist had affirmed to that truth way back in 1899, when Charles Sherrington, wrote that *"positive sciences will never be able to answer the question why, but they will be able to say how or how much!"*

If we were to implement this method we would reduce the medical care budget of every country. All the same an efficient and authentic medical care system is a must under the following circumstances, which covers about 5% of the population at a given time. Emergencies, disaster management, corrective surgeries, judicious authenticated vaccinations, birthing emergencies, congenital problems, and acute life threatening situations need medical help.

The need of the hour is to change our medical education system to incorporate the new philosophy of health promotion, which is never taught these days. The student must be taught that the human body could correct most of its problems without outside interventions but we must create the right environment for that to be useful. Too much intervention might put off the body's immune system. Doctors are trained primarily to keep the public healthy (public health) which is not our present stress. Young doctors should be impressed that they should leave the well alone and they should never try to treat the disease but try and understand the patient better before intervening, and they should see that their interventions do not make the patient worse than his/her original disease! While a good doctor treats the illness; a great doctor treats the patient.

The need of the hour is for *thought leaders* in the field to understand that there are a host of medical care systems in the world, out with our reductionist modern medicine, that have stood the test of time over thousands of years before the advent of modern medicine. But for them human kind would have been extinct like the dinosaurs long, long ago. Modern medical system, developed in the last few centuries', in its present *avatar* of hi-tech stuff is only less than a few decades old. One has to take into account the recent audits in many countries on the impact of modern medicine on human morbidity and mortality. The data is there for all to see and take corrective measures lest we should be left out in the race. Every medical student must be told that while patients could (and did) survive without modern medical doctors; we cannot survive without patients.

We need urgent research to try and scientifically authenticate many of those inexpensive methods in other systems of medicine to put together a future system incorporating the best in all the systems together-call the new system Meta Medicine (after modern medicine) if you like-to help patients and also the world governments to contain the ever mounting costs of medical care which would make people like President Obama to get sound sleep while his people remain healthy and when they fall ill they are well cared for without spending too much of the tax payers' money which should satisfy both sides of the divide. The effort of trying to put together Meta Medicine is already on.

In this deafening cry for better hi-tech medicine let us not forget that the womb of all ills, ranging from common cold to cancer, is poverty. The latter is a double-edged weapon in that while diseases are more common in the poorer sections, diseases further make the sufferer poorer when the breadwinner gets sick the family starves and becomes poorer. The poor people with very little protein in their system suffer from a very serious illness, which I call as Nutritional Immune Deficiency Syndrome, NIDS, which is many times more dangerous than the fashionable label of AIDS! It was a thinking family doctor in the poor coal mining community of Wales, Tudor Edward Harts, who wrote decades ago: *"the poor pay for their poverty with their lives."* This one line tells it all and should be taught to our doctors and politicians alike.

> *"Truth is ever to be found in the simplicity, and not in the multiplicity and confusion of things."* -Isaac Newton

Prof. B.M. Hegde is an Indian medical scientist, educationist and author. He is a retired Vice Chancellor of the Manipal University and the head of the Manglore Chapter of Bharatiya Vidya Bhavan. He has authored several books on medical practice and ethics. A recipient of numerous national and international awards including Dr. B. C. Roy National Award, Pride of India Award, Padmabhushan, he is also the Editor in Chief of the medical journal, Journal of the Science of Healing Outcomes.

www.bmhegde.com

CHAPTER 50

Disinformation in the New Age

Mandy Peterson

As a mighty flood sweeps away the sleeping village, so death carries away the person of distracted mind who only plucks the flowers (of pleasure).
~Gautama Buddha

Disinformation is nothing new, even in the new age. Due to the fact that many of us hold the ancient masters in high regard, it is natural for us, as new-agers, to want to portray or believe that our ancient teachers would support the new-age movement. After all, we founded this movement, in part, based on the wisdom of their teachings. We've done this through taking a little of one masters teachings, a little of another's, and we've packaged it all together as a philosophy that we feel is good to live by. Yes, there are huge differences; but, we circumvent around these differences through rationalizing that we live in different times.

Because we have taken pieces of wisdom from different places, it does not always offer us a complete picture of the masters involved. What many people may not even know is that many quotes that are floating around the internet, and which we believe are the words of our masters, are fake, misworded, or taken out of context (e.g. see FakeBuddhaQuotes.com). While people may see this as a relatively trivial matter, it really isn't. After all, how would we feel if we saw a Facebook banner which displayed an image of Jesus with the quote, "*Ho, ho, ho, Merry Christmas! – Jesus Christ?*"

Many of us, having not studied the works of many of our masters, only see collectively chosen quotes from a small portion of a master's work. These portions may be framed in a way that the master appears to support our new-age sentiments. What we never see is the remainder that would have been in direct conflict or might appear "negative." Unfortunately, this promotes disinformation

Holistic Wellness in the New Age

and misunderstanding as to who our masters really were and what they really taught. To prove this, I even posted a real Buddha quote (from the Dhammapada) on Facebook and someone confronted me that the quote must be fake because Buddha would "never have said" that.

So, keeping this all in mind, it is fair to say, yes, there is disinformation in the new-age. And, it is safe to wake up to it, as well as where disinformation exists outside of the new-age. It is safe to realize that the new-age has an agenda just like every other religion, cult, faction, institution, etc. Even I have my own agenda. So, you must find the Truth for yourself.

The new-age agenda appears to be with distraction, denial, and the repression of "negative" emotions and thoughts, while encouraging individuals to keep up with a consumerist mentality that is destructive both internally and externally. This is not passing judgment here; I'm just dispassionately stating a perception which seems, to me, a fact.

What I've learned through having been part of the new-age for most of my life is that there is something inherent in the path that creates a no-win situation. On the one hand, we are taught to deny "negative" illusions as unreal. On the other hand, we are taught to exhaust ourselves in the pursuit of "positive" illusions (which many masters have discouraged this kind of approach, and excess materialism, though we may not have understood why). Some of us are starting to catch on that living in this way leaves us subtly feeling that we never have or are enough. For, this is another illusion: that we can attain a feeling of completeness if we can manifest this-or-that. However, fulfillment rarely is forthcoming, as once we complete a goal we immediately seek to attain something else.

While not suggesting we live entirely without external striving or material "abundance," what may be labelled as more problematic is our collective approach. Because we live in a world which we perceive as 'normal,' we do not always understand the ways in which we become conditioned, as individuals within a larger society, to have things defined for us; i.e. such as success, failure, abundance, loss, etc. We have so much information coming at us that, "you can shine," "you can succeed," or "you can have unlimited this or that." But, notice how this leaves the subtle impression that we are lacking. So, repeating these kinds of mantras naturally serves as an inspiration that keep us driven. But, toward what end? More illusion and potential suffering?

I am not implying this is right or wrong, merely that many of us may not always be aware of how we are being conditioned, or the effects of such conditioning. After all, how many of us could live a simple unaffected life without worrying what people would think? How many of us get called "lazy" for not being productive enough? How are we conditioned out of taking care of our minds and bodies through being encouraged that we need quick-fixes-because there is not enough time for rest? Many of us are terrified to slow down in ways lest we miss an opportunity for advancement, or let ourselves or others down in some way.

I find it no wonder that so many people end up with "ascension symptoms." Seen from a rational perspective of cause and effect, these symptoms likely arise from the living split between our minds (which tell us to be "love n light") and our contradictory lifestyles (which ask us to be aggressive, striving, competitive, and to not truly care about anything beyond our personal outcomes). Many of the idealistic concepts that we espouse, don't even add up with how we live our lives. For, how can we truly end up manifesting peace, love, and oneness while being taught to be self-entitled, self-oriented, and to climb various hierarchical ladders to "success"?

Looking at how innately aggressive the world is, and how we keep marching and banging our drums like little energizer bunnies trying to get ahead, to me, it makes sense that new-agers feel sped up–ADHD; anxious, repressed emotions surfacing; sleep-disturbed; and intolerant to food, chemicals and geopathic stress (aka "dirty energy"). We seem to lack the wisdom of our masters which was by-passed and which could have advised us on how to bridge the various splits we created in our minds and lives. In fact, it seems many of our present-day gurus can only instruct us on how not to deal with negative realities and emotions as they come up, which come to be treated with distaste and dissociation.

We end up being taught conflicting messages regarding how to find our "off switch." On the one hand, we are taught to practice meditation and to be "in the now;" finding our divine self-worth internally. On the other hand, we are taught that we can have it all, be special, be a "star seed, blue ray, etc.," or can "succeed" or "manifest;" finding approval and self-worth externally.

On top of this, we are taught to withhold judgment. Taken out of context, we come to lose the discriminating ability to identify and address disharmonies or untruths within the world; except those truths we deem "positive." We forget that if we want to manifest things that are "good," there must exist an opposite polarity where things become "judged" as "not so good." We have to be careful not to forget that judgment also implies "karma," which can incur from collectively self-destructive behavior that is continually enabled. Though, there are more and more people waking up to this now.

The main fear seems to be one of being unloving. Though, enabling one another's bad behavior or addictions is not something I would consider loving. The main addiction of this age appears to be one of consumerism and self-indulgence. And, lacking a standard of ethics to follow, we can end up inadvertently and unconsciously acting impulsively, with no restraints and little care for how our addictions affect the younger generations, the environment, etc.

Through the Law of Attraction, we are taught accountability, but primarily when it comes to our personal lives and not the bigger picture. When it comes to the bigger picture we are taught a completely different approach: "Don't think about it or it will manifest."

The biggest truths we miss through the misquoting of our masters are their own realizations that the path to ascension comes through what we release rather than gain. However, we all fear loss and in trying to avoid it, we spin out in the opposite direction of trying to manifest gain (at a cost of loss of resources and vitality of our bodies and environment).

If we can come to understand the true wisdom of Buddha and other masters we will realize that if we wish to deny all negatives based on their being "illusion," this must be matched with denying all positives too, based on the same argument. For, the pursuit of only pleasure brings as much harm, egotism, greed, self-entitlement, addiction, compulsion, destruction and suffering (as evident within Nature) as does the pursuit of negatives.

While the answer is not likely not to be found in any kind of extreme, the dis-informed new-age appears to be split between two ends of the spectrum: an "all spirit" focus on one end (with ideals of love and light) and a hedonistic "all material" focus on the other (with ideals of manifesting "unlimited" abundance, fame, etc.). There is one path we have yet to collectively try yet: the middle path that Buddha was known to speak of. The middle path leads us to a simple path; one not found in remaining dis-informed, but in becoming enlightened.

Mandy Peterson is a Visionary, Empath, EFT Practitioner and Channel for spirit. Her life and passion has always been toward being a voice of empowerment. Her desire is to help empower those struggling within themselves and their relationships, as well as to help others understand a bigger picture which includes the collective and our planet.

www.mysticmandy.com

CHAPTER 51

The Journey of A Seeker with The Power of Gratitude and Birth of A Tarot Reader

Nidhi Chauhan Sharma

I have always been very sensitive. As a child I would quickly sense the energy around me with my very being and how it made me feel and deep down I always knew that I had a gift, which had to be shared. A powerful invisible force always guided me to the right place at the right time. All I had to do was trust and move forward.

It was only after I quit my job that I realized I now wanted to give new meaning to my life. I had many questions about my life and life in general. I just knew I wanted answers to my questions, not from anyone else but from within. I knew that learning Tarot was the first step towards achieving this. I wanted to learn tarot from my early college days but was not finding a teacher. I can't put it in words how deep my yearning was to learn Tarot. I bought a deck anyway and started connecting with the mesmerizing cards. Tarot was not so popular back then and finding a teacher was quite a task. It was only after I completely surrendered and let go of my deep quest for a teacher that I finally met Ma Suraja, my lovely tarot teacher through the New Age Foundation in 2005. And that's when my real inward journey started. During my journey, so far, one thing became crystal clear to me that I have to share my gift with the world. Suppressing it and not sharing will only bring unhappiness to me. This message just kept coming back to me until I finally completely accepted it.

Tarot is a wonderful tool to know and understand where exactly you are in the here and now. It's like gazing at yourself in the spiritual mirror and looking at your truest self. The experience of a tarot reading can be truly liberating. It helps you to let go and gain amazing clarity, which helps you move forward with ease. It leads to these "aha" moments when you really know what your fears are and where they are stemming from and how unreal they can be, losing their power when you know them. And that you are finally able to put your finger on what was bothering you all this while or what you really needed to know or both.

Having the cards read can instantly clear one's foggy mind and help one choose and live life with more zest. The beautiful cards help you to know and understand what you truly feel about yourself and what you want the most which is great in achieving true well being. When you have clarity about yourself, there's an instant positive shift in you which leads to lasting happiness and brings about much needed closure if required. Tarot includes a deck of 78 cards depicting and holding the deeper meanings of the cycle of life, which helps you to simplify your life in today's world.

A session can lift years of burden, pain, misery and other negative emotions and give you the beautiful experience of lightness, expansion and freedom. What better way to simplify your life and bring in the much needed clarity and peace and you can truly empower yourself in the process. As Plato said, *"The part can never be well unless the whole is well."*

When one has mental peace and clarity it can magically open doors to true happiness and help you heal on all levels. I am truly blessed to have learnt Tarot and several healing modalities from some of the best teachers. Their teachings brought about many more positive changes in my life. They were always available with all their love and wisdom. I would then and continue now to appreciate all that they are and the work they do and feel so deeply thankful, loved, cherished and cared for.

That's when I started to realize the true power of Gratitude.

"Be thankful for what you have; you'll end up having more. If you concentrate on what you don't have, you will never, ever have enough." - Oprah Winfrey.

Much has been written and spoken about gratitude and being thankful but I feel that words can't truly capture its potency and beauty. For me, gratitude is this energy, which first leads to self-acceptance, realization of true self worth and self-love. It truly allows me to be in the now. To totally appreciate all that I have and all that is. Also, when I look at the past, I do it with a loving, happy heart feeling thankful with my entire being thanking all the people, events and things that helped me along my beautiful and empowering journey to this day.

Looking at my near future again with gratitude in my heart which then fills my entire being. Gratitude for all that is in store for me. When you are in the process of manifestation you thank the Universe in advance. Thanking magically ripen the seeds of what you are manifesting and transform them magically into reality. Thanking in advance creates so much faith in you and you become this gorgeous shining magnetic vessel, just ready to receive. Being thankful and having deep gratitude opens your heart and rewires your brain. Once you get into the practice and eventually start living in gratitude, life will give you so much more to be thankful for.

I have truly witnessed the power and beauty of having deep gratitude. It makes you more receptive, which further expands your energy and makes you this broad vessel for receiving all the goodness in life. People who struggle with receiving miraculously shift their energy from being hesitant to receiving to being beautifully receptive to receiving once they truly start living in gratitude.

Gratitude is an antidote to many negative emotions and feelings. Gratitude is like a magic potion. Once you have a sip, once you take in its essence, the divine taste nearly consumes your entire being and then the only way is forward with child like wonder. I started by maintaining a gratitude journal where I wrote all that I am thankful for. Now I live in gratitude as much as possible. Living with an attitude of gratitude has made me more receptive to love in all forms. When love and gratitude come together the energy is super powerful.

Here I would like to talk a little about a wonderful Japanese scientist Dr. Masaru Emoto who has written this amazing book called The Hidden Messages in Water. He conducted this amazing experiment where he photographed the water crystals after labeling the water (frozen at a particular temperature) filled glass tumblers with words having positive and negative energy. The images of the crystals formed in water labeled with thank you in several languages were found to be breathtakingly beautiful.

"If the only prayer you ever say in your entire life is Thank you, it will be enough" - Meister Eckhart

I sincerely thank and deeply love and respect Ma Suraja, Sandeep Goswamy, Shalin Kaintal Khurana and Suresh Padmanabhan Sir amongst many others and the magnificent Divine energy watching over me and guiding me. My life is super special and I know I have miles to go, many more lives to touch and empower. Looking forward to being of service and being grateful for much more.

Nidhi Chauhan Sharma is a Delhi Based Quantum Tarot Card Reader, Theta Healer & Energy Healer

nidhi.chauhan@yahoo.co.in

CHAPTER 52

Spiritual Journey with Animals

Ritambhara Nand

*Did you know that our Animal Companion has the power
to lead and bring us in harmony with our own self?*

The idea of existence is simple yet extraordinary for me. The energy exists all around in form of trees, small plants, ants, birds, animals on street, even rocks found around the tree. All we need is a process that fine-tunes our consciousness with Universal Consciousness in a perfect setting.

I always felt the need to understand the deeper dimensions of energy and what leads us from one circumstance to another. Various energy driven therapies will help you come closer to the SOURCE. But finally, one needs to connect the dots and understanding the real essence of synchronicity.

I work as Tarot Card Reader& Body Worker. I blend both of these to give a beautiful synthesis of gross body and subtle body. Tarot as an Energetic Tool helps you receive answers from Universal Consciousness whereas the Dynamic Balancing (Body Work) helps you come in contact with the energetic movements within your body. Now, this is a single unifying point where one feels at ease and bliss.

But my journey was enhanced as a beautiful cat came into my life. She brought along immense discoveries. My connection with her was established from the first moment. But our association led me to discover hidden principles of energy. She was keen to show me the path while I was taking time to open up and receive all the beautiful messages from the Unconscious realm.

When I travelled on the path of interacting with animals, the transformation occurred at many levels. It is not something spiritual or psychological or physiological. Instead we can experience expansion of energy in all the directions simply because we consciously enter into a different realm. Our ability to reconnect with the animal companion restores our spiritual power while we also have a direct access to the wisdom of other compassionate beings!

> *It is said that Man Once Spoke with Animals till he placed himself as the master of Earth, having dominion over all other things.*

We are here dealing with energetic beings that live in glory of nature; they deeply follow their natural instincts. When we travel with them, we work towards making our life as authentic as theirs. There are many times that you feel the need to simplify life. You will find many complexities around. These complexities create all the problems.

To size up, let us say that these problems arise out of contradictions between feelings of heart and the actions that we take, whereas when we see the animals, we see a whole and united being. There is no duality in their feelings and behavior.

I totally believe that the animals are a reflection of your deepest self and also represent qualities you need in this world. Therefore, when you travel on the path of establishing a 'Healing Touch' with Animals, it becomes a part of you for life and reflects your inner-spiritual self!

Some of powerful discoveries that I came across were—

Animals are wondrous happy creatures. They love and defend one another. They even feel sorrow and melancholy. Yet there has never been war between animal species. They know nothing about greed, envy and hate. They live their entire lives without sin. They have many amazing powers and use those only to benefit their kind and not to overcome their opponents.

> *Can we see the reason why Creator put all of us together on the same planet?*

A part of that reason is to learn from one another. Animals are here to teach humans. They have many powerful teachings to give!

They are extremely in-tune with nature and the ebbs and flows of the seasons. They communicate with the sun, with the moon, with the stars – and this communication is communication of energy. They take energy; they give energy.

There is a delicate transfer of energy happening everywhere. All we need to do is simply be 'Available to the Source'.

When interacting with Animals, we are plunging into collective consciousness. A lot of wonderful things can happen. For me, the biggest take-away was being sensitive to warmth, creativity, higher consciousness and awareness!

Honor the process of establishing a bond with Animal Companion. They will help you to be grounded, to be present and establish a delicate balance in the energy systems.

"If the vibrations of existence come within one's grasp, if there is a no-thought state on both sides, then there is no need to talk. The communication takes place on a very intimate level, and this communication goes straight to the heart. there is no explaining because there is no way to explain. Then you also will not waver over whether this or that will be or will not be. Your being will directly know what has happened"

"It is not necessarily the case that only human beings are reached by the vibrations of the fifth body. There is a wonderful phenomenon in the life of Mahavira: it is said that even animals attended his gatherings. Jaina monks have been unable to explain this phenomenon and they never will. Now an animal does not understand human language but it understands the language of being very well".

"If I sit in a no-thought condition near a cat, the cat is already in the state of no-thought. With you, however, I will have to talk. To take you to the cat's state of no-thought is a very long journey. Animals, plants and even stones understand the vibrations that begin from the spiritual body; there is no difficulty in that". - Osho

While traveling the powerful journey with Animal Kingdom, one direction lead to another and the 5-step process came down as a gift to me! 'Veterinary Healing Art' is ourinitiative to establish a sacred bond with animal companion.

- Your ability to connect deeply with animals will restore great balance and harmony in your life.

- As a result of deep association with animals, you will receive sacred messages from the source itself. You will be protected as well as gifted with talents and strengths.

- It will help you re-establish your own relationship with other human companions around you.

The foundation of this therapy is based on the single factor that we all are a part of one Source. Even the current understanding of Physics suggests that anybody who can relax, clear their mind and envision being in different way --- such as successful, healthy, wise – can quantum jump.

Develop a spiritual rapport with pets to overcome the language barriers and have a life-long friendship full of joy and understanding!

Ritambhara is a Veterinary Healing Artist, Tarot Reader & Coach for Conscious Living. She facilitates growth and renewal of all the dimensions that exists within an energetic being such as thoughts, emotions, conditioning, behavior, beliefs, patterns and energy movements within the physical body!

www.veterinaryhealingart.com

AFTERWORD

Behind the veils of consciousness...

My journey starts from 3rd March 2013. It might not be seen as a very long time but till this moment, and as I continue ahead to live each day with immense self-love and appreciation, I feel every moment has been a sheer bliss!

I faced some difficulty to write down this one. My inability to put it across on paper comes from the fact that each moment was such a deep transformation that it surpasses any description through words. I experienced a complete shift in my 'being'.

A Delhi-based girl who intends to have a fabulous lifestyle; shopping freak and a set of friends who were make-believe.In all its uniqueness, I was still just another person living and being influenced by the regular everyday energies that influence the mainstream.How far is it going to go when I sit by myself thinking of all the gap years and endless question marks even after five years of study in psychology? Emotional upheaval and turmoil, loss of loved one, self-depreciation and immense suspicion on how am I going to relate with others. Each experience just added more tussle in mind. It is now that I realize, I was doing nothing but expanding the same state of mind with which I was moving ahead! New jobs, relationships, all caught my attention. *There I was, going for all of it, but doing nothing and finally touching the ground! Now, the only choice was just to move upwards.*

As I write this article, I narrate the beautiful journey with my organization. I witnessed it unfolding for me and within me; not occasionally, not often, but every single time. Just watching itself brought me into a new light. Every organization offers certain traits that one carries ahead in life. My work environment offers a relaxed gentility of power flowing within and beneath the action. The inner purpose emerged as the outer purpose collapsed and the shell of ego began to open. The past few months have been marked by breaking of old structures, dependencies and fears. What remained behind was the unique, undiluted self!

Being a student of Psychology, I came across the whole arena of human behavior. The study, the theories, tests, further evaluations about a particular disorder and the resultant behavior.And then I came across yet another dimension. Study of Mind, Body and Soul in a way that I had never been introduced to! There have been healing forces that can be traced to shape, quality and combination. Past work experience left me with a cloud ofno apprehension, no worry, no passion to follow and no reason to conquer the world!But that almost seems like another lifetime. Today, I work as coordinator for The NewAge Foundation. Our organization has been working towards teaching various alternative healing modalities, conducting self-growth programs and spiritual retreats. I attended calls and laid down description about the programs. It might seem rather confusing but my first step towards an inner growth began while trying to establish a communication with people over the phone. Days passed and eventually I found myself floating on a whirlpool of questions. My insight on human behavior grew deeper as I tried understood their queries, beliefs and reasons for attending any of these workshop. Some were thoroughly distressed and seek help while others were just skeptical or/and under denial and a lot of them just wanted to share their success story. They were all in desperate need 'to be heard'. This is when I could let go off my 'Silence mode' because I finally balanced my belief that it was "ok to be heard". My inability to express was adding more to my trauma. I choked with my own words and uttered some when I felt that *'it is safe to express'*. The reason was an unduly desire to be appreciated and accepted, born out of childhood issues, past life or some other reason that need not be mentioned. I learned that one lifetime was too less to balance out or unlearn or drop the baggage. Therefore, I do not feel tempted to relive the past, unless it's a revelation that will facilitate my growth. Now, my only reason to wake up next morning is to explore more of me as I am the extension of ever expanding *Universe!*

Honestly, there were times when I was tempted to fall back on the old pattern. Connecting to my higher self wasn't a cakewalk but I moved ahead with the only tool called "Willingness". It has been a gradual process and I could feel that light filtering through me. When I looked deep, I saw a scarcity, an unfulfilled expression with my own self that manifested as unpleasant emotions at conscious level. We feel insecure in our relationships, desperate to fulfill our desires/goals, in failure to do the same, we get depressed, judge or push it

Holistic Wellness in the New Age

beneath the carpet. We abide by society yet swear by it when we face resentment. None of the experiments done in college or internships done under psychologist could bring me this clarity over the years! One of my major breakthrough took place in a Workshop that brings you to the core (We call it The Money Workshop). It was flow of mountain stream that surely awakened my soul from heavy labor! Universe works on absolute simple laws; while us being just one of the component of it, complicate our life. That moment I expanded to become the sky, the earth, the oceans and forest too! My Journey began as I lived each moment with complete awareness. There were infinite possibilities and every scope to unlearn and then re-learn. I did not resist as I choose to reprogram myself with a new belief that, "*I have the power to create an effortless life for myself*". I bow down to my Mentors who guided me on various dimensions of Energy. These learning or experiences were not random but instead synchronistic. By paying attention to these synchronicities, I immersed a layer deeper. My learning just went ahead indicating that *there is no beginning and no end, but expansion always*. Presence of Mentors was a blessing as they listened to me patiently, answered to all my questions, kept holding my hand and walking by my side. They showed me the way, yet kept saying that "You are the one attracting all these beautiful experiences". They re-affirmed it again and again till I knew I was open and took 100% responsibility for attracting all to my life. Now, I truly respect my past experiences as they empowered me to be who I am today; bitter and cold experiences turned into rich and abundant learning. I was ready and therefore, what could have been normal experiences for others were producing breakthrough for me! Even though I was vulnerable and falling back to the old pattern, my mentors brought me close to the silent impulse of my heart. They walked up with me, and after a point left my hand, left me to find my own path, my own truth! I saw myself floating. Each day is a new revelation, followed by an action.

Today, I feel blissful as Tarot Card Reader and shaman by heart. My understanding of life is born out of my own clarity and internal stability. I believe in a rope of compassion that connects me to an individual, during a session. This rope eventually takes both of us deeper into our own self where we find our answers. One surely experiences a deep seated Self Empowerment by the end of the session!

Tarot for me is a beautiful tool to look deeper into life and its dimensions. I see it as a 'window to existence'. So, in each session, the client and me will consciously step in to the world of cleansing and transforming Life. Tarot opened the doors to possibilities that I thought never existed! During my journey with tarot, I discovered a process called 'Dynamic Balancing'. It allows body energy to flow, removing the blockages using Himalayan singing bowls and other Shamanic musical instruments.

Finally, I knew that each of this process is opening the door for increasing the 'awareness towards our body'. We feel more sync-in with our emotions and beliefs. We understand the design of Universe and see how our life fits into this Jig-saw Puzzle. A combination of Tarot Reading and Dynamic Balancing has been working as Diagnostic and Therapeutic Device. I intend to do this majestic work till the end of my life!

It is indeed a blessing when you see the world with a little more awareness and consciousness that seeps into your system. The next moment, you see your enthusiasm flowing into different directions bringing new explorations. 'Veterinary Healing Art' is my journey with Animals. A five-step process that intends to establish a sacred bond with an animal companion.

I have deep love, faith and reverence for the Great Master 'Osho' and my dearest Mentors (Sandeep Goswamy and Suresh Padmanabhan). Through them, I got the first glimpse of divinity while traveling through many unknown paths and opening many unknown locks. Thank You.

Ritambhara Nand

The LightWorks Publishing
Spirituality . Wellness . Self
TheLightWorksPublishing.com

The LightWorks Publishing has evolved out of The NewAge Foundation to publish books and multimedia publications in the domain of NewAge Spirituality, Holistic Wellness & Personal Growth. With the objective of encouraging focus on alternative healing, we also encourage & seek to promote research-based books on alternative/ complimentary healing systems and energy medicine. Being part of The NewAge Foundation helps us reach out to a large member database of interested people and directly supply the books on Free Home Delivery basis. Facilitating our customers, we also make the books available in our NewAge Wellness World centres as well as on our own webstore, the NewAge Wellmart.

About The NewAge Foundation: A New Delhi (India) based organization committed to spreading awareness on the power of the self, mind and consciousness, The NewAge Foundation offers a variety of different holistic modalities for an individual to choose from. Services include empowerment workshops, meditations, training programs, holistic retail and much more:

- Meditation Camps
- Personal Growth & Self Help Workshops
- Spiritual Retreats
- Courses on Reiki, EFT, NLP, Psych-K, Meditation, Mind Power, Law of Attraction, Theta Healing, Karuna Reiki, Quantum Touch, Cranio Sacral Balancing, Re-Birthing, Tarot, Feng-Shui, I-Ching, Vastu, Aroma Therapy, Color Therapy, Energy Medicine, Ayurveda and most of the Complimentary & Alternative Therapies.

THE NEWAGE FOUNDATION

Through the above facilitations, the organization aims at providing the opportunity, means and support to discover your true potential as an individual.

For more information, log on to:
www.TheNewageFoundation.com

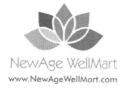

Books & DVD are Available On Our Own Online Retail Store along with many other Products Related to Wellness. All Online Payment Options along with Cash on Delivery makes it a Pleasure to Shop at www.NewAgeWellMart.com

Other Publications

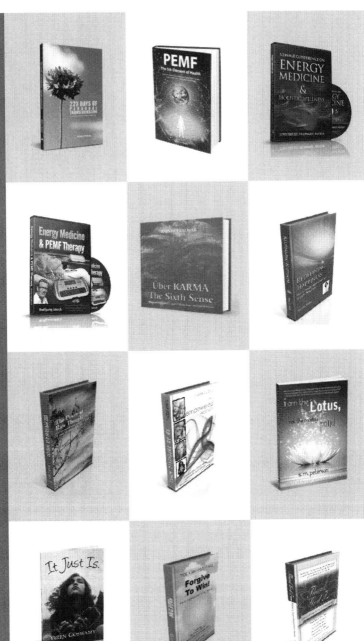

Author's Brief

Sl	Chapter	email	Author Name
	The Wellness Approach		
1	Health, Happiness and Harmony in a Time of Love	www.brucelipton.com	Bruce H. Lipton
2	You are Not Stuck! You can Change your Destiny!!!	www.atmayoga.in	Atmyayogi Shri Aasaan Ji
3	It's a YES Universe!	www.hylindia.com	Lakhwinder B Gill
4	Empower Your Dreams	www.themoneyworkshop.com	Suresh Padmanabhan
5	Willingness	www.janekirby.info	Jane Kirby
6	Ho'oponopono - The Magical Prayer Healing	rashmi_mimi@yahoo.com	Rashminder Kaur
7	The Power of Forgiveness	www.walterjacobsonmd.com	Water E. Jacobson
8	Spiritual Healing Through Storytelling	www.dramitnagpal.com	Dr Amit Nagpal
9	Parenting in New Age	www.salonisingh.com	Dr. Saloni Singh
10	Holistic Education	nehapsychologist@gmail.com	Neha Patel
11	Shifting the Paradigm: Healing Coming From Within	www.mitreawellness.com	Rucsandra Mitrea
	The Belief Approach		
12	Origin, History and Introduction of belief	www.nvlife.in	Naveen Varshneya
13	Journey of Psych-K*	www.psych-k.com	Robert M. Williams
14	PSYCH-K*-The Missing Piece	www.ritasoman.com	Rita Soman
15	Leading-Edge Neuroscience Reveals Significant Correlations	www.psych-k.com	Robert M. Williams
16	Reiki and the force called Motivation	www.paulahoran.com	Dr. Paula Horan
17	ThetaHealing	www.shalinkhurana.wordpress.com	Shalin Khurana
18	Aura Healing	www.biofieldglobal.org	Nishant
19	Emotional Freedom Technique	www.vitalitylivingcollege.info	Rangana R Choudhuri
20	Serenity Surrender (SS)	www.pastlifeconnection.com	Minal Arora
21	Beyond Self-sabotage*	www.archnamohan.co.uk	Archna Mohan
22	Fitness: The Challenge Within	t.khetarpal@gmail.com	Tarini Khetarpal
23	The Four Pillars of Health	www.nandinigulati.com	Nandini Gulati
24	Program your mind to a slim body	www.thoughtfulengagement.com	Preeti Subberwal
25	Allowing the Magic to unfold: Access Consciousness	seemasharma.accessconsciousness.com	Seema Sharma

		THE BODY APPROCH	
26	Ozone – Nature's Detox Doctor & Healing Superhero	www.healyourselfwithozone.com	Dr. Paula Horan
27	PEMF	www.pemfbook.com	Bryant Meyers
28	From the Desk of Hermina	www.pemfassistance.com	Hermina Daniel
29	The Art of Acupuncture	www.holisticmedicare.org	Dr. Ravi K. Tuli
30	Sujok & Acupressure	www.sujokacupressure.net	Amarjit Narula
31	External Counter Pulsation	www.sssibia.com	Dr. S. S. Sibia
32	The Magic of Crystal Healing	www.bindumaira.com	Bindu Maira
33	Breath-Work, The Re-Birthing Process	www.pastliferegressionindia.com	Smita Wankhade
34	Food as Medicine	www.ashishveda.uk	Dr. Ashish Paul
35	Bach Remedy	www.7pathwaysglobal.com	Aryanish Patel
36	Sports and Spirit	www.sportandspirit.co	Theresia Eggers
37	Say Yes to Money	www.themoneyworkshop.com	Suresh Padmanabhan
		THE BEING APPROACH	
38	Healing Through Hypnotherapy	www.suzyheals.com	Suzy Singh
39	Integrated Healing Through Hypnotherapy	www.kalpavrikshakriya.com	Anjali Chawla
40	Transformation Through Past-Life Regression	www.pastliferegressionindia.com	Smita Wankhade
41	Cellular Rhythms in Regression	www.ashawarriar.com	Asha Warriar
42	The Journey™ To Healing	www.vitalitylivingcollege.info	Rangana R Choudhuri
43	Working with Angels	www.godheals.in	Susan Chopra
44	Akashic Records - An Illuminating Healing Journey	www.kindredsoulzs.com	Bhavya Gaur
45	Feng Shui	meenakshijain@gmail.com	Meenakshi Jain
46	Colour Therapy	meenakshijain@gmail.com	Meenakshi Jain
47	Astrology- A Tool For Healing Energies	www.deepikaastro.com	Dipikka Gupta
48	Mantra Healing	www.angrishastro.com	Ashok Angrish
49	The Wellness Concept	www.bmhegde.com	Prof. B.M.Hegde
50	Disinformation in the New Age	www.mysticmandy.com	Mandy Peterson
51	The Journey of A Seeker withThe Power of Gratitude and Birth of A Tarot Reader	nidhi.chauhan@yahoo.co.in	Nidhi Chauhan Sharma
52	Spiritual Journey with Animals	www.veterinaryhealingart.com	Ritambhara Nand

Made in the USA
Lexington, KY
09 February 2019